tending the
heart fire

SHIVA REA

tending the heart fire

Living in Flow with the Pulse of Life

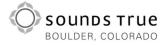
sounds true
BOULDER, COLORADO

Sounds True, Inc.
Boulder, CO 80306
Copyright © 2014 Shiva Rea
Foreword copyright © 2014 Sally Kempton
Sounds True is a trademark of Sounds True, Inc.
All rights reserved. No part of this book may be used or reproduced in any manner
without written permission from the author and publisher.
Published 2014
Book design by Amy Hayes
Printed in Korea

Excerpts and poems by Rumi and translated by Coleman Barks from *The Big Red Book, The Book of Love,*
The Essential Rumi, and *A Year With Rumi,* are reprinted with permission from the translator.

Excerpts from Daniel Odier's translations *Vijnana Bhairava Tantra,* Albin Michel 1998 and *Yoga Spandakarika:*
The Sacred Texts at the Origins of Tantra, Inner Traditions 2005 are reprinted with permission from the translator.

The excerpts by Vasant Lad, BAMS, MASc, from *The Textbook of Ayurveda: Fundamental Principles, Volume One,*
pages 211, 212, 216, 224, The Ayurvedic Press, Albuquerque, 2002, are reprinted with permission from the publisher.

The excerpts by Diane Stein from *Casting the Circle: A Woman's Book of Ritual* are copyright © 1990 by Diane Stein and are
used with permission from Crossing Press, an imprint of the Crown Publishing Group, a division of Random House, Inc.

The excerpts by Brian Swimme from *The Universe Is a Green Dragon,* Bear & Company 1984,
are reprinted by permission of the publisher. Innertraditions.com

The excerpts by Nitin Kumar from *Exotic India* are reprinted with permission from the author. Exoticindia.com

The excerpt by Mechthild of Megdeburg from *The Flowing Light of the Godhead,*
Martino Fine Books 2012, is reprinted with permission from the publisher.

Library of Congress Cataloging-in-Publication Data
Rea, Shiva.
 Tending the heart fire : living in flow with the pulse of life / Shiva Rea.
   pages cm
 ISBN 978-1-60407-709-4
 1. Spiritual life. 2. Yoga. 3. Heart—Religious aspects. 4. Fire—Religious aspects. I. Title.
 BL624.R397 2013
 294.5'436—dc23
                        2013006569

Ebook ISBN: 978-1-60407-912-8
Enhanced ebook ISBN: 978-1-62203-343-0
10 9 8 7 6 5 4 3 2 1

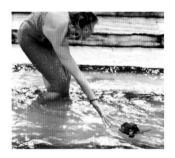

To the Primordial Fire and all
firekeepers past, present, future

For our heartfire—El Corazón
del Fuego—within all

To my Son/Sun, Jai

To my Beloved, Mi Amor

To my heart mandala—family, teachers,
friends, and student mitras on the path

To our ancestors, future generations,
and a renewable energy future for all

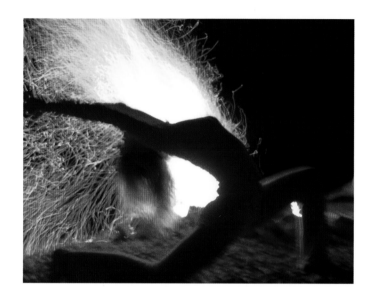

*He encendido el corazón del fuego
y he bebido de su miel*
    I have ignited the fire of my heart
    and drunk its honey

                —ESMERALDA LAMAS, TRANS.[1]

Om Chidagni Kundayai Namaha
    I bow to Shakti, the Goddess that arises
    from the fire altar of consciousness

                —LALITA SAHASRANAMA

CONTENTS

I've been awed by Shiva Rea ever since I first co-taught with her. The year was 2003, and a group of women teachers from different traditions had come together to present a weekend workshop. Most of us had never before taught together. We got to meet in person just two hours before the first class. As we sat together, sharing ideas, I began to feel nervous. Though there was immense good will, none of us seemed to know exactly how we would integrate our very different offerings.

Then Shiva began to share a vision for how we could work together. I watched in delight as she cajoled us into synchrony—suggesting, inspiring, weaving everyone's unique energies so that each person could shine and at the same time support a shared vision. It was a profound demonstration of heart-coherent leadership. I've never forgotten it.

Heart coherence is Shiva's style. She is an integrator, a synthesizer of worlds. Since her teens, she has moved at the cutting edge of yoga, exploring the classical forms and creating new ones. An intuitive with a deep bent for scholarship, a lover of science and a master of flow, Shiva's way is both audaciously original and profoundly respectful of tradition. Many people talk about integrating ancient wisdom and modern science. Shiva lives it. She has practiced asana and devotion in deserts and remote forests. She climbs mountains and meditates in caves. She surfs, practices esoteric martial arts, and has introduced a generation of yogis to ecstatic dance. More than that, Shiva is a natural alchemist of the heart. She has taught thousands of people to take risks, to love intensely, and to live creatively—basing it all on the foundational principles of the ancient yogic texts.

In *Tending the Heart Fire,* Shiva lets us in on some of her secrets. Not everyone can work Shiva's magic. But any one of us can drink from the wisdom she has brought together in these pages.

This book is ambitious, even radical. It captures in words and pictures a set of life-changing principles that let us live in deep harmony with ourselves, the world, and the divine. These principles sound simple: Tune into the light and energy of your own heart. Live in rhythm with the flow of the natural world. Learn to love outrageously. Connect to your body, and bring the energy of the subtle world into every move you make. Discover how to read your own energy, and how to transform it when necessary. And do all this through the living force of inspiration and illumination that the spiritual traditions know as the fire of the heart.

Joseph Campbell used to say that when the ancient humans first discovered fire, they probably didn't cook with it. Instead they worshipped it. To early humans, watching a fire's glow, its leaping tongues, its hot kaleidoscope of color and warmth must have seemed like being in the presence of the divine. It still does. More than any natural element, fire embodies both the power of awareness and the power of transformation. In Vedic times, a young man coming of age was given a piece of sacred fire to tend. When he married, he and his bride circled that fire as they made their vows. The fire became the center of the house. When the man died, a flame from that fire kindled his burial pyre, and was passed on to his son. Was there ever a better metaphor for the inner fire that sustains life?

To tend a fire demands care and devotion. More than that, it asks us to be conscious. If you forget to feed the fire, it dies out. Let it get out of control, and it might burn down your house. But there's a mystery to fire that anyone who works with it knows. Priests who work with ritual fires know it. So do many firefighters. It's this: when you practice with fire, you learn that fire is *conscious*. Fire is not only alive. It is responsive.

In tantric texts, consciousness is often described as a fire, which uses as its fuel the material of what is known. And people who work with fire know that this isn't just a metaphor. Once, in India, I was given the honor of making offerings at a fire ritual. The priests had made the fire very hot by offering great streams of oil and clarified butter into it. Now, it roared horizontally around the edge of the fire pit, leaping so powerfully that it almost licked the faces of the people making offerings. Soon everyone was leaning away from the fire. Some people even backed up to put some distance from it. I didn't want to shy away from the sacred fire. First, because I love fire. But also because (this is a little embarrassing, but it's the truth), I didn't want the priests to think that I was just a wimpy foreigner. So I did something that any fire keeper might understand. I talked to the fire. I said to the fire, "Please cool down a little so I can sit with you." And the fire, believe it or not, responded immediately. The flames, which had been roaring around the sides of the fire pit, leapt backwards when they came to me. They made an arc until they had passed a foot beyond me. Then they roared back to the edge of the fire pit, literally dancing in the faces of the people sitting near. This happened over and over again. It almost felt as if the fire was playing with me.

In these pages, Shiva explains why such a thing could happen. Our inner world is inextricably connected to the natural world. Our bodies contain all the elements in the universe. The rhythms of day and night, and the flow of seasons express themselves through our breathing patterns. The weather outside is reflected in our emotional weather. Our bodies contain the density of earth, but also the infinite subtlety of spirit.

The heart connects all this. Physically, it is the pump that keeps our body running, energetically, its magnetic field connects us to other beings. It is a brain that holds memories. It is a seat of feeling and emotion. And it is a portal to inner worlds. In Western mysticism, the heart is considered the eye of wisdom. In India, it is the seat of the soul. The heart holds the many-leveled mystery of human life.

In *Tending the Heart Fire,* Shiva has given us an indispensible manual for living the wisdom of the heart. Drawing generously from the teachings and practices of several yoga traditions, she offers mudras and mantras, meditations and contemplations that can open you to the experience of the sacred in every moment of your life. This book contains an invitation—and I hope you'll accept it! Play with the practices. Experiment with the postures and mudras. Notice which mantras enliven your body. Create an altar, and explore the ways that ritual can help you embody your aspirations. Explore the principles that let you tune your body to the seasons. And above all, let these practices draw you into an ever-deepening intimacy with your own heart.

Sally Kempton
Author of *Meditation for the Love of It*
and *Awakening Shakti*

When I was seventeen, I left my home in Memphis, Tennessee, and traveled via Belgium, Greece, and Egypt to Kenya. I had saved all of my work money to pay for my expenses on a nine-month volunteer trip in village development before I was to enter my freshman year at New York University. I ended up staying in Kenya for a year and a half, postponing college indefinitely; it was a pivotal period that changed the course of my life. Back in Memphis, the seeds of yoga had first begun stirring in me when I started a little yoga practice in my room from a book I had found in the library, while roaming around to find a book about my name. A burning search for meaning had begun to arise in me. On the news, the horrific suffering of the Ethiopian famine of the mid-1980s moved me to do service work in East Africa.

For the first six months in Kenya, I lived with my coworkers in a three-room earthen hut made of mud, thatch, and dung from our neighbor's cows, deep in the bush near Mount Kenya. We had no electricity or running water. The rhythm of "life unplugged" deeply shook yet soothed my teenage soul, as I had left home disheartened about what I felt was a superficial urban life in the United States. Everything in America seemed to come in packages—food, what to wear, what to do—disconnecting us more and more from our origins.

In my village life as a volunteer, I began to reconnect with earth rhythms. The water I carried on my head from the local stream made my neck strong and my connection to water more precious. Pulling food from the earth and walking a mile to market made food taste more alive. Building rain catchers with one hundred villagers while we all sang the Swahili refrain "Harambe Pamoja Kujenge Kenya" ("Let's work together as Kenyans") began to link my body to a collective body. Going to sleep with the moon and rising with the sun started to shift my rhythm to that of nature and the cosmos.

Although my teachers and friends in the Murang'a Valley had very little material wealth, living on less than $400 a year, the happiness they expressed while living in harmony with the natural world—sitting around the fire together to sing songs and tell stories—was rich and profound.

Even though I had become integrated into daily village life, I questioned whether I was doing anything effective as a volunteer. Was I really helping? Wasn't I receiving more than I was giving?

One day as I walked slowly into the village from my home, I felt a deep malaise come over me— first the chills, then the shakes and a high fever. It turned into a serious five-day bout of malaria that still affects my health today. As I lay in my thatched hut, usually alone, my body wracked with pain, I existed in that space outside time. I was so sick I could do nothing else, so I opened to all the memories of my life that were arising, simply to stay connected to being alive.

I remembered hearing the rhythm of the ocean waves in my first years living in Hermosa Beach

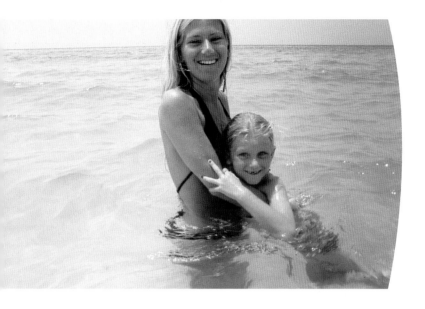

through my body. I didn't know if I was dying or being reborn. This inner force blew away any thoughts or conceptions of what was happening. It was a feeling of intrinsic sacredness—an unmistakable presence of the One, a healing force that was melting within my heart and transforming my whole being. It's a feeling I still experience today whenever I listen deeply. At this eleventh hour, I felt strangely blissful and suddenly without fear as this most intimate heat moved from my heart center to my limbs, filling the room and moving into the night sky. An all-pervasive feeling of gratitude washed through me, because in that moment I knew I was not alone.

I wasn't quite sure at the time what, exactly, was happening, yet I hovered in that state all night, at some point finally falling asleep for the first time in days. When I woke up, I felt transformed. The fever and shaking were gone, and I felt euphoric but incredibly weak. I will never forget walking outside that next morning and heading out into the green flourishing of life: leaves swaying in the early morning wind, the sounds of roosters crowing, the first light on the horizon.

What I'd experienced was one of those mystical moments that often arise during life-turning events—be it a significant illness, childbirth, or standing at the crossroads of a new adventure or life change. Yet this fire, this warmth, that lives in the center of our hearts is accessible in all of us, in any moment. When I was confronting leaving this life, this body, I was reminded of this fire within, and I made a pledge right there that I have followed ever since: To follow my Heart Fire—this energetic inner blaze, the love of life—at the center of my being.

with my surfer father and sun-worshipping mother; the chaotic and colorful years in the Bay Area through the 1970s while my father was at the University of California, Berkeley; my teenage years in downtown Memphis near the blues hub of Beale Street. I remembered all the characters I had met. I exhausted every memory of family, friends, teachers, lovers, loss, and precious joys until all that seemed to be left was the feeling of how rich life had been in such a short span of time.

By the evening of the fourth day, my fever was still so high, despite my taking the medicine, that my Kenyan coworkers decided they would carry me five miles to the clinic the next morning if my fever didn't break. We all started to pray. They said their prayers aloud in Kikuyu, Swahili, and English. My prayers arose quietly between the violent shakes that came and went in waves. There was a strange, sacred calm inside the shaking, a place I had not been before, one of initiation.

Slowly, within the stillness of the night, an intense sensation began to spread from my chest

My heart is burning with love. All I can see

is this flame. My heart is pulsing with passion,

like waves on an ocean. I'm at home, wherever

I am. And in the room of lovers, I can see

with closed eyes the beauty that dances.

Behind the veils intoxicated with love,

I too dance the rhythm of this moving world.

—RUMI[1]

Tending the Heart Fire is an offering from my heart to yours. Through my thirty years as a student of yoga, I have come to recognize the great truth that the human body is a universe—and that it is one and the same with the cosmos itself. Our bodies are literally made of the same materials that surround us—dirt, rocks, plants, rivers, oceans, and sunlight—and the wild and creative pulse of life that actuates the universe exists within the body itself.

The Universe began in fire, an explosion so powerful that we are still basking in its radiance. Our very own bodies contain traces of elements that exploded outward to birth our galaxy at the moment of the big bang, 13.7 billion years ago. Every mineral, every trace of our environment, can be found in our bones, our blood, our sweat, our tears. At the center of this magnificent and elegant universe of the body is our very own sun, the heart, with its electromagnetic radiance communicating with every cell of our body and synchronizing with our brainwaves and the heartbeats of others around us.[2] Just as a reference, the electromagnetic field of the heart is

five thousand times stronger than that of any other organ in the body, and in heart-transplant patients whose vagus nerve has been severed this field is a means of heart-brain communication.[3]

Within this heart burns a fire.

Fire is at the core of our existence. From the original primordial fire of the big bang to the generative energy of the sun, all life depends on light and heat for creation and survival. As we will explore in this book, our Heart Fire, the energetic center of our bodies, functions as a pulse of life, just as the sun functions as the life pulse for our solar system. As the sun radiates the heat that warms the planet and animates all life, our hearts pump blood and nutrients throughout the body and send electromagnetic waves outward that connect to the world around us. There are hundreds, thousands, of examples of how our external environment and our bodies work in unison. As such, the *vinyasa,* or flow, of our bodies—what we eat, when we sleep, when we create, when we rest—seeks to be in harmony with the natural rhythms of the natural world and our source of energy, the sun. Just as the length of days increases in spring and summer and releases a great generative energy that allows for new buds on the trees and a great expanse of green to blanket the earth, our bodies experience windows of potential for creation. And just as the world around us darkens in winter, our bodies seek to move inward, to rest, and to reflect during the season of winter and in the night. The cycles of time are mapped in the body—and when we attune to those internal and external forces, we are able to experience enormous peace, harmony, creativity, and longevity.

In the typical 9-to-5 work world where life has become ever more mechanized and urban, we need to find a new way of being. For those of us in the West, our natural rhythms have changed to one of 24/7 constant stimulation and high levels of stress, both of which contribute to the rise in heart disease—the number-one killer in the U.S. even though it hardly existed more than a century ago.[4] There is great need for a new way to deal with the fragmenting effects of life in the twenty-first century. However, tending the Heart Fire is *not* entirely a "new" way of being, but instead a return to the ways of our ancestors—who placed the movements of the environment at the foreground of their lives. As such, much of what I offer in this book is actually a remembering of what our bodies already know to be true. When we synch our lives with the fire in our hearts, we can access the power of creation and manifestation and letting go. Similarly, we can access the slowing and inward movements that allow us to fall back into the wide, spacious quiet of gestation and rejuvenation, which is critical for finding peace and wholeness in our bodies. Everything in nature, and everything in our being, goes through a process of expansion and contraction. And it is the heartbeat, expanding and contracting, that keeps us alive.

This living in deep attunement to the natural rhythms of the planet is what I call "living in flow with the pulse of life." Yoga is infinitely more than the now well-established world of movement practice that has branched out into studios across the world. Yoga, too, is a universe, and it is a gateway through which we can live in harmony with the solar and lunar rhythms that dominate our biological and spiritual experience in order to find optimal flow in our lives. The word *yoga* means to "yoke," or, in other words, to "unify." Thus, in the yoga of the heart that I offer in this book, we seek to reintegrate ourselves with the natural flow of our bodies, guided by the warm, central wisdom of our Heart Fires.

LIVING VINYASA: THE BACKGROUND AND PRINCIPLES GUIDING THIS BOOK

Tending the Heart Fire is a life-guide book, an offering of meditations centered on the innate wisdom of our heart and the rhythm of the seasons. This book invites you to take a journey into the legacy of meditation connected across deep time to firekeeping, a practice that's more than two million years old—the current carbon-dated evidence of our ability to tend fire[5]. All animals, including human beings, become more focused, reflective, and meditative around a fire. It is here that the earliest forms of meditation such as fire gazing, chant, movement, and music emerged.

This book includes more than 108 such meditations, ranging from sound to movement, and from ayurvedic health practices for balancing our inner fire, or *samagni,* to ritual bonfires for the solstice. These meditations are a tapestry woven from what I have learned through personal experience and from the wisdom traditions I have studied, including yoga, tantra, bhakti, ayurveda, and *natya* (dance). As a graduate of UCLA's World Arts and Cultures/Dance program, I have always been drawn to a universal, big-picture understanding of yoga. As a student, I keep returning to the roots of my path—not just in yogic lineages, but also within the world's indigenous traditions. These pathways of yoga have all informed the body of knowledge presented in this book—but above all, I offer my gratitude to my teachers.

TANTRA, BHAKTI, AND THE INNER FIREKEEPING OF THE HEART

Much of the material in this book is guided by the Tantra, the origin of most of the embodied yoga that we practice today, and has become a central part of my personal practice and offerings. Often misunderstood, nondual tantra is a spiritual movement originating in North India that reached its peak in the ninth to twelfth centuries, primarily characterized by a life and body-positive approach to daily practice (*sadhana*). Within tantra, there is an emphasis on a direct experience of divine reality that has transcendent and immanent aspects, called Shiva and Shakti, respectively. Shiva is primarily understood as the pure consciousness that is the ultimate ground of being, while Shakti is the flowing energy making up the entire manifest universe.[6] A tantric orientation to yoga recognizes that the highest place of realization is not to be found outside of us but within our embodiment amidst daily life.

Within tantra, the cosmology of the universe and the rhythms of the earth are all directly mirrored in the body. All the sacred junctures of the year—the lunar cycles, the change of seasons—have a direct and observable point in the body. Thus when we try to override the body's natural shifts, we create blockage, a stagnation, and the truth of what wants to emerge from our minds, bodies, and hearts is impacted.

Central to tantric meditation is the offering of breath, mantra, and awareness into a living energy of the heart visualized as a fire altar, or *hrd kund*. Here meditation embraces the senses and the entire spectrum of one's life, as we have a direct, transforming experience of the inner source as the fire of consciousness illuminating the way.

Bhakti often refers to the way of the heart, from the root *bhaj* as devotion. Bhakti can refer to the historical movement of *kirtan*, dance, and teachings that blossomed during the fourteenth to fifteenth centuries and led to the contemporary kirtan movement. It can also refer to the mystical traditions within tantra and the devotional texts, sutras, and songs from Abhinavagupta to Lalleshwari, Tirumoolar to Kabir, whose heart realizations are offered in various passages in this book alongside meditations, offerings, and *pujas* dedicated to tending the fire of devotion and liberating the power of love as a living bhakti.

Tantra encourages you to experience your body as your most sacred altar and to honor the cosmos that is your body by honoring the fire that lives in the heart.

AYURVEDA AND THE FIREKEEPING OF OUR VITALITY

Ayurveda, one of the oldest healing systems in the world, is based on a foundation of religion, philosophy, and medicine to balance the natural flow of the body for optimal health and well-being. Native to India, ayurveda is based on the observed wisdom of the body—and it acknowledges that the body, just as the outside world, is a fine-tuned instrument that contains the five basic elements that also make up our planet: ether, air, fire, water, earth. It also takes into account what Dr. Vasant Lad, a preeminent doctor and author of ayurveda, terms the "trinity of life": body, mind, and spiritual awareness. The word *ayu* means "daily living," while *veda* means "knowing." Simply put, ayurveda teaches that our bodies are microcosms of the universe and that disease in the body has a direct relationship to the macrocosm—the environment, the cycles of the seasons and time, and what is around us. We mirror each other. Just as the earth, when in balance, has immense generative and healing power, so too does the body. But again, we must bring it into balance with its gorgeous and wise natural rhythms.

This book is informed by ayurveda because its practices honor the deep relationship between humans and the cosmos. According to Dr. Lad, cosmic energy manifests in all living and nonliving things. Our bodies are no less complex than the cosmos itself. Because ayurveda has long been such an integral part of my life; teacher trainings; annual ayurvedic retreats to Kerala, South India; and my study of *kalarippayatu*, a martial art and healing system that integrates ayurveda, I want to share that which has transformed me. Throughout this book, I thus provide many "living in rhythm" practices and suggestions based on ayurveda that honor the needs of the body in relation to what is happening with the seasons and time of day.

PRANA FLOW–ENERGETIC VINYASA

When I first began teaching vinyasa in 1990, my teaching was rooted in the practice of Ashtanga Vinyasa Yoga taught by Sri Pattabhi Jois and informed by Iyengar teachers and teachers of Desikachar—all students of Sri T. Krisnamacharya

of Chennai, India. Throughout the last two decades, I have been dedicated to a holistic vision of the understanding of "living vinyasa" in its roots and branches. Vinyasa in its original meaning from the early Tantras is understood as the "sequence of consciousness," or how life unfolds from *spanda*—the creative pulse of life.[7]

In nature, vinyasa is any cycle, from the tiniest vibration to the cycle of our entire life. It represents the journey of how a potent seed evolves into a full, branching tree. My father gave me the seed name of Shiva at birth from his love of the sculptural image of Nataraja, or the Cosmic Dance. This name led me to seek out yoga as a teenager, to perform service work in Kenya, and to follow the mystic opening of my heart through the fire of malaria, leading eventually to living in an ashram-orphanage run by yogic nuns in the slums of Nairobi. The fire of yoga had been ignited within me. In the intimacy of self-practice, my organic relationship to the wave of breath, the cellular energy, and the ebb and flow of my heart consciousness has guided me throughout, including saving me from burning out from a fiery yoga practice during my early years of study.

Now I offer vinyasa as living flow connected to the dance of life—a changing and evolving sequence based on the movements of prana (life force) and our energetic body. From my earliest studies in Odissi (classical Indian dance), kalarippayatu of CVN Kalari (Indian martial arts), and my undergraduate and graduate studies in the department of World Arts and Cultures at UCLA, I have become dedicated to a global understanding of movement meditation and *namaskar*, or moving prayer. Going deeper into *sahaja yoga* (spontaneous, natural flow) with my root teacher Daniel Odier as well as within trance dance systems of Jamaica, Haiti, Mali, Ghana, Morocco, Bali, and Kerala awakened the experience of being a vessel of movement. My body could no longer be held in the physical perfection of an asana. The life pulse of the breath and the connection of the heart reclaimed my body. Thus I've chosen in *Tending the Heart Fire* to offer a more universal book of meditations, but I also offer an entire practice companion of Prana Flow–Energetic Vinyasa, featuring a mandala of more than forty namaskars: solar-lunar vinyasa sequences that complement the living vinyasa meditations on these pages.

WHERE TO BEGIN: TENDING THE HEART FIRE

This book invites you to take a journey into the legacy of firekeeping that is more than 800,000 years old. I want to pass on to you the inspiration of the legacy we've been given by our ancestors, who observed the cosmos and created daily practices, rituals, festivals, and celebrations to align themselves with the deeper rhythms of nature. Our whole body is synched with nature to preserve this balance.

When we "tend to our Heart Fire" we center our life-energy into the core of our being, our hearts, which is ever generating. Like the sun, our hearts contain an eternal flow of energy that is life-giving and life-holding. When we tend to our Heart Fire, we integrate the solar and lunar aspects of ourselves—our our inner regeneration and dynamic energy. Much of yoga today does not integrate this tending. Yoga as asana practice is

only part of the picture. Firekeeping is thus the central metaphor for this book. It is a metaphor for the infinite ways we stay attuned and attentive to our core truth. Firekeeping is primal and raw. It requires discipline and deep attention. It demands agility, for life is always changing—externally and internally—and we need to shift and adjust to what life presents us. And it calls us to activism—for we must wake up and live in our highest potential so that we can be a force of good in the world.

This book is divided into four parts: In Part One we explore the cross-cultural meanings of the heart through time among mystics and philosophers, East and West. We trace its fall in Western thought to the status of a mere mechanical pump, and the welcome resurgence of knowledge of the true energetic heart that is taking place today. We explore the deep tradition underlying the tending of the Heart Fire—firekeeping through human history—and look at the effects of our disconnection from this profound history. Through the flow of nature (envisioned as the ecstatic dance of Shiva and Shakti within yoga), we see the creation of the cosmic rhythms and elements of the universe and explore the power of living in synchronization with these rhythms and elements to reclaim our firekeeping power.

We begin our firekeeping practice in Part Two with movement meditations, again visiting the dance of Shiva and Shakti as archetype and inspiration. I will introduce you to simple, accessible, and yet profound forms of movement such as *pranams, mudras, kriyas,* and *namaskars*—movement alchemy. In this part we also look at the influence of time and rhythm, place, and our somatic mood on our practice. In this part, I offer a series of meditations for tending the Heart Fire.

In Part Three we begin to link the energies flowing through our bodies with daily, monthly, and seasonal rhythms, exploring the *sandhyas*—sacred junctures of time—that are highly potent for practice. From the elements created by Shiva's dance flow the principles of ayurveda, which we explore here. Practical ways to live in accordance with these principles are included. We learn to attune to the rhythms of day and night, sun and moon in our firekeeping and to use sacred retreat time and ritual to regenerate our Heart Fire.

With Part Four we apply our knowledge in six-week annual cycles, using a calendar that I developed that integrates the solar and lunar cycles of the sacred mandala of the year. We begin in the fertile darkness of winter, the time of least external light, when we envision and gestate our own renewal, regenerating and rekindling the internal light, the Heart Fire. Then it is on to the swelling of spring, the creative fire of summer, and onward through the letting-go energy of fall. Food, body, and yoga rhythms appropriate to each season are included, and along the way we visit some of the great sacred holidays and festivals that mark each season.

Notwithstanding this structure, my hope is that you can open to *any* page in this book and be inspired by a meditation, a passage, a sutra, or an image. If you are not interested in theory, you can dive right into the practices starting with Part Two. Meanwhile, if you have any physical hindrances or are not a "yoga practitioner," you can still enjoy most of the meditations at any time or place without limitations.

I am grateful to the many teachers and friends on the Heart Fire path as well as to the "Tending the Heart Fire: Living Yoga Sadhana" program within Samudra Global School for Living Yoga, which I founded in 2002. This book is also a multimedia ebook and online resource, in which you can see the practices come alive. Since my first Sounds True CD offering in 2000, I have been dedicated to home-practice tools as a grassroots way to help people tend their inner fire in a direct relationship to the cellular energy that awakens through the breath of yoga.

THE DIRECT AWAKENING OF THE HEART: BHAKTI AND THE MYSTICISM OF THE HEART

Since my beginnings in yoga three decades ago, tending the Heart Fire has been my personal dharma. The direct awakening of the Heart Fire often happens when we are at a crisis point, when we fall to our knees, when the armor of our heart has to crack. The mystic heart is the awakening of direct experience that each one of us can access by tending the fire of any spark of love, bonding, inspiration, truth, or passion. This is the fire we can see in each other's eyes that leads to a waking up and to serving life in all forms—your own sacred activism. In the words of my great mentor and Sacred Activist, Andrew Harvey:

The human race is now in an unprecedented and destined evolutionary crisis— a global dark night. This global dark night is potentially the birth canal for a new, embodied divine humanity chastened by tragedy and illumined by grace . . . The birthing force of the divine human is the force of the Motherhood of God, expressed not only in new and radically evolutionary mysticism but also in sacredly inspired radical action on every level and in every arena.[8]

The teachings and practices of yoga have always held the heart in both practical and mystical ways. So let us return to the power and magnificence of our hearts: heart as fire and heat. Heart as intelligent energy and electromagnetic radiance. Heart as our illuminating guide toward love, creativity, and deep knowing. May the journey begin now, as we awaken our direct relationship to our Heart Fire, both primordial and intimate.

Great Fire of the Heart

Indescribable joy at the
heart of the Real.

Everything becomes free
in the present moment,
Nothing to do or avoid,

Movement and stillness are
luminous consciousness.

Free from seeking and from practice,
The essence of the heart inundates
your whole being.

Your cosmic body is
manifested in totality,

The cosmos tremors within
your own dwelling-place!

The honey of this realization
flows in every glitter of light

Neither matter nor people
are deprived of it,
The sun, moon, the rocks, and
the trees, the sky and the earth

The body and the mind do
nothing but proclaim this Heart
vibrating to Infinity.

—SAHAJANANDABHAIRAVA[9]

PART ONE

tending the heart fire

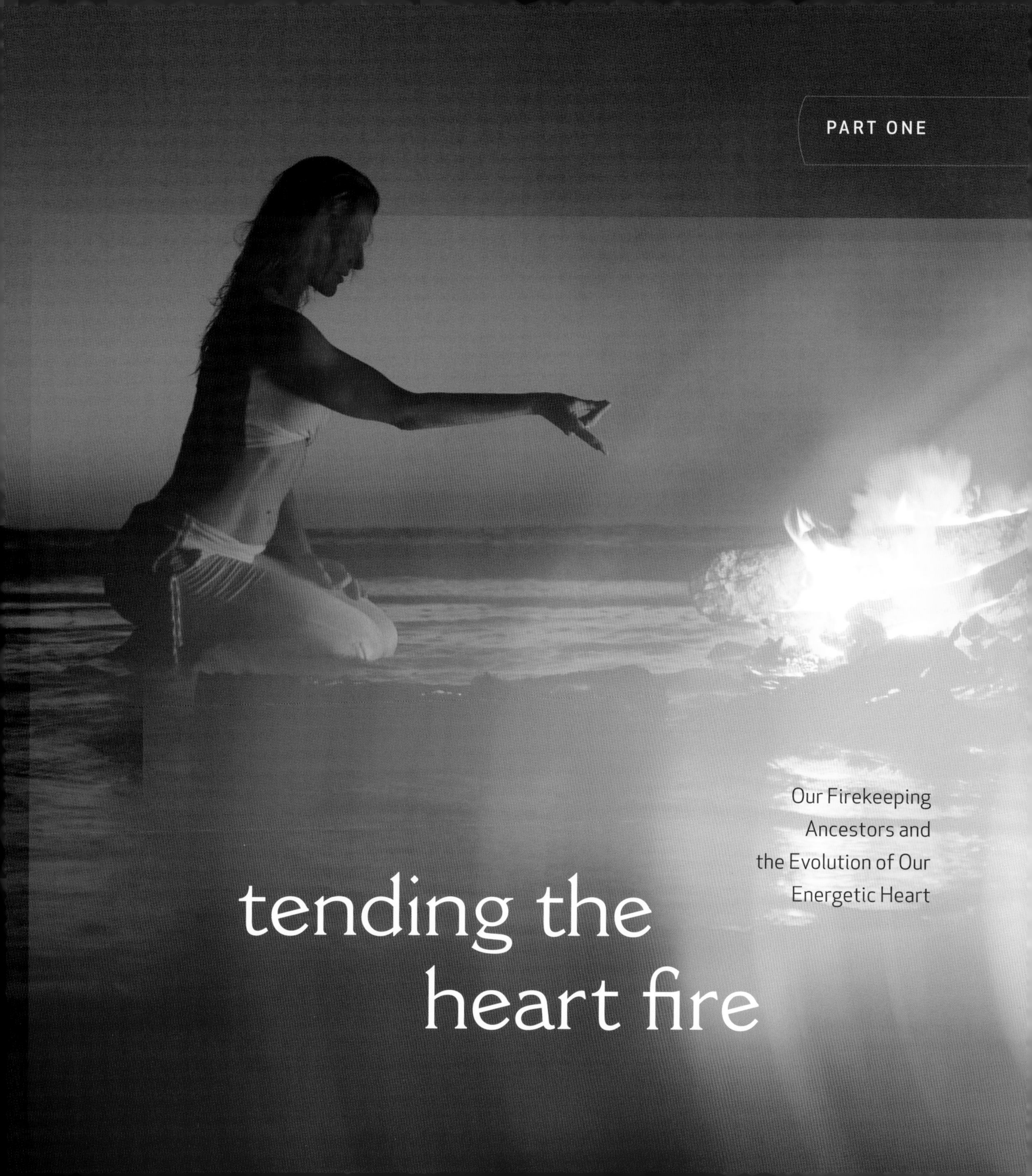

Our Firekeeping Ancestors and the Evolution of Our Energetic Heart

CHAPTER ONE

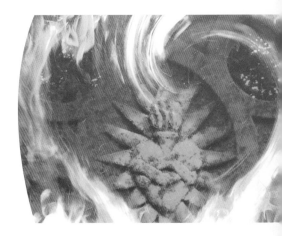

envisioning
the heart fire

From Ancient Wisdom to Cutting-Edge Science

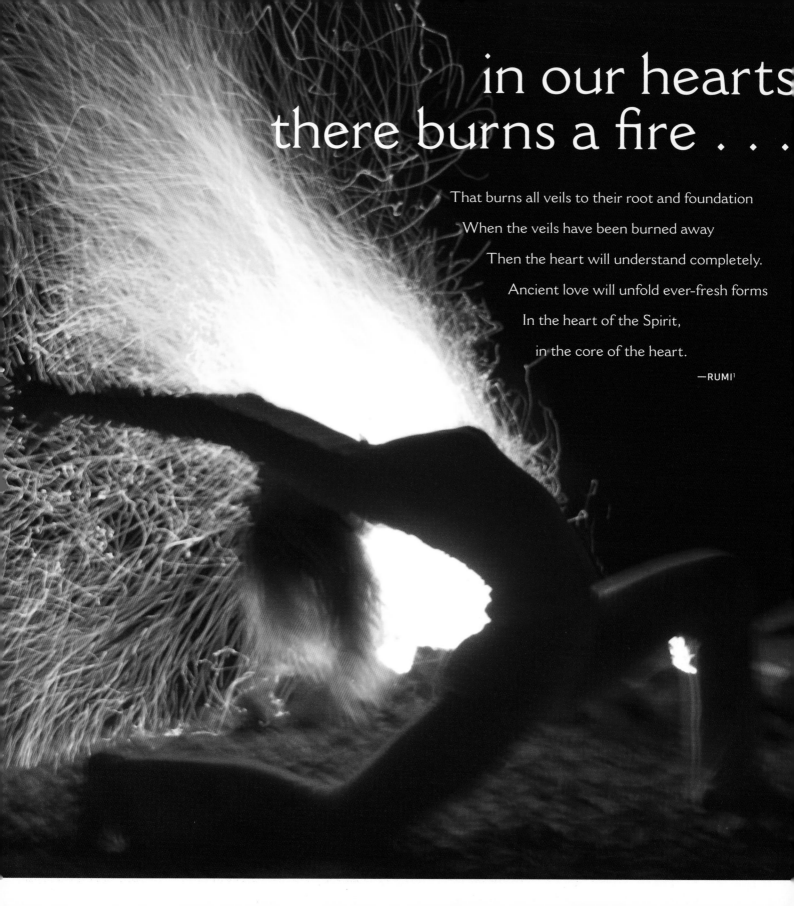

in our hearts
there burns a fire . . .

That burns all veils to their root and foundation

When the veils have been burned away

Then the heart will understand completely.

Ancient love will unfold ever-fresh forms

In the heart of the Spirit,

in the core of the heart.

—RUMI[1]

WE ARE CREATED IN RHYTHM, KEPT ALIVE IN RHYTHM, AND EVOLVE THROUGH RHYTHM.

Tides, breath, and blood flow in rhythm. We are born into a universe of currents, and our heart is the great conductor of the body as it maintains the rhythmic pulse that oscillates to the flow of our lives.

Twenty billion years ago when the universe surged into being, a primordial fireball exploded in a colossal burst of light. Everything in existence today still pulses with original light—including our own bodies.

The Heart Fire within each of us connects us to the beginning of creation, to the *rtam* or cosmic rhythm generated by the blazing *tapas*—generating heat—of this original fire. From this original burst of light, Surya (the sun), Chandra (the moon), all the heavens, and the cycles of cosmic time emerged. Your heart's rhythm embodies the pulse of creation (*spanda*). In addition, our hearts vibrate as the innermost essence of consciousness (*hridaya*), the flow of love (*rasa*), and the light of the true self (*jyotir*). Each of us carries this enormous source of power and love in our bodies.

To live in ways that honor these natural currents, those within and those without, is to live vinyasa, in touch and in alignment with the flowing rhythms of our world.

If we drop into our feeling sensations of our body, we discern a subtle reverberation of this light in our chests as a deep, penetrating heat that ebbs and flows, expand and recedes, dims and intensifies. While we may not often pause to think about it, this intimate connection and truth in our hearts is reflected in our speech by how we counsel one another: "Listen to your heart." "Trust your heart." "Follow your heart." Our heart feels "heavy," or we are "lighthearted." When we affirm the truth, we "swear upon" our heart, instinctively making the universal mudra of connecting hand to heart. When we open to our heart's deepest knowing, we have a "change of heart."

While we can think of the heart as the extraordinary circulatory-system pump we learned about in school, we know in our bones that it is so much more than this. All of the world's spiritual traditions—and now recent scientific discoveries—have revealed the Heart Fire as a radiant field of connection and inner wisdom that transcends time, space, and culture.

the mystic heart fire
across cultures

The mystical foundations of all the world's spiritual paths meet in a single, sacred place—the heart of the seeker. Whether the tradition is Sufi, Christian, Buddhist, Hindu, Jewish, Muslim, or shamanic, all of our ancient paths recognize the universal pulse of the heart, the source fire within that connects us to the mystery of being.

Mystics of all traditions—those who seek their own direct communication with Source unimpeded by priests or other intermediaries—are drawn to the Heart Fire as to a bed of glowing embers in the night. They attune to the sacred pulse that helps them see through the veils of illusion, hear the truth, and feel unity present in the heart: a presence that transforms all differences, transmutes all poisons, and cultivates the nectar of unconditional love. That the heart is a reflection of the divine is a universal mystical understanding that has always threaded through disparate cultures around the world. From the Christian Sacred Heart to the Celtic vision of the heart as a cauldron, this wisdom is found in imagery and metaphor across traditions.

Lie down in the fire

see and taste

the flowing One

through your whole being;

Feel the Holy Spirit

moving you within the flowing

fire of the One.

—MECHTHILD OF MAGDEBURG[2]

CHRISTIAN MYSTICISM— THE FLAMING HEART OF LOVE

The flaming heart of Jesus—sometimes shown disembodied and wrapped in thorns, at other times depicted blazing in Christ's chest—has been a source of mystical realization for countless saints and devotees, releasing the light of divine love that transmutes the pain of suffering. Also known as the Sacred Heart within Roman Catholic worship, it is the core transformation and realization of divine love that has sustained Christians for millennia.

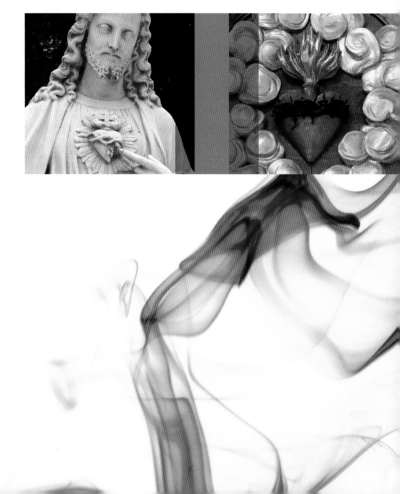

The heart is like a candle

    Longing to be lit.

Torn from the Beloved

    It yearns to be whole again,

      But you have to bear the pain.

    You cannot learn about love.

      Love appears on the wings of grace

                — RUMI[3]

JUDAISM—KABBALAH—AISH: THE SACRED FIRE OF THE HEART

In the Hebrew tradition and in the Old Testament, the heart has its own power to see, and all prayers are generated by and held in the heart. In the Kabbalah, the mystic branch of Judaism, a name for the heart is *leve*—which sounds, when pronounced in Hebrew, like "love." The Talmud Sotah teaches that the Hebrew words for man and woman both contain the word *Aish,* meaning "sacred fire." The heart is viewed as an innermost altar where the Aish rises as the Heart Fire of eternal love.

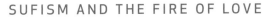

SUFISM AND THE FIRE OF LOVE

In Sufism the heart is the sacred space within where we encounter God as the Beloved. Here the fire of love melts away any separation—the coverings or masks of the soul. Through meditations including chanting, movement, and prayer, a burning love that was lived by the great saints of the path such as Jelalluddin Rumi and Rabia— is stoked to realize the One.

TAOIST ALCHEMICAL FIRE

Taoists see the heart as an alchemical fire that is nourished by water. Together these two elements create the eternal quality of love. The Heart Fire is considered the natural "governor" or organizing intelligence that refines one's eternal spirit. Taoist alchemical practices carried out in the heart center focus on regenerating energy through the combining of male and female essence, respectively symbolized as fire (sun) and water (moon).

When the inward and outward
are illuminated, and all is clear,
You are one with the light
of sun and moon.

— LIU I-MING,
AWAKENING TO THE TAO[4]

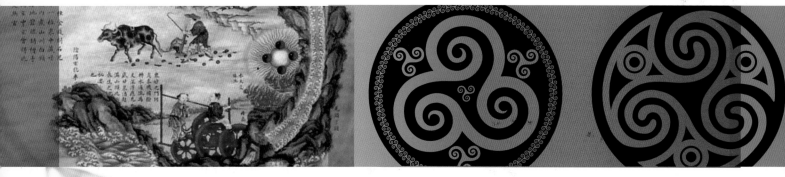

CELTIC CAULDRON OF THE HEART

In Celtic tradition, the heart is envisioned as a cauldron, an image that evokes the home hearth and the light of what is known as the *nwyvre,* or sacred fire. At eight sacred points on the wheel of the year, the community bonfire and the central fire in each home are reignited as an act of rekindling this Heart Fire to reconsecrate and bless land and family.

Fire in the head to quicken us.

Fire in the cauldron to heal us.

Fire in the forge of the heart

to temper us.

— CELTIC POEM
BY HEDGEWYTCH[5]

SHAMANIC AND INDIGENOUS TRADITIONS

Shamanism is a worldwide spiritual practice that transcends religions and schools of philosophy, one that has been adapted to modern life and is still practiced in ancient forms in indigenous communities today. The core pan-shamanic ritual is a fire ceremony that recognizes the fire within all beings drawn together from the fire of the earth-womb (mother) and the fire of the sun (father) into the fire of the heart.[6]

VAJRAYANA—TANTRIC BUDDHISM AND BODHICITTA

In the mystical practice of *vajrayana,* also known as Tantric Buddhism, clear seeing becomes possible when we cultivate *bodhicitta,* limitless love and compassion toward all beings. To develop bodhicitta we must nurture the most pristine expression of wisdom and compassion, and this lies in our heart center. In other words, the path to liberation begins in the heart—the original light of consciousness. In this tantric tradition, there is an alchemical meditation in which the yogi visualizes a glowing red sphere of feminine heat at the navel center; this point of heat bursts into flames and rises up

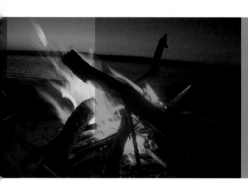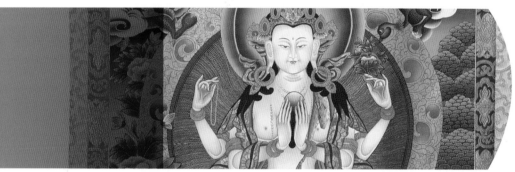

Your heart is your first teacher.

— CHEROKEE SAYING

the central channel toward the crown of the head. The crown holds a visualized seed syllable of the masculine, which begins to melt and drip downward. Thus these psychic energies are drawn toward one another and meet in the heart—where they join in an explosion of bliss and emptiness that radiates throughout the body, purifying it of toxins and activating bodhicitta, the "heartmind of awakening."

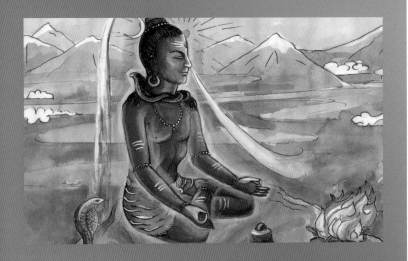

THE HEART FIRE IN THE YOGA TRADITIONS OF INDIA

Within the ancient traditions of yoga, the heart has been known as *hridaya*, a source of universal light and human consciousness. Drawn from the root *hrd* meaning "center," *hridaya* refers to the heart organ itself, as well as to the field of energetic consciousness that is present in every part of the body and in all creation. It is also connected with the heart chakra, *anahata*.

In this view, the microcosm of the heart is the central altar of the body and all macrocosmic bodies as well: the "heart" within the hearth of the home; the Heart Fire within the "body" as a fire pit—the inner sanctum of the temple; and the heart of the cosmos as the sun. All of these elements breathe and pulse together. When we bow to the outer fire, we bow to the fire within; and when we bow within, we are also connecting to the heart of creation. Yoga is the process that allows us to see and experience all of these different levels of extraordinary interconnectedness, a practical transmutation of the tensions that create separation and disconnectedness.

Hridaya—The Light of the Heart in the Vedas

> It is the heart which enables a human being to penetrate into deep secrets and mysteries.
>
> — VEDAS[7]

The Vedic texts, the oldest scriptures of Hinduism, offer our earliest glimpse into the extraordinary relationship between sacred fire and the cosmic body. The heart as hrd and hridaya—a light of consciousness—is prevalent throughout the Vedas, a means of deep insight (*dhi*) that leads one to become a *rsi* (seer). The Rig Veda correlates the sacrificial fire altar (*vedi*) to the human heart, considered the *axis mundi* between the microcosm and the macrocosm.

The Upanishads—Loosening the Knot in the Heart

> The shining self dwells hidden in the heart. Everything in the cosmos, great and small, lives in the Self—the source of life.
>
> — MUNDAKA UPANISHADS[8]

Within the foundational Hindu scriptures of the 108 Upanishads, the heart is continually invoked as the secret locale of the immortal soul or the Self (Atman), ultimately understood to be an expression of the Absolute (Brahman) in microcosm.[9] The Upanishads prescribe that ignorance of one's own immortal Self must be sacrificed to a transformative, subtle fire kindled within the altar of the heart. All yoga practice is described as a means to loosen the knot in the heart. Once the Self is revealed and experienced within the lotus of the heart through this internal fire ritual, the pure Self is liberated.

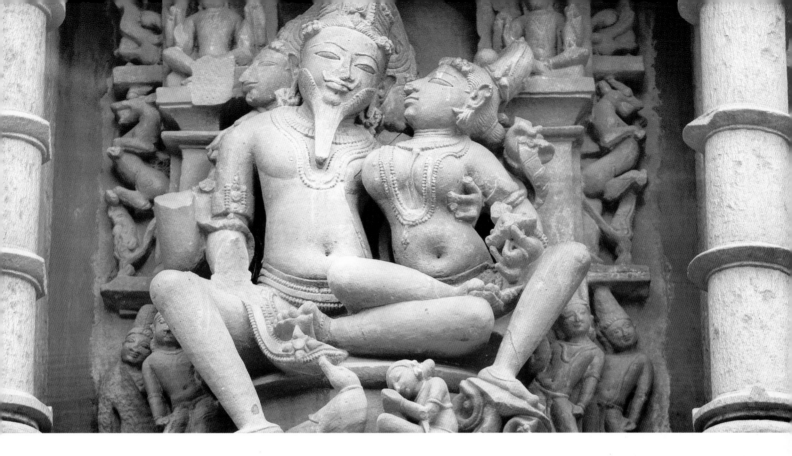

Tantric Shaivism and the Inner Heart Fire

> One is to visualize the fire of the union
> (*samghattam*) of the sun, moon, and fire as
> a single-pointed focus in the heart.
>
> — SRI ABHINAVAGUPTA[10]

The tantric tradition also teaches of the realization of the inner Heart Fire as a fire altar that can be experienced as the omnipresent source of divine consciousness in the union of Shiva and Shakti. Shiva (the Auspicious One) is seen as the ultimate ground of the dynamic universe.[11] The timeless rhythms of the universe, the limitless cycles of expansion and contraction, are the play of the Goddess, known as Shakti (energy/power). She is the continual pulsation of the universal heart, manifesting as the innumerable wavelike expressions that arise and dissolve back into the "ocean" of Supreme Awareness (Shiva).

Tantra views the soul and the elemental body as expressions of the one divine consciousness that manifests itself into myriad infinite forms—only to dissolve these forms back into itself in a continual pulsation encapsulating the cycle of life and death.

The dance of Shiva and Shakti is known as the great *sphuratta*, the "pulse" or "heartthrob" of the Supreme Light that continuously delights in its own blissful radiance. The cyclical rhythms of the macrocosmic universe exist in the microcosm of the human being, experienced as the pulsating cycle of breath connected to the fire altar in the heart where Shiva and Shakti are united, or *yamala*.[12]

the energetic heart
throughout western history

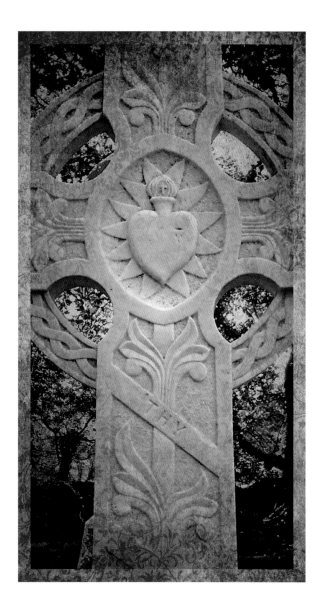

The mystics who have always walked among us have not been the only people to investigate and contemplate the heart's many meanings. While theirs is a direct experience of the Heart Fire, philosophers, artists, scientists, and others have considered the nature of the heart as well, and perceptions of the heart have evolved through time.

Since before the ancient cultures of Egypt and Greece and through the Renaissance, the human heart was known as a light of guiding wisdom and a source of love. This had been human understanding for thousands of years. Then came the disembodied philosophy best expressed by seventeenth-century French philosopher Rene Descartes—"I think, therefore I am"—and that notion that our thinking, not our feeling, drives our existence has now persisted for hundreds of years. The heart has been conceptualized as a mere mechanical pump, and the brain has been elevated to dominion over the entire being.

But a seismic shift of perception is occurring. We are reclaiming our understanding of the heart as the center of the human body—and of human life and experience. Through science, medicine, and the introduction of myriad forms of yoga and spiritual practice, we are being reintroduced to the rhythmic beat that animates us, the pulsing force that connects us to one another, the planet, and the cosmos.

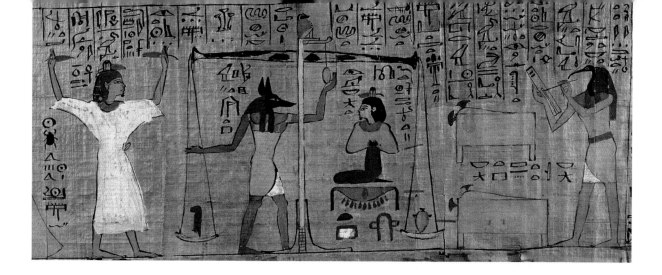

ANCIENT EGYPT: THE ETERNAL HEART

Mention of the heart first appears in writing in Egypt around 2000 BCE. The Egyptians believed that this primal throbbing in the body belonged to the heavens, and that it was its own living force, eternal and separate from the rest of the body. It ignited all life, all thought, all emotion—and it was created from a single drop of our mother's blood.

ANCIENT GREECE: THE HEART OF COURAGE

For the ancient Greeks, the heart was the body's center of strength, courage, and loyalty. It was the great furnace of the body—the force of heat that generated all thought and action. It was also home to the body's "humors," the fluids that kept the body in balance.

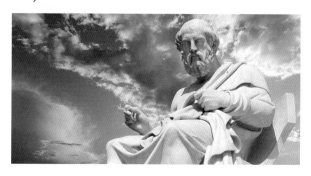

The great Greek philosophers invested considerable energy in contemplating the heart. Plato deemed it the organ of passion, the center that fueled human ferocity—anger, love, pride, and determination. Yet he saw it as second to the higher-functioning brain, theorizing that love became nobler, more high-minded, more true, when it traveled from the heart to the brain.

Plato's student Aristotle disputed this claim and pronounced the heart to be the most important organ in the body—the locus of all our intelligence, wisdom, and sensation. He described it as a "hot" organ and believed the other organs of the body existed to serve it.

It wasn't until Hippocrates, considered the father of Western medicine, became curious about the heart that its exploration became a more scientific investigation.

THE MEDIEVAL HEART

During the Middle Ages, the body was viewed not as a vessel of beauty and goodness but as an object of fear and shame.[13] Medicine aimed to cure disease by clearing the body of sin. But even during this time, light and spirit in the body were considered centered in the heart. There, one could connect to one's goodness and ascend to God.

In the late twelfth century, Master Nicolaus deemed the heart the primary "spiritual member of the body." St. Augustine of Hippo, who wrote extensively about the heart as a path to God, wrote, "By your fire, your generous fire, our hearts are filled with fire."[14] During medieval times, the heart was the very center of spiritual experience.

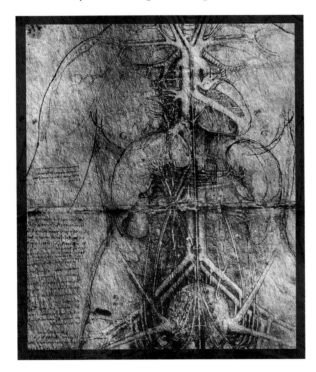

THE RENAISSANCE AND LEONARDO DA VINCI: THE FOUR-CHAMBERED HEART

During the Renaissance, physicians practiced human dissection and discovered the four chambers of the heart. The human body became a popular subject of artwork during this time, and many artists—most notably, Leonardo da Vinci—honored it through drawings and paintings. Da Vinci created intricate depictions of the heart's

valves and surrounding arteries, and through such detail, also provided by other famous artists and dissecting physicians, it became clear that the heart was involved in the flow of blood through the body by means of a circulatory system.

It was at this point that a great rift emerged: the heart began to be divorced from spirit.

RENE DESCARTES: THE HEART AS AN ENGINE

Descartes adopted an idea that the heart was the "sun" or "king" of the body and then took it a step further by describing it as the great combustion engine driving the body. He also saw the heart as an automatic mechanical pump, "an automaton whose movements followed the same principles as a clock."[15] In his view, spirit was not present in the heart—and the new and radical split between mind and heart became a chasm in Western thought.

THE INDUSTRIAL REVOLUTION: THE HEART AS A PUMP

During the Industrial Revolution, advances in technology led to more accurate representations of the anatomy of the heart. Now its transformation into a limited and purely functional organ—as a pumping machine in service to the brain—was complete. With this strictly mechanical view, the mind and body were split by the barriers in the heart, which was now devoid of intelligence, emotion, and sentience.

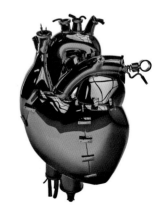

THE ENERGETIC HEART RETURNS—THE NEW FIELD OF CARDIOENERGETICS

Extraordinary discoveries in cardiology over the past century and in recent decades have reaffirmed the energetic heart through the development of devices to measure heart rate, electrical activity, and the heart's electromagnetic field. Further insights have come from the experiences of patients who have had heart transplants. The heart is now described as a "heartbrain" for the ways in which it communicates within the body neurally, hormonally, and energetically. The discovery of the electromagnetic field of the heart, which is five thousand times stronger than that of the brain[16] and radiates outside the body to connect with other "heart fields," is parallel to the metaphorical descriptions of the experience of the heart held within the world's spiritual traditions.[17] The heart's heat and radiance, intelligence and intuitive power can now be understood within the scientific discoveries of the heart's energetic knowing, which we will explore in Chapter Three.

Organizations such as the Institute of HeartMath have taken this a step further by developing heart-based educational and stress-relief tools and making them available to a wide population. Projects like its Global Coherence Initiative are measuring and activating the collective energetic field of the earth and human beings around the world.

So through scientific evolution, our view of our heart is coming full circle, transforming to encompass many of the ways in which our ancestors experienced the heart: as a seat of organizing intelligence, a light of consciousness, and a transforming locus of the rhythms of love.

ancestral firekeeping
and our energy future

The universe bestows on us fire from the
beginning of time, simultaneously evoking
our profound reverence for this fire.
This is the central fire of your self, the central fire
of the entire cosmos: it must not be wasted
on trivialities or revenge, resentment or despair.
We have the power to forge cosmic fire.
What can compare with such a destiny?

— BRIAN SWIMME,
THE UNIVERSE IS A GREEN DRAGON[18]

OUR ANCESTORS TENDED FIRE FOR TWO MILLION YEARS BEFORE THE ADVENT OF ELECTRICITY[19]

This ability to tend fire is often considered to be *the* turning point in human evolution. Furthermore, the harnessing of electricity drastically changed our relationship to the living flame—we now had the ability to summon or banish light and heat with a simple switch. We have gained this ability so recently that it occupies barely a blip on the continuum of human history: Less than a hundred years ago, only 15 percent of the population of the United States had electricity. It has only been about forty years since electricity was made available virtually everywhere in America.[20]

This means that, for all our recent technological achievement, we are only a generation or two removed from a connection to the living flame and a rhythm of life based in the natural ebb and flow of light, of activity and rest. Consider this striking fact: worldwide today, a billion people on earth still tend a living flame. How has our relationship to convenient light affected our soul and our relationship to energy resources in this last century of unprecedented waste and ecological destruction?

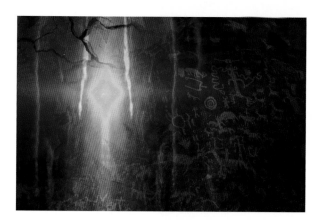

Can the living flame reconnect us to our own inner fire and help us realize the miracle, mystery, and call of our times—to replace toxic fuel sources with renewable sources? We must wake up to our legacy of two millions years of firekeeping, reclaim our sacred relationship to our inner and outer fuel, and pass it along to future generations of firekeepers.

EMERGENCE OF MEDITATION AROUND THE FIRE

One thing we can all agree upon in our history of firekeeping is that all beings become quiet around a fire, particularly an open-air bonfire. We seem to remember fires past as we enter into a natural meditation. We can sense the shift of consciousness the flames induce in us as the fire calls forth in cellular memory the reverence and passion of untold generations. The living flame in the candle on our altar or in a fireplace or bonfire contains the same energy as those that illuminated prehistoric shelters, ancient home hearths, and the eternal flames of temples and sacred sites. Fire is at the center of time, our solar system, the atoms that compose our cells, and our energetic heart. It is no wonder that we gather in its presence.

The meditations arising from the fire are the yoga of our collective cultural heritage. Whether we remain in quiet contemplation, gazing at the flames against a deep night sky; unleash primal sounds in the form of mantra; or embody the fire's activity through the moving meditations of asana or dance, we touch the lives of our ancestors, who responded just as we do to the fire's call. Instinctually and through time, we have always recognized it as an outward manifestation of the fire burning at our core, a reflection of the fierce energy of the heart.

the loss of the living flame

When we have no open flame in our lives, when we cannot ignite or tend a living fire, we become disconnected from our essential primal nature. The impact of this disconnection is profound and is experienced both individually and collectively:

> Our vitality and passion fade

> We experience widespread heart disease, depression, and anxiety unheard of in our ancestors' worlds

> We disturb the very rhythms of the earth and witness the destruction and poisoning of the natural world that has sustained us

Before 1900, very few people in the world died of heart disease.[21] But since then we have been living with the consequences of our disconnection from natural rhythms—our electrified world—and heart disease has become the number-one killer in the United States: one out of three Americans and more than 50 percent of American men die from it.[22] The same changes in technology that ushered in the mechanized view of the heart as a pump automated human activities, leading to sedentary, indoor lifestyles; making available diets high in processed foods; and creating stress, 24/7.

At the turn of the twentieth century, one-third of Americans lived and fed themselves on farms; a century later, only 1 percent of our population lives in a rural environment.[23] We used to spend 90 percent of our waking hours outdoors. Now that figure has been upended: we spend 90 percent of our waking hours indoors.[24] This marks a drastic change not only in natural physical activity but also in our relationship to the natural rhythms of rest and activity, light and darkness. This creates imbalances in the anahata chakra.

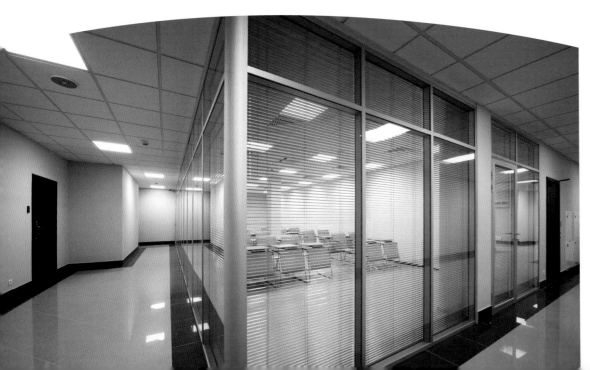

A FIREKEEPING / ENERGY-FUTURE TIMELINE [25]

> **20 billion years ago**—Estimated date of primordial fire (big bang)

> **5 billion years ago**—Formation of the solar system

> **4.5 million years ago**—Oldest human ancestral remains in Ethiopia

> **2 million years ago**—Fire used by precursors of *Homo sapiens* at sites in Kenya and South Africa

> **790,000 years ago**—The earliest known traces of controlled fire at Gesher Benot Ya'aqov, Israel

> **400,000 BCE**—Widespread evidence of fire-making in caves and rock shelters in Africa, Asia, and Europe

> **250,000 years ago**—The first known cooking fire in East Africa

> **34,000 to 23,000 years ago**—The first hearths, charcoal, burnt bones, and burned wooden objects appear in southern Greece

> **8000 BCE**—World's oldest sun temple in Bulgaria is built

> **Circa 5000 BCE**—At Mohenjo Daru in present-day Pakistan, fire altars appear at the center of the community and homes

> **Circa 2600 BCE**—Egyptian sun temples: Pyramid of Djoser (Zoser) built

> **Circa 1200 BCE**—Passover candles are lit for Jewish Sabbath

> **Eighth century CE**—India's oldest sacred fire continually burning is brought from Persia as a sacred fire within Zoroastrian religion

> **Twelfth century CE**—The development of chimneys

> **Eighteenth century CE**—Coal begins to displace other fuels

> **1820s**—The industrial revolution begins

> **1860**—The first solar-powered system is developed in France to produce steam to drive machinery

> **1882**—The first electric plant is built by Thomas Edison in New York

> **1901**—The beginning of the modern oil industry

> **1920**—Only 15% of United States has electricity in urban areas

> **1950**—Petroleum becomes the most-used fuel in the United States

> **1978**—The world's first solar-powered village is created on the Tohono O'odham Reservation in Arizona

> **1980**—The world's first wind farm was created in New Hampshire

> **1994**—The United States began importing more petroleum than it was producing

> **2005**—The U.S. House prevents oil drilling in the Arctic National Wildlife Refuge

> **2008**—The National Biofuel Action Plan was announced

> **2009**—The Kyoto Protocol was revoked after committee members failed to reach agreement about the future of its role in regulating international greenhouse gas emissions as global warming is brought to the forefront of the world's attention

> **2010**—Energy use analysis shows that Americans waste 54% more energy than they use

> **2012**—An estimated 16% of global final energy consumption comes from renewable resources, including biomass (10%), hydroelectricity (3.4%), and newly developed sources (3%) such as wind, solar, and geothermal

> **2066**—It is estimated that solar-powered generators will be the primary provider of the world's electricity needs, significantly decreasing harmful greenhouse gas emissions

Imbalances in Anahata Chakra

Excessive imbalances relate to the reactive emotions that arise through stress, triggers from the past, attachment, drama, and too much heat. They include:

> Excess attachment and controlling energy toward material possessions or relationships

> Obsessions and ruminating about unfinished business, emotions, or conversations

> Entangling energetic bonds and emotions across space in an unhealthy way

Deficient imbalances include:

> Loss of joy or pleasure in life, which can lead to apathy or depression

> Numbness and a lack of feeling, emotion, love, appreciation, gratitude, or empathy

> A damming up or suppression of unresolved emotional or thought patterns or experiences from the past, either by "shutting down" through disconnecting from the heart or "stuffing" the emotion or thought rather than dealing with it

> Apathetic, cynical, or overly intellectual or analytical outlook to avoid feeling

> Shallow breathing, contracted ribcage, and sunken chest

OUR HEART'S CALL— HEALING THE SOURCE OF STRESS

Only by reclaiming our fire-tending—on the altar, in the hearth, and in the pulsing fire that burns in our center—can we reconnect to natural rhythms within and reverse these modern trends. And it is not hard to do. Light a single candle and watch the small flame dance for a moment. You have begun.

Beat by beat, our hearts are patiently requesting that we return to the natural flow of life. The message is clear. Sometimes, in fact, the heart speaks more clearly than we are ready to hear, sparking the brain's expert ability to rationalize and resist change. Yet the heart's mystic force continues to invite us to inhabit our core selves: our truth, our longing, and our deepest passions. Even if we have distanced ourselves from its rhythms for a long time, the moment we place our attention there, it will always welcome us again.

When the power of love overcomes the love of power, the world will know peace.

— JIMI HENDRIX

tending the fires of primal love

At the very, very beginning, the universe comes into existence and these various forms of matter experience an attraction for each other. ...by responding to that, they complexify and over time gave birth to galaxies and then living beings and humans. So that very attraction is what gave rise to our existence in our consciousness. We are becoming aware of the attraction that actually gave birth to us. That would be the way to summarize the whole story in terms of attraction or love.

Using love now as a word that refers to the whole cosmological dimension of attraction, love brought forth complexity in the universe and then burst into awareness of itself. So we are the place in which the original primal love of the universe is aware of itself and we're aware of that every time we fall in love.

—BRIAN SWIMME[26]

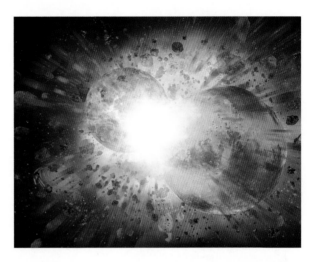

One of the most powerful forces in the heart is the force of love. Physicist Brian Swimme describes love as gravity, a primary force of attraction and bonding found in the creation of the universe. We are part of this original primordial fire and the force of love. The discovery of fire and our destructive use of energy on the planet are two sides of our human legacy. Modern firekeepers tend their lifeforce in many forms. They are artists, activists, teachers, musicians, scientists, healers, and entrepreneurs. They are mothers, fathers, sisters, and brothers. Love, devotion, and skill are required to keep such fires flourishing. We must embody fuel, fire, and firekeeper all at once to realize the extraordinary creative force that burns within us. What do you love intrinsically? What do you live for? What would you die for?

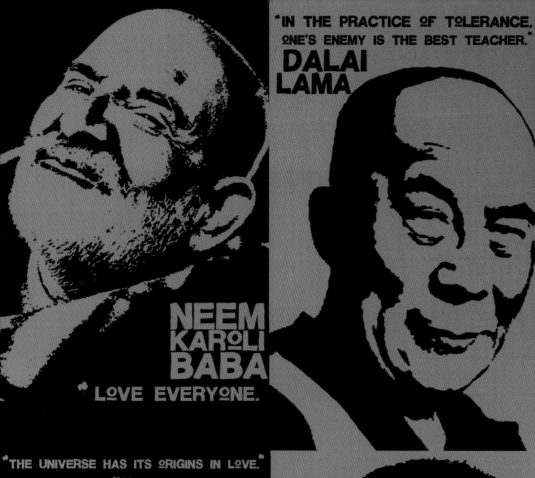

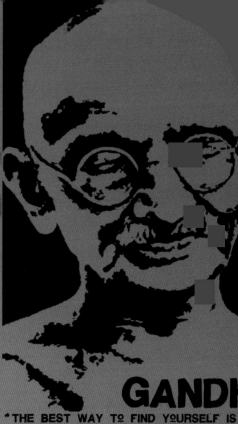

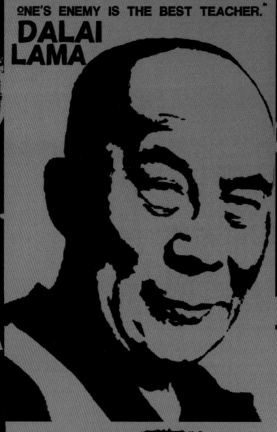

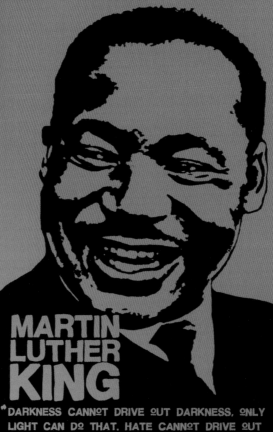

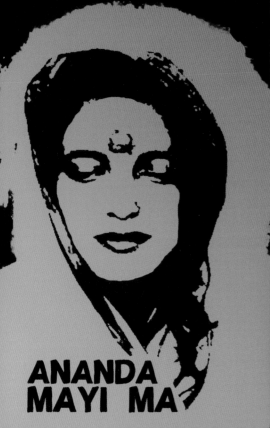

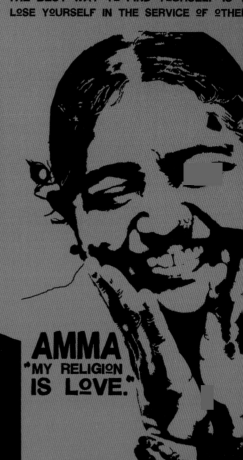

"IN THE PRACTICE OF TOLERANCE, ONE'S ENEMY IS THE BEST TEACHER."
DALAI LAMA

NEEM KAROLI BABA
"LOVE EVERYONE."

GANDH
"THE BEST WAY TO FIND YOURSELF IS T LOSE YOURSELF IN THE SERVICE OF OTHER

"THE UNIVERSE HAS ITS ORIGINS IN LOVE."

ANANDA MAYI MA

MARTIN LUTHER KING
"DARKNESS CANNOT DRIVE OUT DARKNESS, ONLY LIGHT CAN DO THAT. HATE CANNOT DRIVE OUT HATE. ONLY LOVE CAN DO THAT."

AMMA
"MY RELIGION IS LOVE."

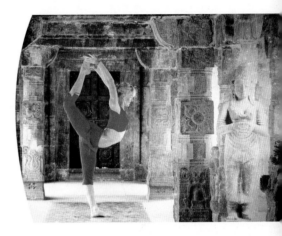

embodying
the cosmos

From the Primordial Fire to the Inner Heart Altar

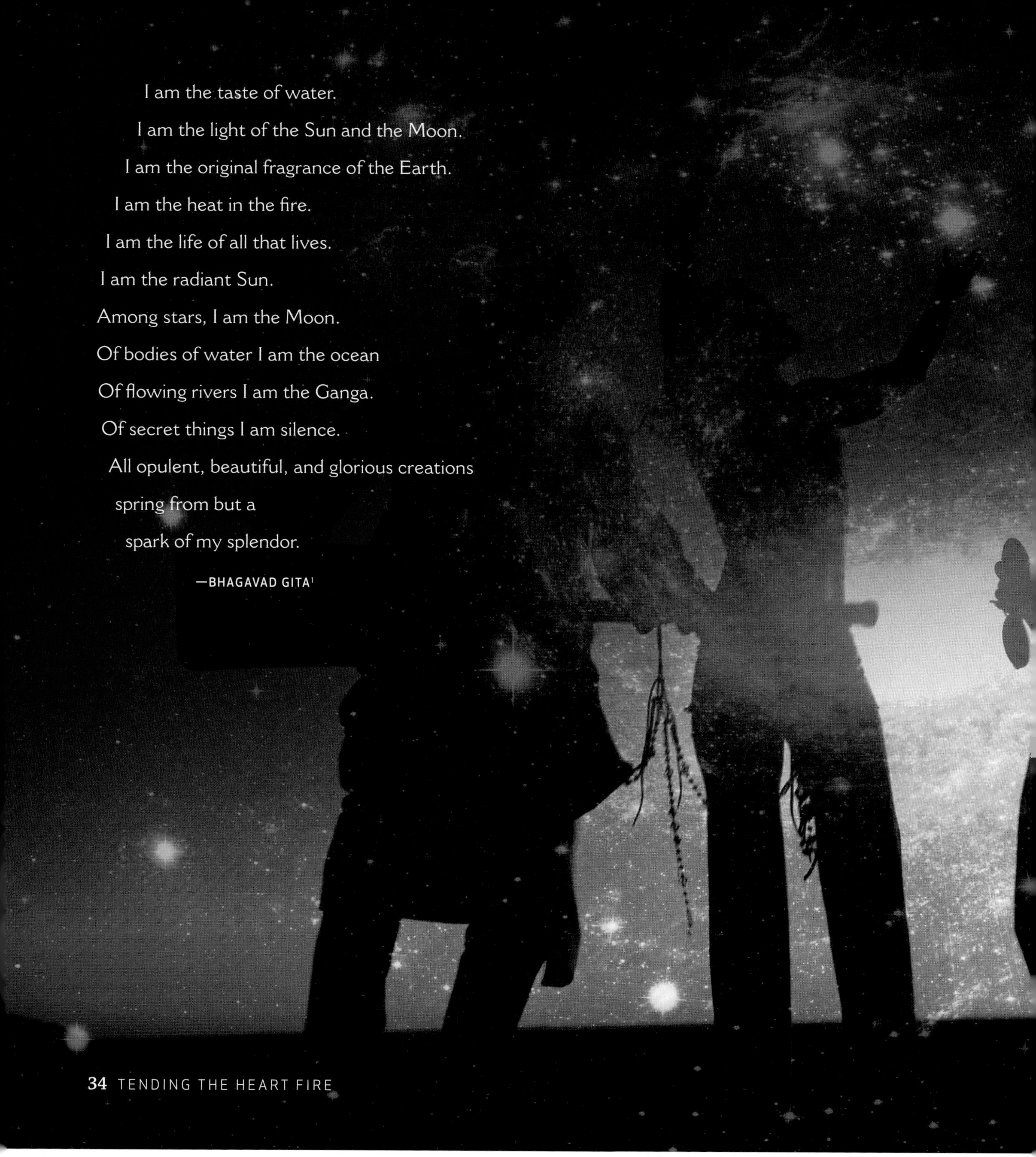

I am the taste of water.

I am the light of the Sun and the Moon.

I am the original fragrance of the Earth.

I am the heat in the fire.

I am the life of all that lives.

I am the radiant Sun.

Among stars, I am the Moon.

Of bodies of water I am the ocean

Of flowing rivers I am the Ganga.

Of secret things I am silence.

All opulent, beautiful, and glorious creations

spring from but a

spark of my splendor.

—BHAGAVAD GITA[1]

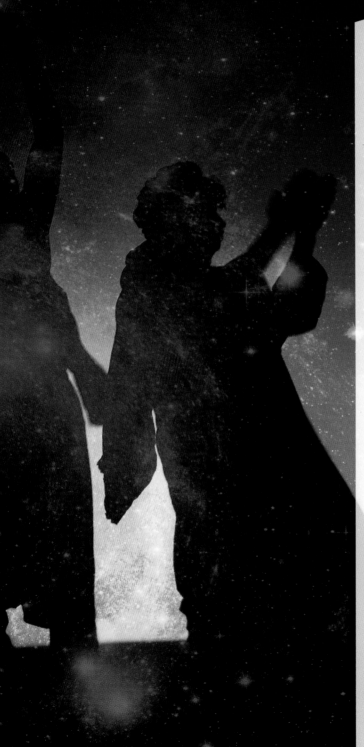

As is above as is below.

The body is the microcosm of the cosmic macrocosm.

— SHIVA SAMHITA[2]

WITHIN THE SPIRITUAL CULTURE OF INDIA FROM WHICH YOGA EMERGES,

the human body is seen as a manifestation of the sacred, all-permeating source: a reflection of the cosmic body. That the human body is a reflection of cosmic life is a central tenet in many of the world's traditions. Temples found around the world serve a dual extraordinary purpose: as observatories of the massive awe of the cosmos—the alignment of the sun, moon, planets, and stars—and as sacred ritual space built in this cosmic reflection that is activated by these alignments. This view first appears in the fire altar of Vedic tradition, where the sacred flame of Agni was tended with reverence under the star-filled sky. It flowers in tantric tradition with the inner fire of the cosmic body found within.

Throughout this evolution, the subtle energy body was increasingly viewed as a microcosmic map of the earth, the elements, and the cosmos. The currents of energy within us were rivers flowing through the vast landscape of the body; the spine was a mountain cradling the cave of the heart where the fire of consciousness burns. The sun was the vital energy of the body, and the moon was the inner nectar.

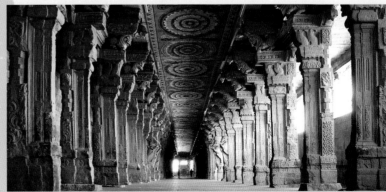

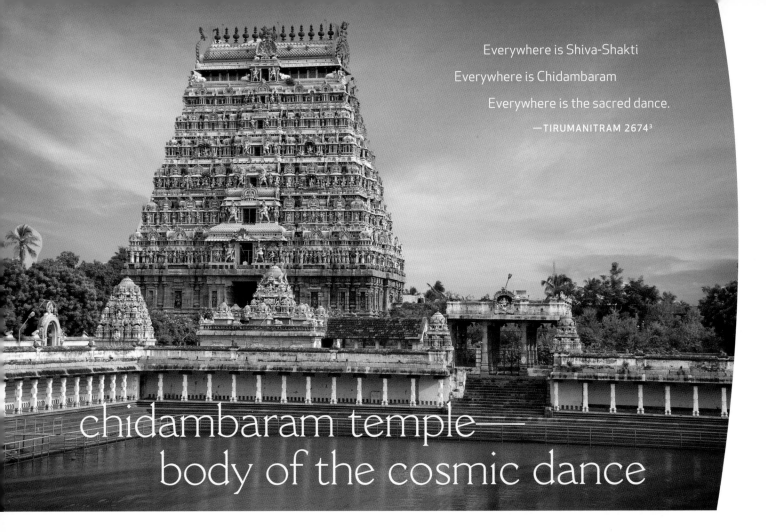

chidambaram temple— body of the cosmic dance

Located at the center point of the world's magnetic equator, Chidambaram Temple in the Tamil Nadu state of India, is considered the "heart of the universe." It is built on the plan of the divine body, *vastu purusha,* and dedicated to Nataraja, the cosmic dance of Shiva and Natarajika or Shakti that brought the world into being. The word *chidambaram* translates as "sky of consciousness."

The inner sanctum of the temple is the heart of Shiva's body, represented as a crystalized *lingam* in union with Shakti as *yoni,* near large statues of Shiva and Shakti as the cosmic dance. Other structures in the temple are also symbolic of the body.[4] Crossbeams represent blood vessels. Some 21,600 golden tiles,

symbolizing the number of breaths in a day, are fastened with 72,000 golden nails—the number of *nadis* (energetic pathways) that exist in the human body. On each of the four *gopuras,* or heads of the temple, depictions of the 108 *karanas* (flowing postures) that express the connection between the human body and the divine are carved on the walls. The image of a dancing universe gives rise to embodied practices that respond to the universal pulse, such as yoga karanas (asanas), namaskar (ritual movement or salutation) and *natya* (dance forms), and *kirtan* (music and chanting). Images of the yogic sages Patanjali, Narada, and Aghysta are carved within Chidambaram Temple as mythic witnesses to Shiva's dance.

PILGRIMAGE TO CHIDAMBARAM

Chidambaram is a pilgrimage place or *tirthas* that has transformed my experience of sublime embodiment. The first time I visited, I became the mudra of Natarajasana in the middle of the mandala of the Devi temple. I felt completely open without warming up. In the living temple, limbs lift from the heart. Freedom of movement is a reflection of the inner current.

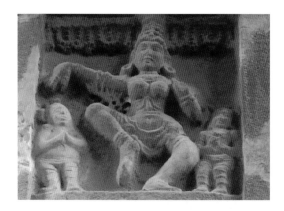

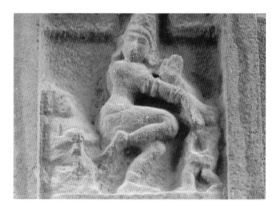

I heard the teachings echoed through mantra, sutras, devotion, *nyasa* (the activation of mantra-mudra-meditation) piercing my body. All the tirthas—places of pilgrimage—are found within the body.

Chidambuda manim budha hridambuja

ravim para chidambaranatam hridi bhaje

(Adore in the heart—the supreme Dancer of Chidambaram)

—PATANJALI FROM THE SHAMBHU NATANAM[5]

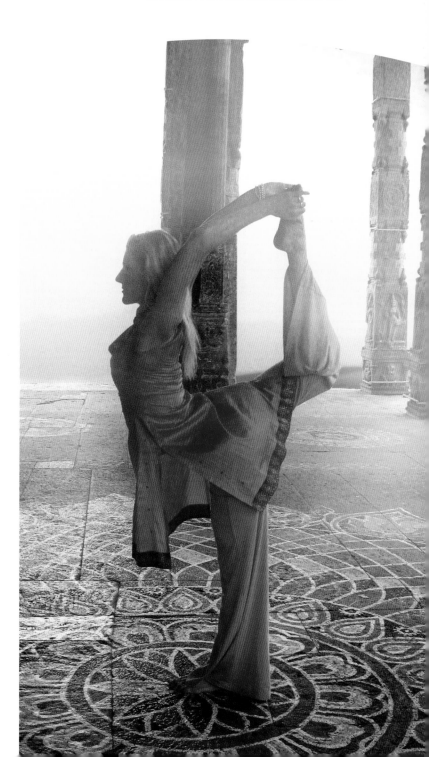

vastu-purusha—fire altar as the cosmic body

From his mind the moon was born,

And from his eye the sun,

From his mouth Indra and the fire,

From his breath the wind was born,

From his navel arose the atmosphere,

And from his head the sky evolved,

From his feet the earth, and from his ear,

The cardinal points of the compass:

So did they fashion forth these worlds.

—PURUSHA SUKTA OF THE RIG VEDA[6]

The *mahavedi,* or "great fire altar," is an altar that is built in a manner that reflects "the cosmic body," which honors all of the elements, directions, limbs, and divine currents. According to ayurvedic physician Vasant Lad, the five elements of the universe correspond to those that constitute the human body: *akasha* (ether), *vayu* (wind/air), *tejas* (fire), *apas* (fluid/water), and *prithvi* (solid/earth). These are considered to be the building blocks of all creation.[7]

The Vedic fire altar is constructed according to an elaborate plan that expresses the cycle of the year and the elements of the universe, incorporating many meaningful, symbolic components. In a complex form, it contains 360 border stones, representing the number of degrees in a circle and the flow of the days of the year. A central pillar, called a *stambha,* is raised near the altar to represent the unity of above and below, heaven and earth. Five

layers of bricks correspond to five seasons of the year. Fire sticks used to kindle the fire represent the friction of creation.[8]

The basic square structure of the fire altar evokes the containment of the earth element, or *prithvi,* while the empty center of the fire altar is "space," or *akash.* When ghee is poured in the fire ceremony, it is liquid nectar, or *apa.* The sacred fire at the center is *agni.* The eight cardinal directions are linked to the directions and planets, which are revered as divine and which recreate the cosmic "body" within the fire altar. The human body (*purusha*) is symbolically mapped onto the fire altar so that the center fire burns at the heart or navel (see below). Root

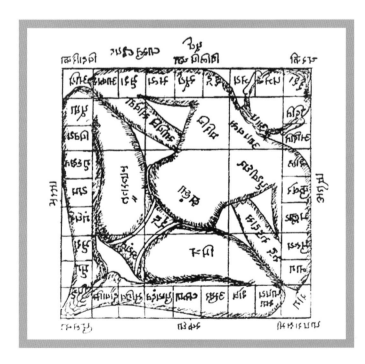

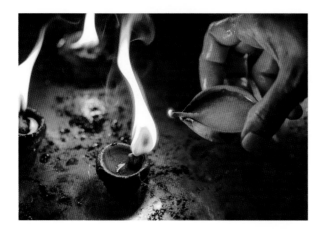

and limbs extend around the altar. The purusha represents the eternal Self, visualized as the divine fire of agni.

The person who tends the fire supplies the final element, exhaling to start the fire and thus bringing in the element of air, or vayu.

The lineage of firekeeping begins to crystallize in the Vedas, which view the fire altar as a way to connect to the cosmic rhythm of nature's cycles. Thus Vedic firekeeping allows us to remain connected to the rhythmic transitions of day and night as the earth journeys around the sun. We know that the sacrificial fire ritual of *yajna* has been performed in an unbroken flow for at least thirty-five hundred years, in synch with sunrise, midday, and sunset as well as during lunar cycles.[9] This is invoked in the Vedas as the *sandhya vandanam,* the practice of synchronizing our own rhythms with the sacred junctures of time.

On most householder altars, the space for the fire offering now takes the form of a *dipa,* or lamp. This represents the eternal flame of consciousness. The waving of the lamp at the end of the ritual, called *arati,* is an offering of the blessing of light.

AGNI HOTRA

Imagine living your life with the rhythms of a *yagna* or fire offering, This daily reminder of cosmic rhythms is reflected in the householder fire ritual known as *agni hotra,* conducted just before sunrise or sunset. The fire altar is reconstructed in a smaller version, usually in a copper fire vessel described as a *kund,* or womb. Traditionally, this fire is never to be extinguished; the fire of the daily offering is lit from the father's fire and passed on to his children, generation after generation. All of the important life-passage ceremonies occur around this central fire ritual, and there are special yajnas for the new and full moon and other important holidays throughout the year.

Om Agnaye Swaha
I Offer to the Fire of Consciousness

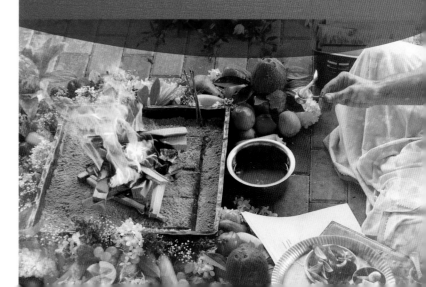

tending the inner fire—
the cosmic heart of tantra

The day is the upward
moving exhale,
and the night is the downward
moving inhale.

— KALOTTARA TANTRA XI.9 [11]

IN TANTRIC TRADITION the inner fire altar is alive within the body: we are embodiments of the divine. Every inner movement is experienced as the flow of Shakti, every breath a reflection of the cosmic pulse. The macro-rhythms of the cosmos are echoed in the micro-rhythms of the heartbeat and breath—and in myriad other movements and processes (spiritual, mental, emotional, and physical)—within. Our very heart is the alchemical meeting point of sun, moon, and fire.

The One who impels the universe is the Source of Consciousness (Shiva) to be discovered within the flow of one's own vital breath.

O Beloved One, Shiva gives rise to the year, the month, the half-month, and the day.

Find Shiva within time through Shakti, who is the cyclical flow of breath-time in the body.

— SVACCHANDA TANTRA [10]

COSMIC TIME CYCLES OF THE BREATH—SUN, MOON, AND FIRE

Within tantra, as practitioners, we place our focus on the realization and *embodiment* of the cosmic rhythm as the flow of consciousness. The pulsation at the heart mirrors the pulsation of life: the rhythmic cycles of expansion and contraction that create our experience of duality. Inhale and exhale, systolic and diastolic blood pressure—filling and emptying the heart—birth and death, young and old, night and day are experienced as a continuum of the Divine Power (Shakti) of Shiva, worshipped as a goddess or Devi in her own right. She is the vehicle by which Shiva manifests joyfully and creatively into the countless forms of the universe, or Shiva's "body," experienced as the field of time (*kala*) and place (*desa*).

Thus the Universal Soul (purusha) is embodied within the form of all beings and located in the heart: always one with Shiva and Shakti, consciousness and creative expression, the two within one that is found in all the world's spiritual traditions as the divine masculine and feminine. Shakti, as the creative manifestation of Shiva, is experienced as the vital force (prana) that follows a rhythmic cycle of creating, sustaining, and dissolving the microcosmic body with the flow of breath (*prana-cara*).

In the tantric tradition, every breath is a reflection of all such cycles, referred to as vinyasa or *cara*—movement or flow. External cycles of time—the day, the lunar cycles, the passing of seasons as we circle the sun—are mirrored in the phases of the breath, creating a "procession of internal time." Thus we internalize time itself by observing the flow of breath (time) within the body (space) in a single round of breath, a reflection of the cosmic rhythm.

O Beautiful Goddess, I have taught that there is a single twenty-four-hour day in a round of breath. Now I will explain how it contains the two halves of the internal month (waxing and waning moon)…

— SVACCHANDA TANTRA VII.64[12]

Arising through Capricorn from the winter solstice in the heart, the breath circulates in the bodies of all beings through twelve months (before returning to the heart).

— SVACCHANDA TANTRA VII.119[13]

sri yantra: essence of the heart bindu

From the fivefold Shakti comes creation
and from the fourfold Fire, dissolution.
The union of five Shaktis and
four Fires causes the chakra to evolve …
When she, the ultimate Shakti,
of her own will (*svecchaya*)
assumed the form of the universe,
then the creation of the chakra
revealed itself as a pulsating essence …
From this pulsating stream of
supreme light emanated the
ocean of the cosmos …
—YOGINI HRIDAYA, I 6–16[14]

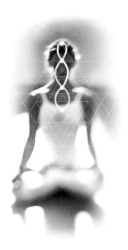

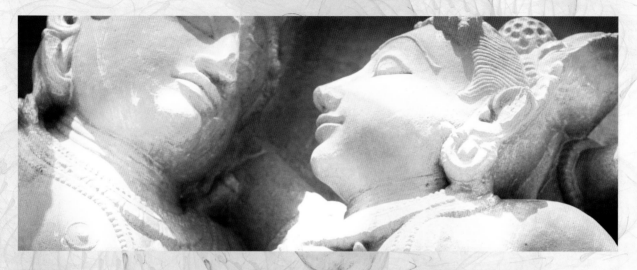

A *yantra* is a sacred pattern of the Divine. Sri Yantra as the sixty-four-point interpenetrating triangles expresses the pattern of the human body and the cosmos emanating from the pulsating *bindu* (center point or seed essence) at the heart of consciousness. This yantra also mirrors the cosmic body created from the union of Shiva and Shakti. And the bindu of the great yantra is mirrored within our hearts as the point of creation and dissolution, the receiving of new breath and the release of the out-breath.

Tantra views this oscillating motion as the lovemaking of fire and water, the interpenetrating of downward and upward, inward and outward, Shiva and Shakti united in the bindu of the heart of our own body and the universal body.

At the very heart of the bindu of Sri Yantra is *kamakala*, containing the three bindus or potentials. One is red, representing the ova of the Divine Mother; another is white, representing the seed of the Divine Masculine; and a third is mixed as the union of Shiva and Shakti, the individual body emerging from Sri Chakra. The three bindus are the essence of the sun, moon, and fire, unified in the heart of a human being like a single cell from which a human being grows. From this bindu of Sri Chakra, the cosmic body emerges, containing the constellations of the solar cycle, phases of the lunar cycle and the twelve months of the solar year, and more frequent cosmic rhythms.

Once again, we see the pulsation of the heart linked to the totality of creation and the cycles of time.

The father form gives four alchemical *dhatus,* or tissues, to the child, represented as the four fires or upward-pointing triangles. The ova of the mother form gives five dhatus to the child, known as the five *shaktis,* or downward-flowing triangles. Consciousness enters into form through the explosion of love from the eternal orgasm that is reflected throughout all of creation.[15]

kundalini shakti—heart fire as creative power

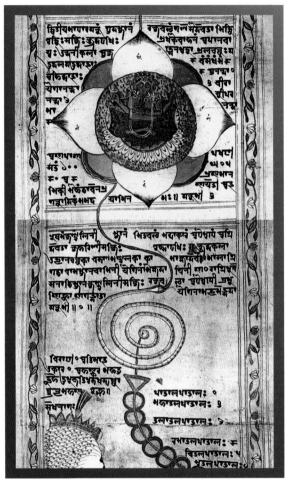

vibrating light that pulses the heart, coiling and uncoiling as the yogi or yogini's inner Heart Fire.

Beautiful sutras and poems from the great tantric sages confirm this understanding of the inner Heart Fire as kundalini shakti, and in them we learn to tend this fire by offering mantra, breath, and *bhakti* devotion to the heart. Just as a fire in the hearth is nourished and flourishes from fuel, the fuel of a practitioner's offering kindles and stokes the brilliance of consciousness.

Knowing this, as practitioners we can draw the moon and sun into our bodies through the in-breath and out-breath, as expressed in this passage:

> The Source manifests into form before
> the yogi, who in continual devotion
> is unwavering in his one-pointed focus
> as his awareness is drawn toward the
> emergence within the heart of Kundalini
> Shakti who, as the embodiment of
> pure consciousness, arises as a spark
> generated by the fire stick (*arani*) formed
> through the fusion of the lunar in-breath
> and solar out-breath as they are
> merged together in the heart.

> — SHRI KSHEMARAJA,
> ELEVENTH-CENTURY MASTER[17]

In the earliest tantric scripture, *kundalini shakti*, the creative life force and the kinetic aspect of consciousness, was always located within the heart. Though this is not well known today, it was not until the thirteenth century that the first written record appeared saying that kundalini rests coiled at the base of the spine.[16] Kundalini shakti is the

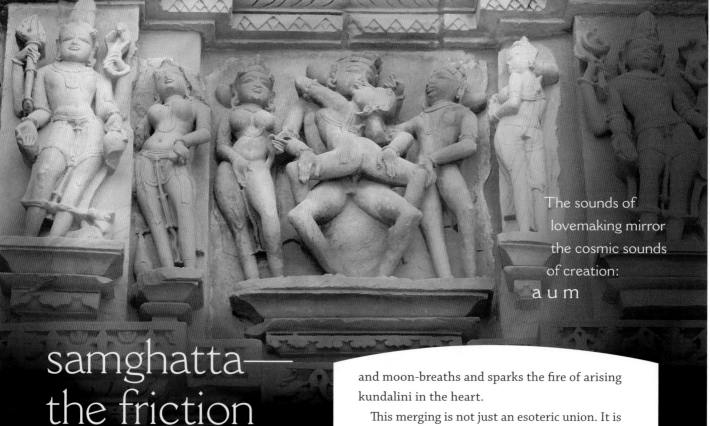

The sounds of lovemaking mirror the cosmic sounds of creation: a u m

samghatta— the friction and fire of lovemaking

The meeting of sun and moon can be found in the friction that starts the ritual fire, with the churning of lovemaking symbolized by the back-and-forth movement of the fire-stick in the "womb" of the sacrificial altar. This ritual reenacts the fire of creation in the heart of the cosmic body and within our own hearts in meditative practice.

In tantric practice, the sun- and moon-breaths are fused in the heart in *kumbhaka,* the stillness between in-breath and out-breath, and the mantra is "seeded" there into a coil. The friction of the pulsing mantra combines the radiance of the sun- and moon-breaths and sparks the fire of arising kundalini in the heart.

This merging is not just an esoteric union. It is experienced in every moment, particularly in heightened states when the heart and brain are in coherent flow and a meditative consciousness can arise within the fabric of everyday life. When we are in these states, we are able to perceive the extraordinary beauty and mysterious truths of life: *shivam satyam sundaram*—consciousness is truth and beauty.

The Heart Fire is alive with the energetic potency of the life force. We can hear and feel it in the pulse and life-giving energy of the breath. The heart center is the embodied nexus of tantric meditation, the vision of the dancing universe—our continually pulsating quantum field of life—embodied in the movements of yogis and yoginis and the dancing mystics through the ages.

Mantra, too, connects the sound of the pulse of life with the heart of consciousness as the origins of all form. The mantra is a sound body representing the sonic signature of the divine body.

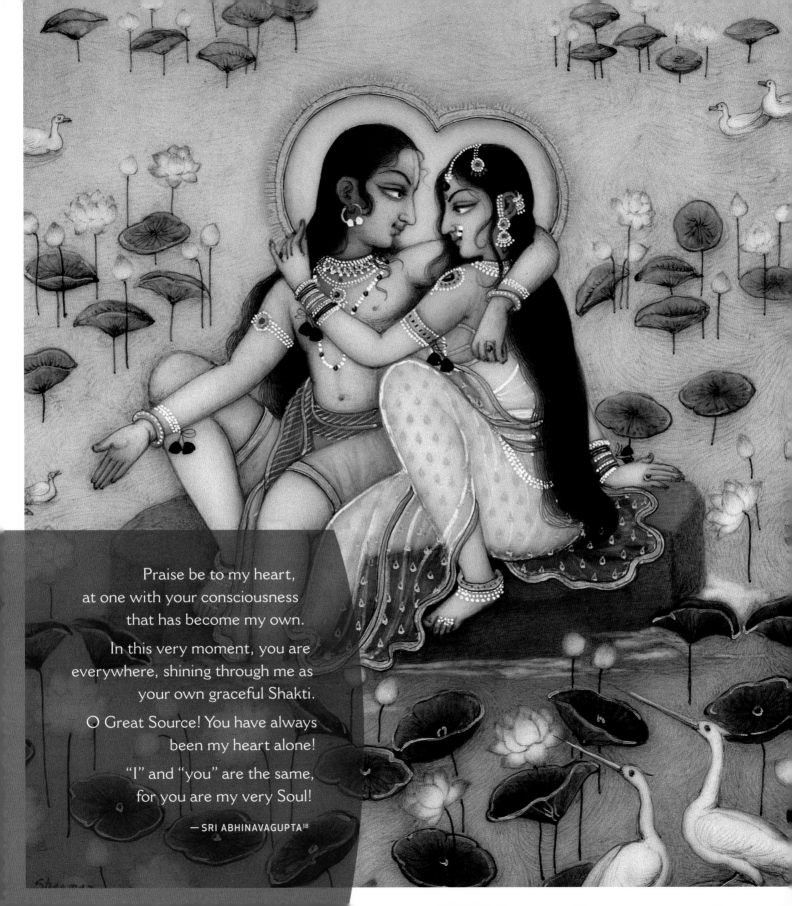

Praise be to my heart,
at one with your consciousness
that has become my own.

In this very moment, you are
everywhere, shining through me as
your own graceful Shakti.

O Great Source! You have always
been my heart alone!

"I" and "you" are the same,
for you are my very Soul!

— SRI ABHINAVAGUPTA[18]

the heart fire of bhakti

The Sanskrit word *bhakti* originates from the word *bhaj,* meaning to "belong to" or "share in" as well as "to worship." Its meaning is often interpreted as "devotion," but the full meaning is beyond definition, as it is the igniting of a natural feeling of devotion, an inner realization of the fire of love that has been core to yoga from the beginning. It was first described as a path of realization through love of God in all forms and all ways, or *bhaktimarga,* in the Bhagavad Gita (500 BCE).[19] Central to bhakti is an emphasis on a mystic and loving experience with the Source, a relationship that is often seen as beloved-lover, friend-friend, parent-child, or God-servant.

The Heart Fire in the form of bhakti ignited a revolutionary change in yoga when bold ones on the path were transformed by their direct experience of the Source. The transforming fire of bhakti lit a flame across India. It is characterized by the dissolution of all caste and wealth restrictions; equality of men and women as the true vision of Oneness and love; and the writings of its poet-saints, male and female—from the Tantric Siddhas, Sri Chaitanya, Basavanna, Kabir, Mirabai, and others. Their writing extolled passionate devotional love for the Divine that released barriers of caste, religion, and gender so that all beings could be seen and respected as manifestations of the One.

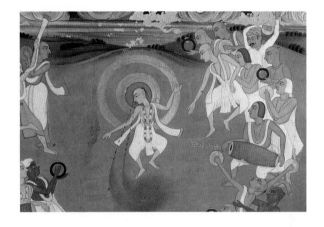

The rich will make temples for Shiva.

What can I, a poor bhakta, do?

My legs are pillars, the body the shrine,

my heart the inner sanctum,

my head a tower of gold.

Listen, O Lord of the meeting rivers,

the things standing shall fall,

but the moving shall ever stay.

— BASAVANNA[20]

awakening the inner heart guru

Our Heart Guru is our visceral encounter with our inner source. Heart Guru is "the one who transforms darkness," an emanation of the transforming fire of connectedness and love, an intimate teacher that speaks in a language beyond words. This is our internal guidance system, a living connection to the source within that enables us to find yoga everywhere.

THE HEART GURU IS

> **The fire of Consciousness**
> that guides us through the matrix of life: the sacred and mundane, this world and beyond, the ordinary and extraordinary

> *Ishta devata*
> our personal connection to God, the divine current

> **The master Teacher of all teachers**
> who have ever existed or will ever be

> **The mother rhythm**
> pulsing in the heartbeat and all of the body's pulsations, connected to the cosmic rhythm

> **Our inner navigation system**
> in speech, thought, and action

> **Our beloved refuge**

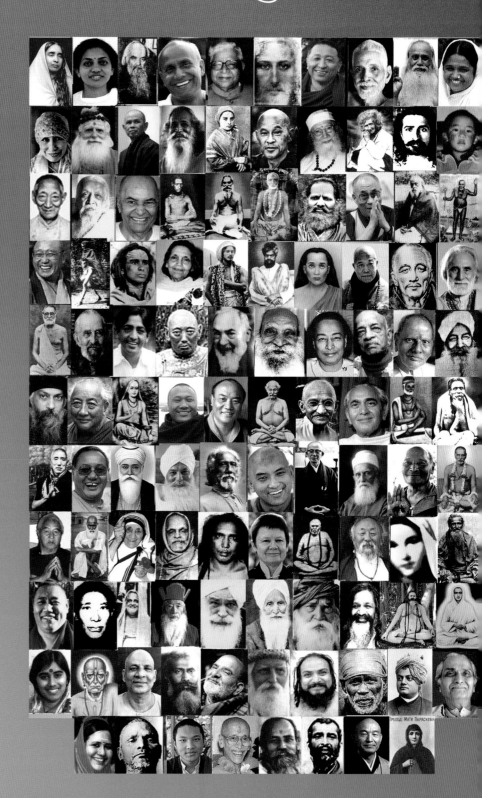

REFLECTION

The heart of the universe
pulses in all hearts,
There is One who is the life in all forms.
There is One who is joyful in simply
existing—in all bodies, as all bodies.
Explore the life that is the life
of your present form.
One day you will discover
it is not different
From the life of the Secret One,
And your heart will sing triumphant songs
of being at home everywhere.

—SRI ABHINAVAGUPTA,
BHAIRAVA STOTRA[21]

O Guru, pierce my eye with
the needle of discernment
so that I may see the light.

—BAUL SONG[22]

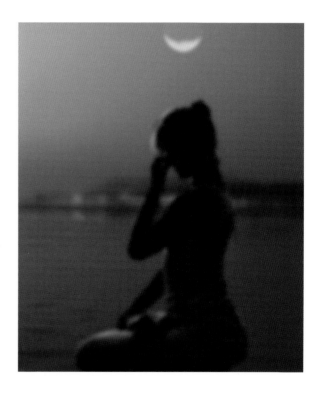

Close your eyes and awaken your inner gaze by
letting your awareness stream downward from
the back of your eyes into your heart center. Feel
the sensations in your heart region and open to a
sacred connection, a living presence felt within.

Open your "inner ears" and listen for an internal
language beyond words.

Dive into your center. Bathe in the regenerative
love in your heart, stronger than any dissonance
on the surface. As the One that is sometimes "two,"
experience the inner sanctum of your heart as a
place of refuge. Completely surrender there.

As you melt into this fire, feel a sacred presence—
your connection to the One. This is your Heart
Guru, inseparable from your very essence: the
inner friend, Beloved.

Feel your relationship with the One who
has been with you since your first breath,
alive in the altar of your Heart Fire.[23]

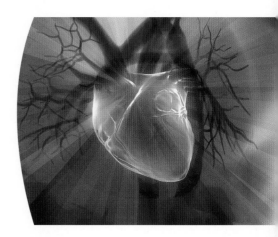

embodying
the heart fire

The Science of the Energetic Heart

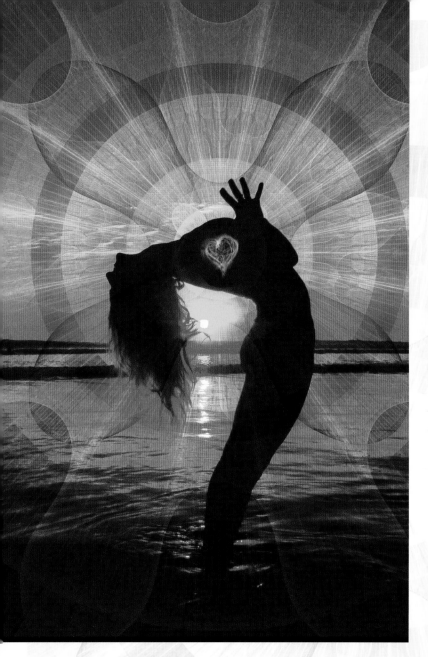

OUR BODY MIRRORS OUR
CULTURAL EVOLUTION.
HOW WE SEE OURSELVES
LIMITS OR LIBERATES OUR EXPERIENCE.
OUR EXPERIENCE SHAPES HOW
WE ENGAGE IN THE WORLD.

We are engaged in a planetary shift as we re-embody our energetic heart and retrieve the fire from within.

Our bodies and our lives are regulated by the cycles of the earth and the rhythms of the cosmos. As day flows into night, and as night gives way to dawn, our bodies synchronize with the solar and lunar cycles even when we attempt to override their rhythms. The human body's core physiological functions are tied to the oscillations of the sun and moon, from the most obvious—sleep cycles—to the pineal gland, which for optimal functioning depends upon the full-spectrum light of the sun.

The great conductor of the body's rhythms is the pulse of the heart. The heart is the only organ made of specialized cells—cardiac cells—with the unique capacity to create a pulsing electrical charge. This charge in turn creates a vast electromagnetic field of energy. As the most powerful "rhythm maker" of the body, the heart has the ability to govern all of the body's other rhythms.

the heart as the
pulse of life

The pulse of the heart links us to our earliest development inside the womb. The *dum-dum* of our mother's heart, its two-part rhythm, is the first mantra we hear, reflecting the very nature of the heart as the rhythmic conductor of consciousness. If we meditate on our own heartbeat, we find unbroken continuity with our mother's heart, our grandmothers' hearts, and back in time to the heartbeats of our most distant grandmothers.

Our hearts begin pulsing in the womb around five weeks from conception without any signal from the brain, which is still in formation—a mystery that science still does not understand. Then, for several weeks in the womb, our heartbeat entrains with (matches) our mother's heartbeat, creating a bond that is reinforced by the sonic nature of the heart's pulse; we can hear this beating for about five and a half months in the "surround sound" of the womb, perhaps feeling the pulse much earlier than our capacity to hear it develops.

The heart is—yes—a pump, but one of extraordinary power. It moves two thousand gallons of blood through sixty thousand miles of the circulatory system every hour, with a hydraulic power that could push water into the sky some thirty feet.[1] But this is far from the whole story—even from a purely scientific standpoint. The heart also radiates an electrical field that communicates with all other cells of the body through the fluid medium of the blood, which transmits vibration three times faster than air. Its "language" is its oscillating rhythm, ranging from slow and peaceful to hurried

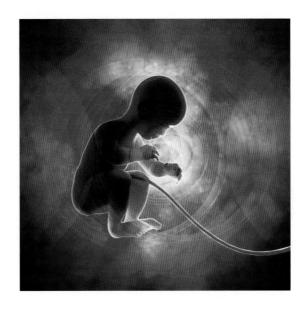

and excited. This rhythm is present in tension or relaxation, in stress or joy, in conflict or love. The electromagnetic field is such a force of communication that in heart-transplant recipients the heart and brain communicate through the energetic field rather than through the nervous system—specifically the vagus nerve, which is severed during the transplant surgery.[2] This is just one example of the power of the heart's energetic field.

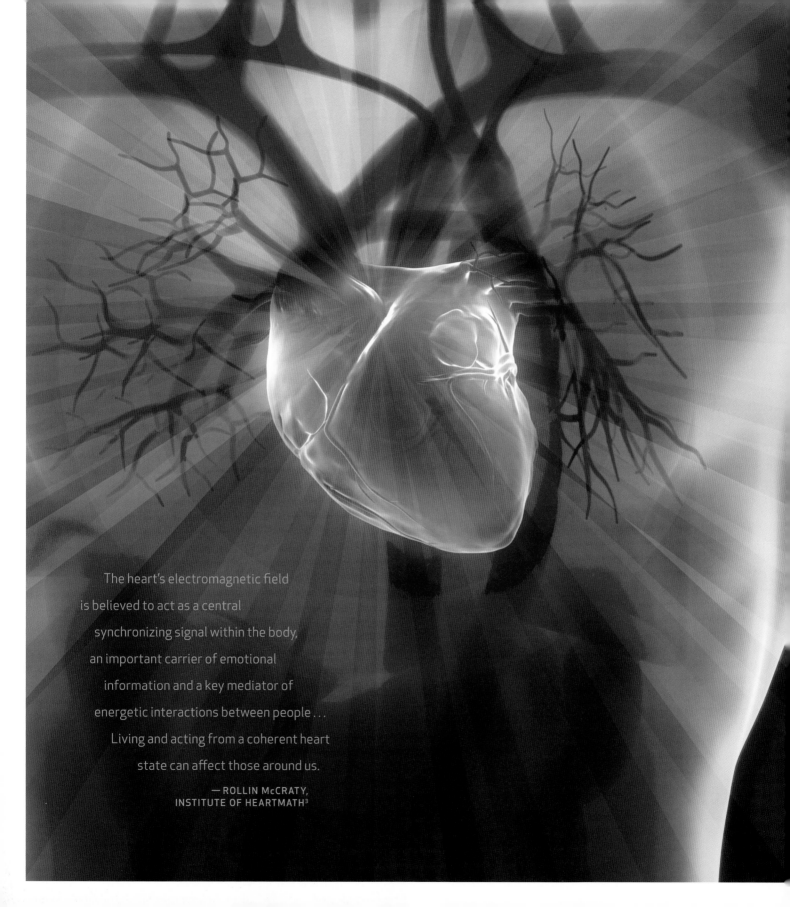

The heart's electromagnetic field is believed to act as a central synchronizing signal within the body, an important carrier of emotional information and a key mediator of energetic interactions between people... Living and acting from a coherent heart state can affect those around us.

— ROLLIN McCRATY,
INSTITUTE OF HEARTMATH[3]

the sun in the heart: the heart's electromagnetic field

The heart's electromagnetic field is five thousand times stronger than the brain's,[4] radiating forth from our core like the body's own fiery sun. When we understand some of the key energetic functions of the heart, it becomes easier for us to experience this sunlike radiance, so let's take a look at how the heart works.

While the blood carries chemicals and cells, it also carries electromagnetic signals that travel to every cell of the body. The entire body, in fact, is held within the heart's electromagnetic field, which can be measured as far as ten feet away with a magnetocardiogram, a device that shows fluctuations of the heart as it responds to both internal and external environments.[5] As we shall see, this "heart field" strengthens and weakens according to our inner connection to our heart, a quality we can sense in the heart fields of others, those who radiate positive energy and those who telegraph some disconnection from their hearts.

The heart transmits pulses of electromagnetic energy—and receives them. Thus it is an *organ of perception* and can decode the information embedded within the electromagnetic fields it senses.[6]

Take your heart into vast fields

of light and let it breathe.

— HAFIZ[7]

ANAHATA CHAKRA AND THE ENERGETIC FIELD OF THE HEART

Anahata chakra is best understood as the electromagnetic field that emanates from our energetic heart. The experience of the heart chakra is perhaps the most tangible in the body when feeling strong emotions of love and the sensation of the warmth that expands and radiates from the heart region. We sense in ourselves and in others when the energetic field of the heart is dim from loss or stress. Many forms of yoga—from movement practice to mantra, prayer, music, and karma yoga—could be viewed as being ways the electromagnetic field of the heart increases. Saints and great beings are living examples of the power of the heart field of anahata chakra. Regardless of external circumstances, in sickness and health, war and peace, the heart can remain in a coherent electromagnetic field and radiate like the sun.

heart entrainment—synchronization through rhythm

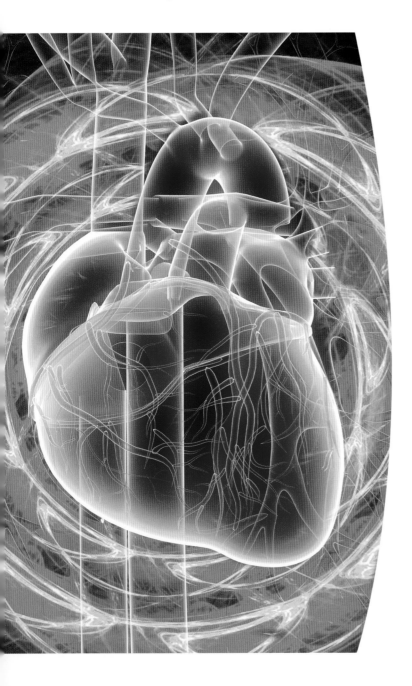

The average adult human heart, weighing roughly eleven ounces, beats seventy-two times a minute, or a hundred thousand times a day.[8] That's 37 million times a year. As the heart rate changes with the energy demand of different activities, the volume of blood it pumps changes accordingly.

A healthy heart responds to what is called heart rate variability (HRV); its rhythm is not fixed. Even the resting heart dances in myriad fluctuations. One of the vital signs of a heartbeat found in young, healthy people is a highly adaptable, ever-changing rhythm, becoming more fixed with age or if the heart becomes diseased. So HRV is a sign of health.[9]

The heart has a direct vibrational influence on every cell of the body—and beyond. It influences other organs or organisms through entrainment, a phenomenon in which two or more processes or organisms synchronize with one another's movements. This is a state of yoga, or joining together, a coherence between multiple rhythmic patterns.

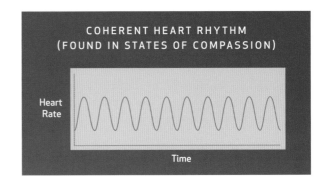

**COHERENT HEART RHYTHM
(FOUND IN STATES OF COMPASSION)**

Heart
Rate

Time

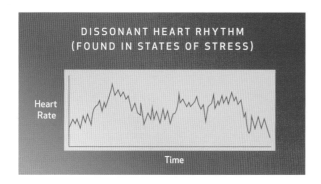

DISSONANT HEART RHYTHM
(FOUND IN STATES OF STRESS)

Heart Rate

Time

The cells of the sinoatrial node entrain, or beat together, and the rest of the heart cells beat in response. As the heart develops in the womb, once the first pacemaker cell begins to beat spontaneously, each new pacemaker cell synchronizes with it, until millions of them create one beating, synchronistic unit.[10]

Laboratory experiments offer great insights into the nature of entrainment. If a single pacemaker cell is removed from the body and kept alive, it will lose track of the rhythmic beat, pulse erratically, and ultimately die. If two pacemaker cells are placed close together, their beating patterns will synchronize—they will beat in unison. If an erratically beating cell is placed next to a regularly beating one, the one that is "off" will begin to beat in synch with the healthy cell. The cells do not need to touch in order to have these effects on one another because as they beat, they generate electric fields that connect the one with the other.[11]

Together these patterns create an unbroken stream of energy, or coherence—a state that brings all of our systems into their optimal flow for creating, sustaining, and regenerating life force.

Dissonance, by contrast, describes a state in which connected rhythms become separate and disordered, and this is usually caused by turbulent change or stress. Dissonant rhythms can have a degenerative, debilitating effect on the functioning and flow of life force.

When you are aware of the forces of entrainment and dissonance, you can begin to see how every experience, every relationship, every moment of your life has a direct effect on your heart.

ENTRAINMENT WITHIN THE HEART: PACEMAKER CELLS

Within the heart, specialized cells called pacemaker cells directly control the tempo of the heartbeat. A reflection in miniature of the essence of the heart organ, they actively create a healthy, rhythmic flow in the body and respond to the dissonant rhythms of stress. Collectively called the sinoatrial node, these cells are located in the walls of the upper part of the right side of the heart.

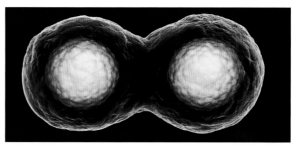

cell mitosis

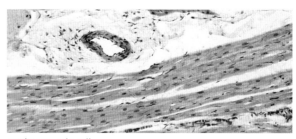

cardiac muscle cell

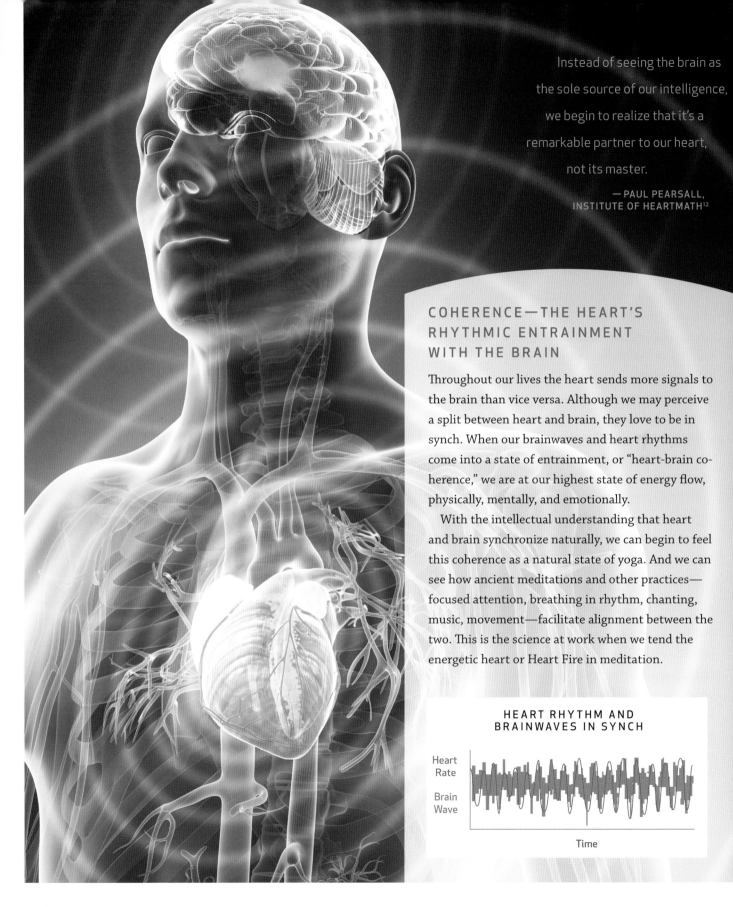

COHERENCE—THE HEART'S RHYTHMIC ENTRAINMENT WITH THE BRAIN

Throughout our lives the heart sends more signals to the brain than vice versa. Although we may perceive a split between heart and brain, they love to be in synch. When our brainwaves and heart rhythms come into a state of entrainment, or "heart-brain coherence," we are at our highest state of energy flow, physically, mentally, and emotionally.

With the intellectual understanding that heart and brain synchronize naturally, we can begin to feel this coherence as a natural state of yoga. And we can see how ancient meditations and other practices—focused attention, breathing in rhythm, chanting, music, movement—facilitate alignment between the two. This is the science at work when we tend the energetic heart or Heart Fire in meditation.

HEART RHYTHM AND BRAINWAVES IN SYNCH

Heart
Rate

Brain
Wave

Time

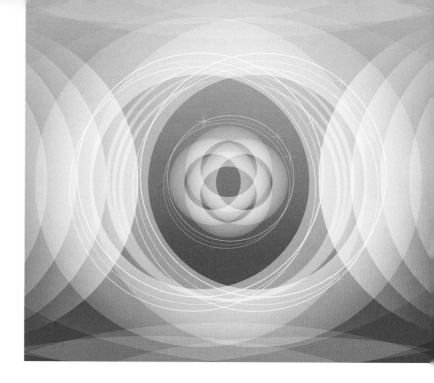

The heart is where the body senses new information first. Then, with every beat, it relays a burst of neural activity to the medulla, located at the base of the brain, via the vagus nerve and nerves in the spinal column—the same pathways that carry pain and other feeling sensations to the brain. Energy, or information that vibrates, constantly flows between heart and brain, assisting us in our emotional processing, sensory experience, ability to derive meaning from events, and reasoning.

When we shift our focus to the heart and away from the brain, large populations of cells in the forebrain entrain to the heart's rhythms. There is a tremendous ripple effect that we can noticeably perceive as the first sign that our awareness of our heart's energy has begun. Mental dialogue is reduced. Messages flow freely and directly between the heart and brain through the sympathetic and parasympathetic nerve pathways, as well as the baroreceptor system (sensory nerves in the arteries). Connectivity increases between brain and body, and neuronal firing increases. Greater heart-brain entrainment allows a person to function at higher states which can be consciously practiced through intentional focus on the heart.

OUR BREATHING UNIVERSE— ENTRAINING THE BREATH AND THE HEART

We receive each breath as part of the extraordinary "breathing universe" in which we live. And every breathing creature on the planet inhales molecules of all other creatures; in this way, the breath connects us all.

It is your heart that brings the breathing universe to every cell of your body. Think about this important point for a moment: your heart, through its deep, pulsating rhythms, distributes your life force—prana—throughout the complex network of bone, muscle, ligaments, skin, nerves, and other tissues. The heart radiates life into every part of you. And it does this quickly: it takes just over a minute for a single breath to circulate throughout your body. Now consider that the heart responds to every little nuance of your inner experience, changing its action in accordance with your moods and thoughts. This means that what you think and feel affects your ability to distribute your life force through your body.

The interlinking rhythms of breath and heart give us the primary embodied experience of the pulse of life. This in and out, rising and falling, contracting and expanding, is mirrored in all of life, from the subatomic pulse of the atomic-quantum world to the pulsing vibration of stars.

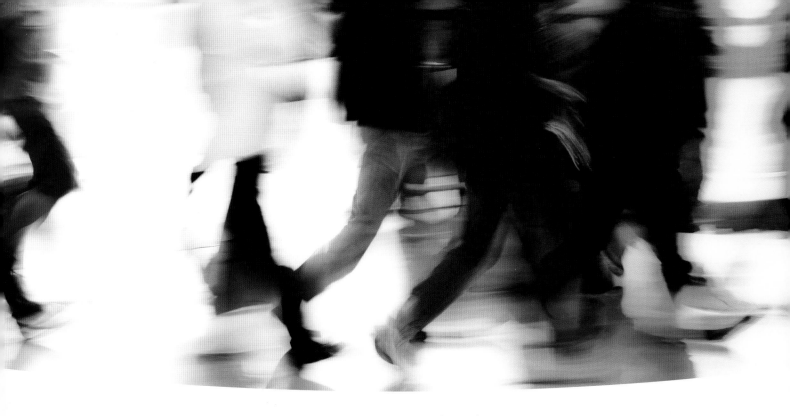

stress rhythms and the
healing power of attention

We often experience stress when we've lost our ability to navigate transitions in a fluid and healthy way—a key teaching that we will revisit when we explore living vinyasa in Part Three. With any transition there is a natural fluctuation, a healthy chaos, a variation to the flow, a change in the fire. Fluctuations are actually positive things; they have the ability to reset the vibrational patterns in our hearts. But they also create a vulnerability that we must tend to on all levels so that these transitions don't agitate or dim the flow of our life force. We need to feel for signs of disruption in the heart field affecting our emotions, insights, actions, or speech.

When brainwaves and heart rhythms are out of synch, inefficiency is introduced into the system and the entire body experiences further stress. But we can bring consciousness to this cycle. Pay attention to the arising dissonant rhythms in your heart—experienced as tension, emotional stirring, pressure, impatience, or a sense of holding, being overwhelmed, or out of synch. These are often the first signs of negative stress, and whether these sensations are large or small, they signal that something needs to change to bring you back into balance.

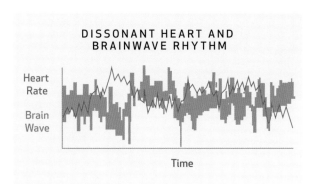

DISSONANT HEART AND
BRAINWAVE RHYTHM

Heart
Rate

Brain
Wave

Time

When we attune to the pulse of the heart, we become able to sense subtle movement toward stress and we can make a conscious shift toward balance. We can develop our own unique healthy heart rhythms and shift into more "solar" or "lunar" modes of being, from fully expressive to quiet and reflective. By tuning in to the heart in this deep and nuanced way, we can create the openness and flexibility that remove constrictions around the heart.

Slower heart rhythms alter brainwave frequencies in such a way that deeper states of being can occur. At the deepest levels of entrainment, our brainwaves and heart rhythms are in synch with every other cell in the body, creating a field of energy that extends beyond it. The strength of this field literally depends upon how aware of and connected to the heart we are. At the end of this chapter, I provide a meditation to help you become more connected to your energetic heart as the key to living in rhythm with the pulse of life.

If we are aware of how damaging "disconnected stress" is to our system and, in contrast, how powerfully regenerating the state of love is for our whole being, we will be more aware of which "fire" we are fueling.

FANNING THE FIRES OF STRESS HAS PROFOUND PHYSICAL REPERCUSSIONS

> The body's stress response encompasses more than fourteen hundred known physical and chemical reactions and more than thirty different hormones and neurotransmitters.[13]

> Chronically elevated levels of cortisol have been shown to impair immune function, reduce glucose utilization, increase bone loss and promote osteoporosis, reduce muscle mass, inhibit skin growth and regeneration, increase fat accumulation (especially around the waist and hips), impair memory and learning, and destroy brain cells.[14]

> Common emotions such as frustration and sadness can trigger a drop in the blood supply to the heart. In daily life, these emotions more than double the risk of myocardial ischemia, an insufficient blood supply to heart tissue that can be a precursor to a heart attack.[15]

> The daily accumulation of stress does the most damage; the little stresses add up. With unrelenting adrenaline and cortisol arousal, our system begins to weaken.[16]

The toll stress takes on our health, relationships, longevity, and quality of life is a consideration for all ages and backgrounds across the globe. Love in its many forms has an unbelievable power to heal and transform stress—as we have known across time and cultures. Knowing some of the science behind the power of love generated through the heart may help some who are cynical or hardened to trust what is naturally available to us.

heart-brain entrainment and the healing power of love

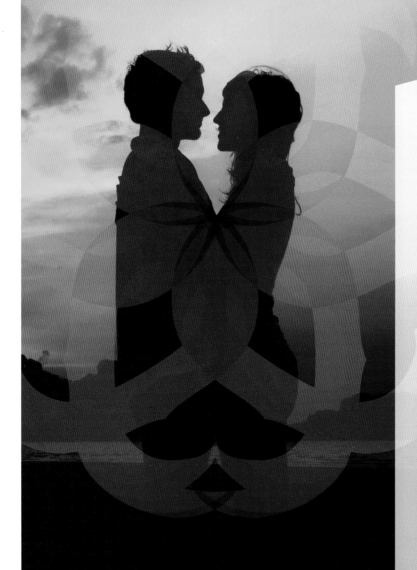

The word *emotion* literally means "energy in motion" and is derived from the Latin verb meaning "to move." When you experience stressful emotions such as frustration, agitation, and impatience, your heart rate variability—your heart rhythm—becomes erratic and disordered. When you tend your fires with regenerative, core heart feelings such as gratitude or tenderness, you effectively intercept the physiological stress response that drains and damages your system, and you allow the body's natural regenerative capacities to work in your favor. Instead of being taxed and depleted, your inner system—your mental, emotional, and spiritual dimensions—is renewed through your own inner yoga or coherence.[17]

When your heart is in a state of coherence with your brain, you more easily experience meditative states, optimal flow, and a connection to life. Stressful reactions are more likely to occur when the head and heart are out of alignment.[18]

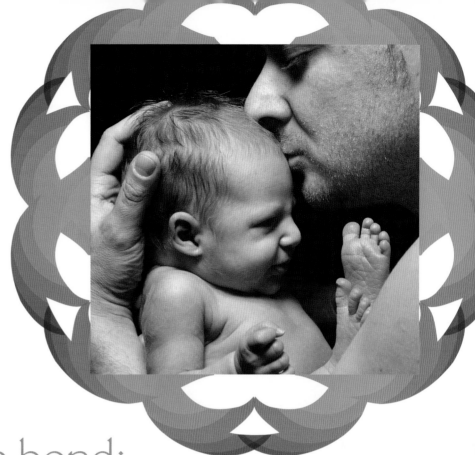

the energetic bond:
heart-to-heart entrainment

Science is in its infancy concerning the complicated energetic connections that take place between people, but it's already clear that if we touch someone while feeling an emotion such as tenderness, we're transmitting a signal to that person's body that promotes their well-being and health. Caring for someone or something has an uplifting effect on us as well, one that goes directly to our hearts. It is a regenerative experience that we can pass on to someone else.[19]

One person's heart rhythms can entrain with those of another person; this has been seen in spouses who live and sleep together and in people who work closely together physically over time. Just as pacemaker cells can detect and synchronize with one another to establish a beat, the electromagnetic field generated by one person's heart can be detected in another person, both when they are physically touching and when they are only nearby (measured up to ten feet away). The more interaction two people have, the stronger will be the patterns imprinted in their hearts and other cells.

the collective heart—
the power of music, movement, chanting, and meditation

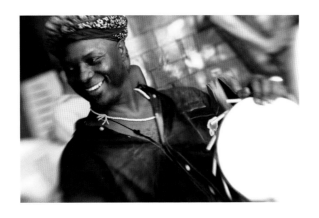

At the root of all power and motion
is music and rhythm, the play of patterned
frequencies against the matrix of time.
Before we make music, music makes us.

— JOACHIM-ERNST BERENDT [20]

HEART RHYTHM AND MUSIC

Science is now coming to an understanding of what yogis and indigenous cultures have known through the ages: that we live in a rhythmic universe and our whole being responds to its music.

Music is medicine, whether we use it for simple release or to enter the mystic states of communion that are the peak experiences of life. Recent studies have tracked how heart health can be enhanced through the power of music as our heart's rhythm literally entrains with the rhythm of the music. Music not only has a positive effect on our heartbeat, pulse rate, and blood pressure; it does much more. It affects respiration, equalizes brainwaves, reduces muscle tension, regulates stress hormones, boosts immune function, stimulates neural pathways, and increases our emotional bonding.

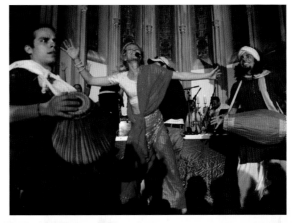

UNIVERSAL MANTRA
Chanting, in all languages, has a positive effect on inner well-being as it activates the body's natural healing process, even including a reversal of heart disease.

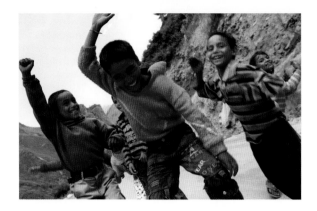

RHYTHMIC MOVEMENT

Our innate response to rhythm is an inborn reflex that every parent on the planet has observed in his or her toddler. A recent study by the National Academy of Sciences found that the only type of sound that babies and toddlers respond to universally is rhythm—they shake and move their bodies to the rhythm naturally and without any other stimulus.[21] When it comes to collective rhythm—making music, moving, and chanting together—the worlds of science, art, and spirituality are now in agreement: bonding in these ways is a gift that can heal our bodies and lift our spirits. Experiencing yoga, dance, and music together re-attunes us to our core rhythms, freeing us from stress and fragmentation.

My heart is burning with love.
All can see this flame. My heart is pulsing
with passion, like waves on an ocean.
I'm at home, wherever I am. And in the room
of lovers I can see with closed eyes the
beauty that dances. Behind the veils
intoxicated with love, I too dance
the rhythm of this moving world.

— RUMI[22]

COLLECTIVE HEART MANDALA— THE "HEART-CHARGING STATION"

In a world where we too often devalue affection and community bonding in the ways of our ancestors, "heart charging" is one of the most radical and effective ways we can recharge our energetic heart. I begin most workshops, retreats, and yoga trance dances this way, and you can feel the tangible shift among separate individuals of thinking mind into an almost instantaneous collective bond. It's possible to reach out and experience the power of heart bonding through the collective by gathering anyone—friends, family, students, team members—spontaneously every time you connect physically. Keep one hand on your heart and extend your other hand outward to the space behind the heart at the back of the person next to you until you have created an interconnected circle or mandala. You will literally feel a heat guiding your hand to the correct position behind the heart. Suspend any skepticism or cynicism and be open to your experience.

With the circle connected, follow what is natural—be it pure silence, offering primal sounds, chanting, or medita-tion—perceiving the collective energetic field. You can keep this formation for anywhere from five minutes to an hour. (People can change hands on their own or with guidance.) Experience the heart charging and the intensification of the electromagnetic field.

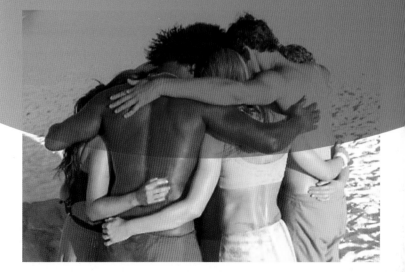

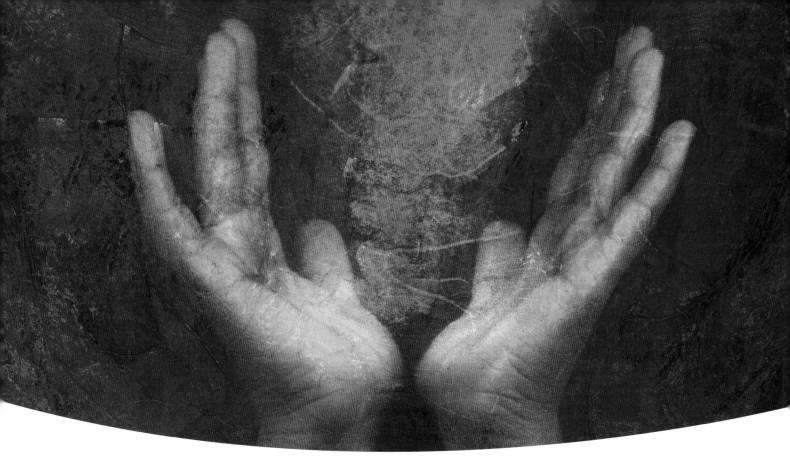

and understood some of the
science behind our ancestral knowing, we can embrace the importance of embodying our energetic
heart, not just for our own well-being but for our
evolution as human beings.

As we feel into our own embodiment, we can
sense the potency of our heart's energetic field—
within our body and beyond. We can feel a sensation, a stirring, an emanating sunlike energy that
we can now understand as the perception of our
heart's electromagnetic field. We can begin to
sense oscillations of the pulse of the heart from
the agitating effects of stress to the calming power
of love through sensing our heart rhythm. We can

relate to our heart as the rhythmic conductor of
all our sacred intelligences—belly, brain, cells, and
energetic fields.

We sense in deep time how the rhythms of
breath, heart pulse, blood flow, activation, and
relaxation create a tidal movement that mirrors the
cosmic rhythm. The ancient vision of our ancestors
that is reflected in the yoga practices that connect
the body with the cosmos does not seem so strange
now. We can find the sun in our heart as the radiant field, the moon in our heart as the hormonal
nectar of love. We can become embodied firekeepers, practical household alchemists. Meditation
becomes natural as our whole being reattunes itself
to our inner fire—the living fire that is the expression of our energetic heart.

embodying your energetic heart— a five-part universal meditation

The following meditation is a meeting of the science and spirit of the heart, forming the basis for deeper explorations in Part Two.[23]

1 FEEL-TOUCH, SENSATIONS, AND YOUR "HEART MUDRA"

Take a moment and feel who you are right now. Bring your hands to your heart, open palms. Experience the subtle shift that comes through this touch, a centering and a settling of your awareness. Feel the sensations in your experience of your heart region. Whether the sensation is of numbness, a dim presence, or a shimmering radiance, it offers a kind of barometer to sense fluctuations in your heart center; notice when it is closing down, and know when it is time to add more "fuel" in the form of awareness, feeling, or presence.

2 LISTEN TO YOUR HEART'S PULSE—HEART MANTRA

Bring your fingertips to your pulse—underneath your jaw or at your wrist pulse point—and feel the rhythm of your pulse. This creates the sonic sensation of also hearing that pulse within. Feel and hear this, the *dum-dum* of your heart. Allow the sound to bring you into the first mantra of your heart. Feel your inner ears open as if to listen to an intimate knowing deep within you, a truth we often resist, a calling to slow down, a wisdom unique to this moment. Allow yourself to merge with the source by simply being, quieting the outer mind, and opening to your intimate experience of your Heart Fire.

3 STEADY YOUR GAZE— HEART DRISTI

Draw your awareness inward to connect with your heart center. Awaken your inner gaze, or "heart *dristi*," by streaming the energy at the backs of your eyes toward your heart center. You may visualize this energy as an inner fire or simply feel your way, guided without any images. You will begin to feel an energetic quality that increases with your awareness, like a fire that can be tended and amplified through the fuel of your awareness. Even your downward-streaming gaze may feel like a river of light pouring into the fire of your heart. This downward flow brings great relief from excess energy to the head as the higher-frequency brainwaves begin to shift and "melt" downward through a loving gaze. This is the yogic way of inviting heart-brain coherence. Steady your gaze around this inner fire as you open to your inner firekeeping.

4 TEND THE HEART FIRE— UNIFYING INNER RHYTHMS

Drawing on the science of the energetic heart, explore your state. What dissonance is arising? What rhythms feel disconnected? How is the flow of your breath—smooth, jagged, tense, restricted, calm, flowing, deep? What is your mental-emotional state? Are your thought waves present and connected, or are they fragmented and disjointed? Do your emotions feel turbulent, repressed, confusing, frustrating, flowing, vital, present, connected?

You will learn yogic practices in Part Two to bring your inner rhythms into entrainment, but you can apply a few simple techniques now that are accessible to everyone:

For one, slow your breath rhythm into a tidal flow of six to eight beats, counting on the inhale or the exhale. This begins to change your heart and brain rhythms into a more synchronized state. Exhale through your mouth to relax and let go. Feel your heart rhythm and brain waves beginning to entrain as you experience fewer thought waves and more presence. As a second practice, bring one hand to your heart and one hand to the crown of your head, and cultivate any healing emotion that arises for you, such as compassion, love, or tenderness. The Institute of HeartMath suggests gratitude is the greatest emotion to create "heart-brain coherence." This manner of tending your Heart Fire offers what is needed to bring your energetic heart into balance.

⑤ EXPRESS YOUR HEART FIELD

Bring your hands in front of your heart with your palms facing inward. Begin to sense the energy that is subtly radiating from your heart to your hands. Allow your arms to expand outward slowly from your heart like the rays of a sun radiating in all directions. In Part Two, you can go deeper with other arm movements or *mudra vinyasas*.

Emanate from your Heart Fire. Feel the pulsing vibrations radiating from your center. This is the state of your energetic heart sent through your electromagnetic field to every cell of your body and beyond. Stay connected to your energetic heart and explore moving through the world with heart-centered awareness of your internal coherence, and experience the difference within the flow of your life.

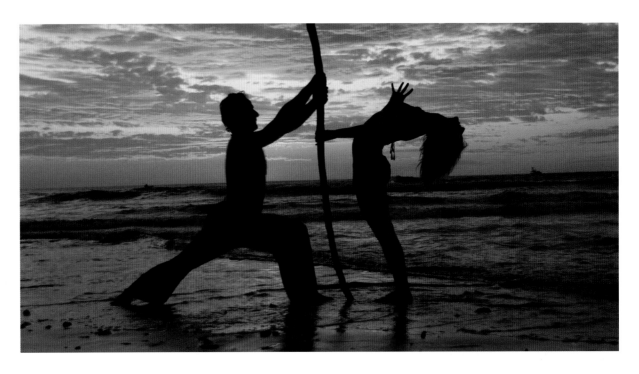

meditations for
tending the heart fire

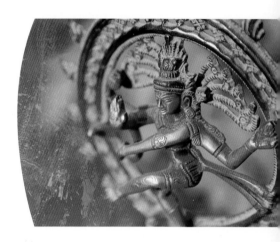

movement meditation

Connecting to the Source of Movement

all of me is on fire

Voice, Spine, Heart, Hands.

I tremble with the desire to express.

With the Earth, my body emerges.

From the Water, creative energies flow.

In the Fire, I transform.

Out of Air, I breathe new life.

In Space, I open to the Source.

The essence of truth and beauty.

My body is the field of my expression.[1]

MOVEMENT MEDITATION IS DEEP ENTRAINMENT

of all of the body's rhythms—the experience of embodying the flow. Breath-induced movement meditation is our original form of meditation from as early as our oscillating movement in the womb to the rocking motion of our father and mother's arms. Movement is life and therefore reconnects us to a natural flow where we are unbound, uninhibited, and alive with a creative current.

There are many other forms of movement meditation within yoga, including temple dance forms, the devotional movement of kirtan, kriyas, and spontaneous movement meditations in tantric *sahaja*. Although less known in the Western world where asana is the predominant identity of yoga practice, all of these forms of movement meditation in yoga have a similar deep intention: to realize and embody the sacred current within.

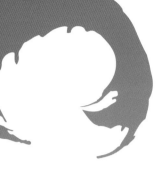

movement meditations across cultures

Like this universe coming into existence
the lover wakes and whirls in a dancing joy
then kneels down in praise.

—RUMI[2]

If we look to the world's ritual movement meditations, we find a spectrum: from the energy activation of Kodo drummers' ritual running to Taoist qigong to trance-dance forms such as Kecak from Bali and Candomblé Orisha dances in Brazil to sublime meditations of the Sema ceremony of the Whirling Dervishes to the davening of Jewish prayer. Movement meditation is any embodied form that brings us into the state of flow—from pure energy to sacred immersion. In every case the dancer experiences effortlessness—time outside of time—and the movements are always generated by an inner source.

Perhaps the simplest and most pervasive movement is the ritual movement of prostration or *pranams,* stemming from the root word *namah,* meaning "to bow," "to realize the essence." This *sharira* (body) mudra creates a natural shift as our heart, forehead, and whole body surrender upon the earth—a simple yet profound movement found in ritual meditations across the world's spiritual traditions.

There are many examples of movement meditations found in traditions around the world. Here are just a few:

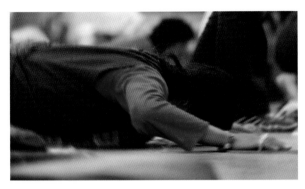

PROSTRATIONS

From the one hundred thousand prostrations of Vajrayana Buddhism to the five-times-per-day prayer of Muslims facing Mecca to the prostrating walk of Christian pilgrims, this whole-body bowing is the gateway to receptivity and humility of the heart.

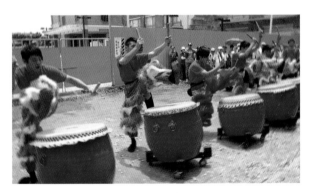

RITUAL RUNNING OF THE KODO DRUMMERS

The Taiko drummers of the group Kodo (meaning "heartbeat" in Japanese) live in the traditional communal way and drum together as a form of movement meditation as the sun rises on the Island of Sado, Japan.

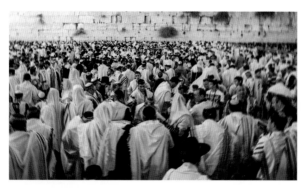

DAVENING

The spontaneous rocking movement of Jewish prayer

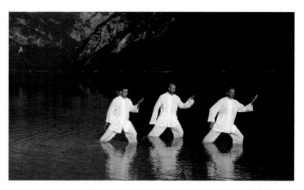

QIGONG

A system of embodied healing through Taoist postures that connect the flow of energy in nature and in the body.

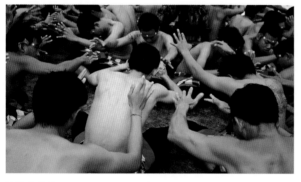

KECAK

This communal form of movement meditation has roots in the oldest Hindu trance meditations of Bali, in which the reenactment of Hanuman's monkey army is expressed in rhythmic sound and movement that builds to a powerful crescendo.

ORISHA CEREMONY

The Orishas of the Yoruba pantheon (the spiritual tradition of the West-African diaspora) are evoked through dance, music, and chanting as participants are "mounted" by the spirit of the Orisha.

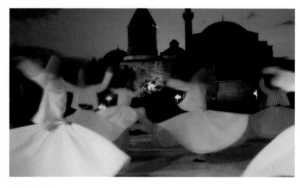

SEMA

The whirling meditation of the Sufi Dervishes, Sema originated eight hundred years ago with the great poet-teacher Mevlana Jelalluddin Rumi, who created this practice to transform his grief at the loss of his teacher.

SHAKERS

The first members of this American Christian group were known as "shaking quakers" because of the ecstatic movements of their worship services.

movement meditations
and origins of the asanas

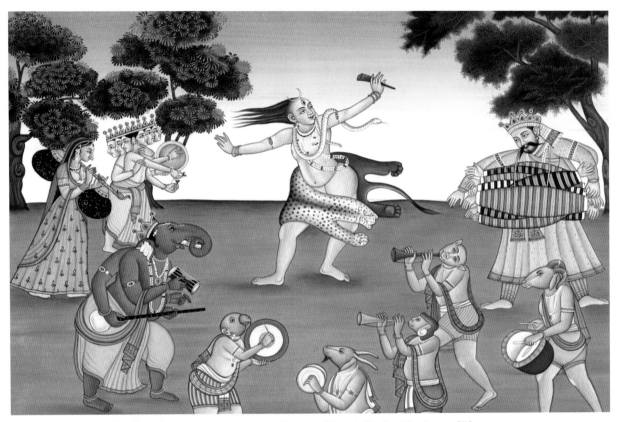

Shiva dancing Sandhya Tandava, the supreme movement meditation of Cosmic Rhythm, the dance of life.

THE DANCING DIVINE—
THE SAHAJA ORIGINS OF
MOVEMENT MEDITATION

Within the visions of yoga, the Supreme dances the world, all of creation, yoga, and us. God as Krishna dances intimately with each devotee, in the Rasa Lila, Ganesh dances over obstacles, and Shiva and Shakti dance the world into creation in the Sandhya Tandava and Lasya. This natural flow of *sahaja* is described as *samavesha*, or "immersion" into the divine current—the goal of yogic practice that transforms our ordinary, stiff, and limited experience of ourselves into a fluid expression of the "mover" moving through us: Shiva and Parvati realized within.

Just as our breathwave is the primary source for the movement of our life, yoga arises from the divine movement of Shiva and Shakti. Within the myths of yoga, the origins of asanas, mudras, dance, and music are found in the ecstatic expression of Shiva, the *mahayogin,* and Parvati, the mother of the universe.[3] It is said that all of these movement arts arose spontaneously from their meditations, and as such, music, sound, dance, mudras and yogasana are viewed and experienced as divine mediums of consciousness.

This vision of Shiva and Shakti in creative movement is reflected in myths, paintings, and oral transmissions from teacher to student. The great tenth-century Maha Siddha Matsyendranath offers a meditation on the body in which each cell is alive with the movement of Shiva and Shakti, whom he describes as being in union within their sport of love for several eons. In between their lovemaking, creative pastimes arise spontaneously, such as the poetic meditations Shiva offers to Parvati (found in the Vijnana Bhairava) and the creation of the *veena,* a musical instrument inspired by the beautiful movements Shiva witnessed arising from Parvati's breath.

Yet the dance of Shiva and Shakti—known as the *tandava* (his movements) and *lasya* (her movements)—is the heart of their creative expression. There are seven forms of tandava attributed to Shiva, with several expressing the loving rhythm of *ngara rasa* that forms the creative cycles of the universe, while other forms, such as *raudra tandava,* express the fierce dissolution that comes with the *samhara,* or the death cycle. Parvati's lasya represents the fluid nature of the feminine and is composed of circular, spiral, and swirling movements. There are 840,000 asanas attributed to their ecstatic dance.

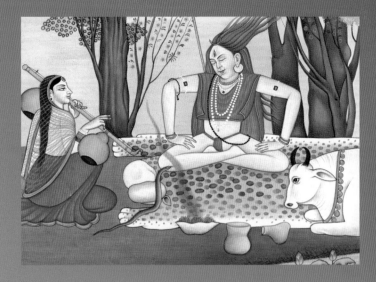

THE MUSIC OF PARVATI'S BREATH

There is a beautiful myth of how the musical instrument, the veena, was created. Once, Shiva came upon his beloved Parvati resting in sublime beauty. As he gazed at his beloved, he listened to her breath like beautiful music, and he saw the flow of her beautiful bosom rising and falling with the breath. As author Nitin Kumar writes, "Shiva was intoxicated by this ravishing vision and watched her for a long time in silence. Such was the impression created in his mind that he found no peace until he discovered a way of making a permanent record of the beauty observed. The result was the veena, a musical instrument whose long neck represents the straight lithe form of Parvati, and the two supporting gourds her breasts, the metal frets her bracelets, and the most expressive of all, the sound generated by this instrument is said to recreate Parvati's own rhythmic breathing."[4]

the evolution of asanas

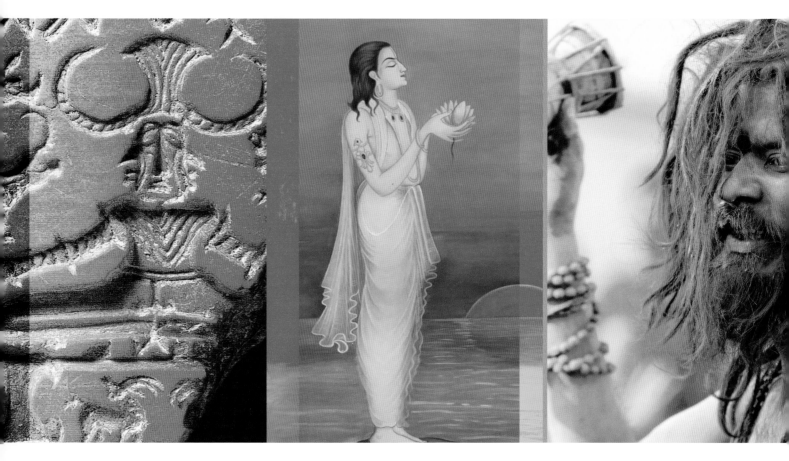

HARAPPAN SEAL OF SIVA (3500 BCE)

The earliest archaeological records of the yoga culture of India are found in the Harappan Seals of Mohenjo Daru. These show postures that indicate the possibility that movement meditation was taking place in Harappan culture more than five thousand years ago.

THE VEDAS—*SURYA NAMASKAR* MOVEMENTS AND MANTRAS (1500 BCE TO PRESENT)

The ritual invocation of *surya namaskar,* the movement meditation postures that evolved into the present-day Sun Salutation, is found in the Rig Vedas. The mantra offering has been practiced in an unbroken chain of daily ritual in Vedic culture ever since.

EARLIEST EVIDENCE OF RITUALIZED POSTURES

Evidence of a postural vinyasa appears in the earliest tantric scriptures. The fifth century *Pashupata Sutra* refers to a sequence of dance-like poses to be performed by initiated tantric practitioners (*sadhakas*) as a specific ritual for healing others.

Movement meditation is a form of embodying the divine, and as we look back through the sources of yoga teaching, from prehistory to the present, we can see an underlying transformation of the body as a vehicle of divine expression.

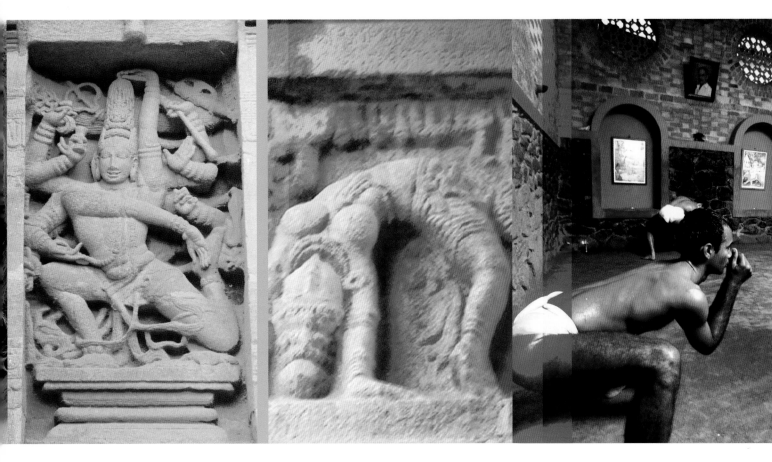

FLOWING VINYASAS IN EARLY TANTRA

The oldest known vinyasa, or sequence of physical poses, prescribed in detail is found in the fifth century *Nishvasa Tantra,* called simply the "50 Bodily Poses" or *Shatardha Shariraga.* The eleventh century Jayadrathayamala Tantra describes the effects of an ecstatic ritual alluding to postural yoga practice: "Some assume series of mudras. Some begin to dance with the playful gestures and postures (*karanas*) taught in the Kaula scriptures. Others, who are warriors, commence the tandava dance of nataraja." The memory of this ecstatic postural movement survived in the tantric-based Hatha Yoga manuals (thirteenth century forward) who traced themselves to a tenth-century Kaula guru known as Matsyendra Natha. The ritualized practice of yoga asanas still performed by sadhus and sadhvis (male and female ascetics) largely draws from this Natha tradition.

KARANA—FLOWING POSTURES

Karana, or pose, is the term largely used in the tantras to describe the sacred postural forms engaged in tantric sadhana, later replaced by the word *asana* in Hatha Yoga texts. "Karana" was most famously used to describe the sacred forms in Indian classical dance forms, such as Bharatha Natyam. Many of these are the same as yoga asanas, requiring the depth of flexibility and strength within contemporary yoga asanas. In temples such as Chidambaram and Kailasanatha Temple in Tamil Nadu, Shiva is shown dancing in asana-like forms.

VAIDAVUS—POSTURES OF KALARIPPAYATU

Vaidavus are the name for postures that are cultivated in the flowing martial art form of Kalarippayatu. Named after animals, these energetic forms awaken the inner energy (shakti) and flow of prana with a shared stance and alignment base with many yogasanas.

MOVEMENT MEDITATION **79**

asana as mudra

> My body is my temple
> and asana is my prayer.
> —BKS IYENGAR

YOGA ASANAS—
ELEVENTH CENTURY TO PRESENT

Late Tantric texts such as the Goraksha Samhita, Hatha Yoga Pradapika, Gheranda Samhita, and Shiva Samhita mention that there are 8.4 million asanas taught by Lord Shiva. Eighty-four, or sometimes thirty-two, are considered essential. Instruction on the practice of asana is included as part of a complete practice for the purpose of embodied realization and for health, vitality, awakening, balance, and integration of the subtle body. The current rise of yoga centered around asana—literally meaning "seat" but usually translated as "posture"—is another wave in continuity in the evolution of yoga asana.

The sahaja origins of yoga and other forms of sacred posture, such as karana and vaidavu, are not yet widely known in the West, but if we open to a direct, living current of the life force, we can feel the underlying flow that creates the liberating and balancing effect of asana.

Sacred hand gestures, or *hasta mudras,* contain inherent states of being. When one simply brings one's hands to the heart or opens to the sky, the form of asana can be experienced as *sharira mudra,* or whole-body mudra. Instead of doing an asana for purely physical effects, we can receive the reverberation all the way to our energetic heart and our feeling mind. Asana as mudra activates an experience of natural alignment, an excavation and awakening of the energy that brings us back to the inner state from which it was created.

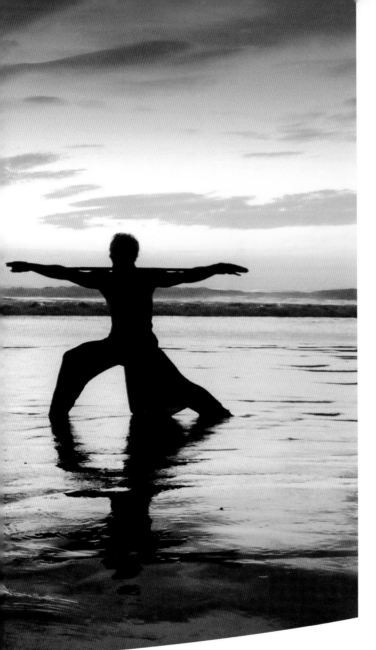

EXPLORATION OF ASANA AS MUDRA

Bring your hands to your heart and bow your frontal brain to your heart. As you inhale, from your inner feeling, feel your spine rising and arching back slowly. Feel the energetic state that arises inside the uplifted heart, the inherent energetic pattern of "backbends." Slowly bow your head back toward your heart and feel the inherent centering and inward movement connected to "forward bends." Oscillate between the two as if the rhythm of the heart in its contraction and expansion was the source of your movement, or explore the arising of other forms or whole-body mudras. Liberating our spine and heart region is key to experiencing the energetic heart.

Feel connected to millions of people around the world and across time who are spontaneously coming into this movement in openness, in quietude, and to the original yogis and yoginis who experienced the source of movement and breath within the flow of the body. Feel the body as mudra and the inner origins of the asanas as the flow of consciousness.

namaskar—
devotion in motion

Namaskar is a special type of vinyasa, a ritual offering in the form of a synchronized sequence of mudras or asanas that can be offered to more than just the sun, as in *surya namaskar*. In the following examples, the "namaskar" can be for the earth (*bhumi*), sacred river (*ganga*), or an altar. This is a kind of movement alchemy designed to awaken and transform the mover to realize the source of their meditation.

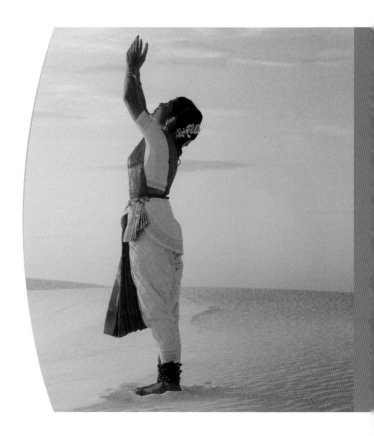

Samudra vasane devi
> The Goddess within whom the oceans reside

Parvata sthana manchite
> Who is decorated by mountains
> Whose breasts are the mountain peaks

Natyam karishye bhudevi
> Dancing upon that goddess of the earth

Pada sparsha kshama sva me
> Please receive me with each step I offer

—BHUMI PRANAM PRAYER[10]

BHUMI PRANAM—AN OFFERING BEFORE AND AFTER PRACTICE

In the temples, the devadasis were the primary conduits for the *pujas* (ritual offerings) performed in front of the sanctums for the audience of the Divine. When the devadasi danced, she became the embodiment of the divine; every posture, every expression was an invocation to the Divine to incarnate, to be felt as a presence in the here and now of the dancer's body.

Just as surya namaskar (Sun Salutation) honors the sun, *bhumi pranam* honors the earth. Bhumi Pranam is a *namaskaram* form done before and after every dance practice and every dance performance.

Nartaka Atman —

The Self Is the Dancer

—SHIVA SUTRAS[11]

Om Hrim Gangayaye

Om Hrim Swaha![12]

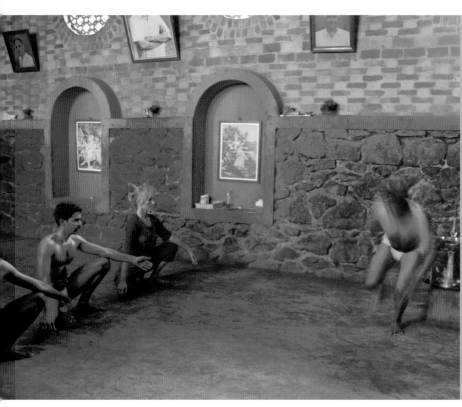

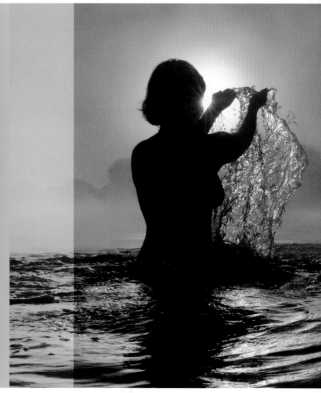

PUTTARA VANDANAM— KALARIPPAYATU NAMASKAR

Ancient martial art forms such as *kalarippayatu,* from Kerala province, include a movement namaskar as part of the honoring of the *puttara*, or shrine dedicated to Shiva and Shakti. This fluid form is practiced facing the altar to connect the practitioner more deeply to the Kalari—the sacred space for practice that is consecrated on special earth that is contained by shrines at all four corners, and that is left uncovered to feel its raw energy. The namaskar anchors the warrior practice by aligning one's energy to the deeper flow.

GANGA NAMASKAR—RITUAL MOVEMENT OFFERING WITH SACRED WATER

The rivers of India are filled with people beginning their day with a ritualized namaskar honoring the purifying element of water, visualized as the great mother goddess Ganga. All forms of water are seen as coming from her source, which begins in the Himalayas in Gangotri. Movements involve individual variation of mantras, *slokhas*, and prayers that are combined with submersion in the water three times.

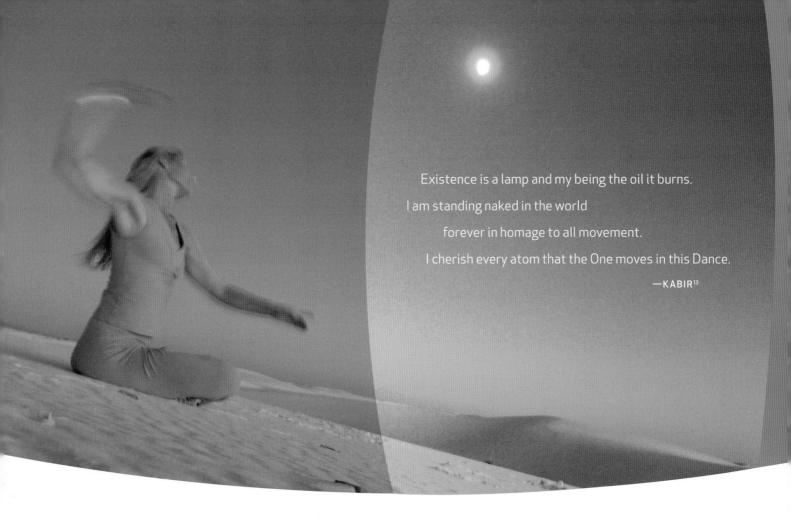

Existence is a lamp and my being the oil it burns.
I am standing naked in the world
forever in homage to all movement.
I cherish every atom that the One moves in this Dance.

—KABIR[13]

movement meditation practice

Now I invite you to your own experience of movement meditation. We will start very simply with a spontaneous movement practice. Then I'll introduce you to several forms of movement meditation: pranams, or prostrations; mudra vinyasa; and heart rhythm–based kriyas. We will close with surya namaskar, often mistakenly translated as "Sun Salutation," as well as *chandra namaskar,* which is connected to the fourteen phases of the moon as the embodiment of the cosmic rhythm.

Wander or dance . . . in utter
    spontaneity (sahaja).
Then, suddenly, drop to the ground
    and in this fall be total.
There absolute essence is revealed.

—VIJNANA BHAIRAVA TANTRA[14]

The sahaja element of such movement—its spontaneous nature—transforms the doing of meditation or yoga into a natural communion with a deeper source. We are released from overthinking, self-consciousness, instructional language, and the external focus on reaching for a particular goal as we surrender to the sublime current moving through us.

SAHAJA MEDITATION PRACTICE— SPONTANEOUS FLOW

Whether you are seated or standing, lying down or on hands and knees, begin to let your body respond to the pulse of life as you find it in your breath; let the breath coax you into movement. Feel the base of your spine begin to rock very slowly with the flow of your breath. Release any tension in the body, particularly in the deep lower belly; this will invite the experience of being moved by the sacred current. Slowly allow the subtle unwinding and meandering movements that arise from within. Feel how these movements flow as the breath in freedom, an inherent intelligence slowly guiding your movements without plan. You may find yourself moving in circles or spirals, rising up or sinking down. Your movements may be subtle or slow and may remain that way, or you may feel a pouring of movement as a wave or serpentine spiral pattern that ebbs and flows in simplicity and complexity. Let the current arise without controlling it or trying to make something happen. Allow the subtle creativity of prana to pour through you in ease and freedom.

Beneath all you are sensing, you may begin to experience the intrinsic joy all creatures express as they embody their true natures. Know that you can experience this at any time, in any space, in any position, without limit.

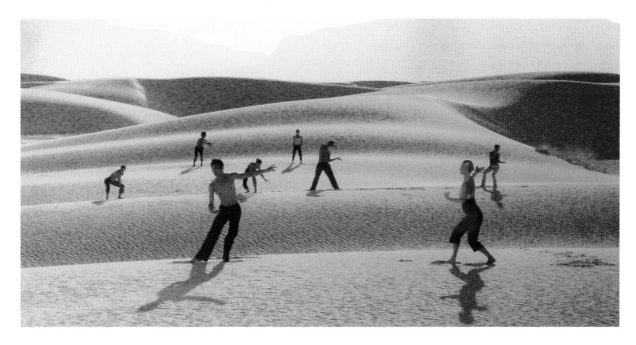

pranams—
whole-body invocation

Whole-body prostration, called *pranam,* is one of the most universal of movement meditations for creating an inward shift on all levels: body, mind, emotions, and spirit.

Begin by bringing your hands to your heart connection as you open yourself before your altar, the sunrise or sunset, or anyplace you consider your sacred space. Begin to open your heart bhava through your feeling mind. Slowly draw your hands together overhead to connect with the macrocosm, and then draw this connection down through your crown, third-eye center, into your heart, and then into full-body surrender (or just to your knees) upon the earth. Feel the release and bond from the point of contact in the frontal brain, heart, belly, and base of the body in a natural way that is deeply grounding and relaxing. With your hands connected overhead, make an offering through feeling, prayer, mantra, or visualization.

Prostrations may be offered once or three, nine, twelve, eighteen, fifty-four times—or in a continuous, moving prayer of 108 rounds. Some pilgrims will flow with prostrations as a means of moving around a temple or sacred mountain. Prostrations are a full-body expression of total release, intimacy, and surrender. You can offer prostrations as a practice all its own or to transition between the rhythms of the day. Feel the power of prostrations as a heart sadhana.

> To do pranam (obeisance) means to put one's
> head where it should be—at the feet of God.
> His feet are everywhere and therefore one
> may do namaskar (salutation) everywhere,
> remembering the feet of God.
> To do pranam means to open oneself
> to the divine power, which is always
> streaming down on everyone.
>
> —SRI ANANDAMAYI MA[15]

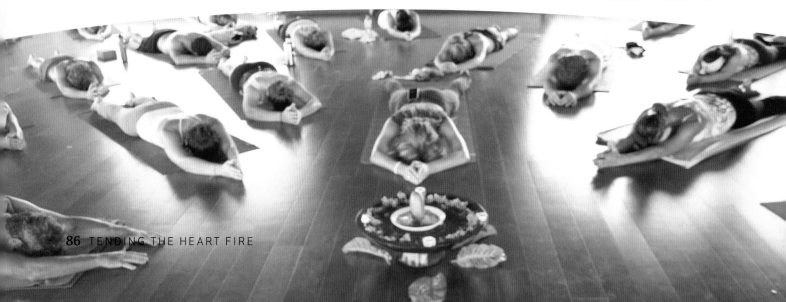

expanding the heart field— mudra vinyasas

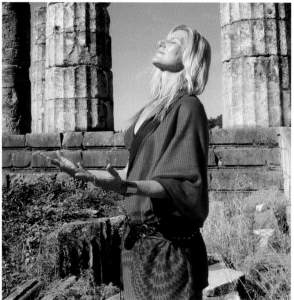

Mudra vinyasas are *mudras* (sacred gestures) that move with the flow of breath as well as mantra. I have cultivated the following mudra-mantra vinyasas (the term I use for flowing hand gestures with chanting) as a means to consciously expand the energetic field around the heart, particularly at the beginning of practice. As you move, the transmission of wisdom that you often need arises through the inherent quality of the movement, such as the healing that arises as the arms expand in generosity or draw inward close to the heart. This is a way of dropping into a nonverbal knowing where we can listen to the heart's wisdom.

All bodily movements, created spontaneously
from awakened consciousness, pure in essence,
become sacred gestures, or *mudras.*
—SAHAJAYOGINICINTA, EIGHTH-CENTURY YOGINI[16]

MOVEMENTS OF PRANA

The movements of prana are the movements of creation: the breath, the cellular pulse, the quantum shimmer, the ocean tides, the leap of a tiger, the expansion and contraction of the heart. Invoked in sacred texts from the Vedas to the Tantras, Yoga Sutras to Hatha Yoga Pradapika, these five movements (*pancha vayus*) are all aspects of the one flow of prana. Prana Flow–Energetic Vinyasa is dedicated to the embodiment of prana as brought forth in this invocation chant:

Om Pranaya Swaha
I honor the "in-drawing, rising energy"
as the essential Self [Swaha]

Om Apanaya Swaha
I honor the "downward, rooting flow"
as the essential Self

Om Samanaya Swaha
I honor the energy that "contracts
to the core" as the essential Self

Om Vyanaya Swaha
I honor the energy that "expands
omnidirectionally from the core"
as the essential Self

Om Udanaya Swaha
I honor the energy that "rises and
moves outward" as the essential Self

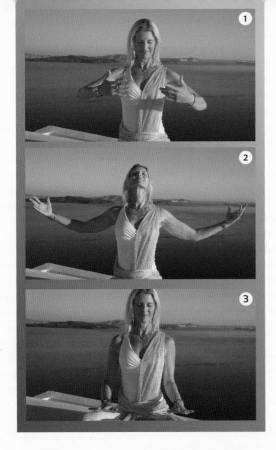

SAMANA-VYANA MUDRA VINYASA— EXPANDING AND CONTRACTING

This meditation cultivates the awareness of the core pulsation—inward (*samana*) and outward (*vyana*)— that connects us with the rhythm of life in every cell and heartbeat.

With your hands upon your heart, inhale into your heart's center. Receive the breath as an offering to your core fire. As you exhale, slowly move your hands away, palms facing your heart (1), feeling the electromagnetic field radiating into your hands with a palpable quality and slowly expanding outward (2). Continue to breathe with this inward and outward movement, to move into a meditative heart rhythm. Then rest (3).

PRANA-APANA MUDRA VINYASA— ROOTING AND RISING

This meditation connects you with the two primary movements of prana, the grounding force (*apana*) and the rising force (*prana*), which helps you integrate the vertical alignment of your heart with your brain and belly as well as heaven and earth.

Feel your roots as you exhale down into your pelvis (if sitting) or feet (if standing).

As you inhale, sweep your arms overhead, either bringing your hands together or keeping the palms open and receptive (1).

As you exhale, slowly draw your hands down the centerline of your body, connecting with the energy centers of the chakras on the way down from your forehead to the base of your spine (2).

As you inhale, begin the cycle again. Allow the flow of this movement to redistribute your energy between the upper and lower poles, brain and heart, heart and belly, belly and roots. When you are done, rest (3).

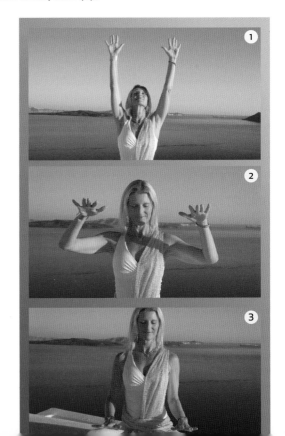

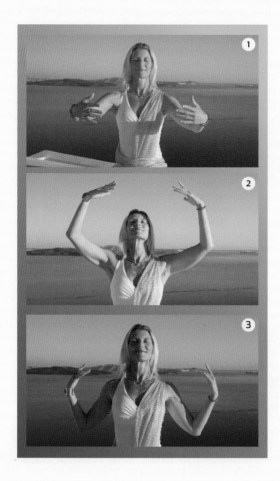

SAMUDRA VINYASA—WAVE FLOW

The wave creates a natural feeling of the ocean *(samudra)* washing over you.

As you inhale, draw your hands straight up to the sky. As you exhale, release your spine and your arms like the crest of a wave across the shore; bend your elbows and draw your open arms forward (1) along with your entire spine toward the earth. Inhale, and draw your spine and your arms back and up like a wave coiling from the shore (2). Continue these movements in an undulating rhythm (3).

> The worshipper utterly inebriated
> drinks from the cup of the inbreathings
> and the outbreathings of love.
> —KABIR[17]

ANAHATA HEART CHAKRA MUDRA VINYASA WITH MANTRA

Bring your hand to your heart, either with open palms or together in *anjali mudra* (see page 135). Integrate the heart gaze and feel its effects deepen your awareness as you open your heart. To integrate chanting with the mudra, circulate the chant as you exhale and the hands come through your heart in offering.

On an inhale, slowly draw your hands in front of your heart.

As you exhale, begin to offer the vowel sounds of *om ahhh ohhhh mmmmnggg,* or any mantra from your spiritual tradition, or just primal sound as you extend your arms open (1) and feel the emanation of the radiance in your heart.

When you reach the full extension, inhale and wrap your hands behind your back (2) as if drawing and integrating a deep, core truth within yourself. Circulate this movement for several rounds (3).

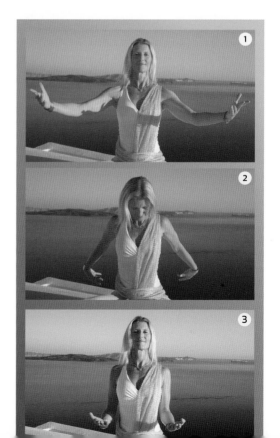

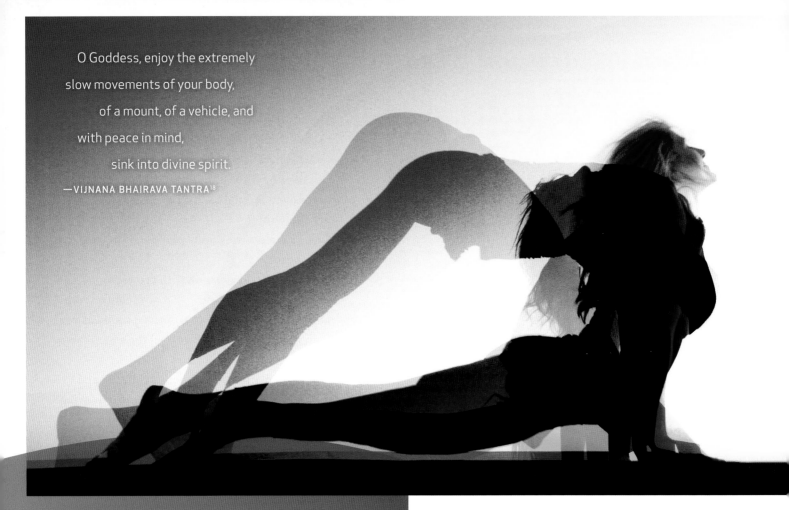

O Goddess, enjoy the extremely
slow movements of your body,
of a mount, of a vehicle, and
with peace in mind,
sink into divine spirit.
—VIJNANA BHAIRAVA TANTRA[18]

HEART RHYTHM–BASED MOVEMENT MEDITATIONS

Kriyas are movement meditations that circulate simple energetic patterns throughout the body. Inner kriyas are often linked with the breath and mantra through the flow of prana in the spine. Outer kriyas are simple, rhythmic movements that create a meditative state of heart-brain entrainment.

ANAHATA (HEART CHAKRA) KRIYA

You can practice this fluid, circular movement in the heart-chakra region to liberate the ribcage.

Begin in a comfortable seat. Take a long, slow in-breath. As you exhale, bow the crown of your head toward your heart so that your spine rounds and the back of your heart expands.

On an inhale, draw your heart through in a wavelike motion that now expands the front of the body and continues to circle now in any direction right or left in a fluid *sahaja* (spontaneous) flow. Feel the region around your heart begin to subtly open in freedom. Breathe through this circular and spiral motion of the spine. Let yourself be guided by this tidal rhythm as it entrains your heart, breath, and brain waves into a receptive state.

AGNI KRIYA— LIBERATING THE INNER FIRE

Agni kriya is a more energized version of *anahata kriya* and is practiced while standing firmly rooted. This kriya liberates the entire system and has the added benefit of toning your core and digestive system.

Stand with your feet hip-distance apart. As you become rooted, visualize earth energy rising through your feet and into your pelvic floor (*mula bandha*), then into your belly (*uddhiyana bandha*).

Bring your hands in *agni mudra* to your heart or overhead in an upward rising. Slowly begin to twist from side to side in a rhythmic friction. Maintain your feet and pelvis connection to the earth and listen to your sacrum and lower back so that every twist feels liberating. Gradually, begin to increase the friction and churning of the spine. In that simple twist you can feel what the Upanishads invoke as the loosening of the knot of the heart. Your upper body will become freer, generating a transforming inner fire and heat, as your base supports your movement. As you move with this kriya, let go of all extraneous thoughts and feel the solar, stimulating quality of positive friction igniting your energy field.

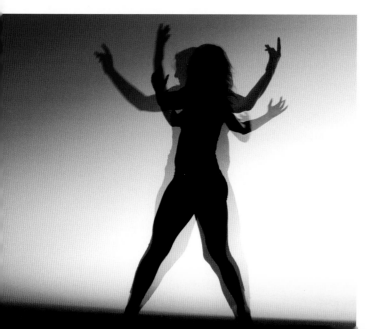

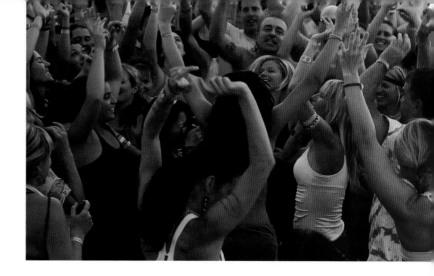

TALA KRIYA—RHYTHMIC MOVERS AND SHAKERS MEDITATION

Shaking is one of the oldest meditations on the planet. We are born knowing instinctually how to vibrate our bodies, from root to crown; toddlers and young children do this naturally. Music is not required, although it can generate inspiration for shaking meditations.

Either standing or sitting, root your feet to the earth. Either in silence or with rhythmic music, begin to start your engines. Feel for the pulse in the core of your body. Follow the rhythm instinctually, moving as the music, in whole-body entrainment. Feel the rhythm of the pulse rising up from your feet into your pelvis. Starting with your hands, begin to send this ripple of whole-body pulsing through the shoulders, heart region, pelvis, knees, and feet. Shake with your whole being in all rhythms that arise. Let your whole body shake from feet to crown in a regenerating movement.

> The dancing foot
> The form assumed by your dancing Guru as Shiva
> Find out these within yourself
> and your fetters shall fall away.
> —TIRUMOOLAR, PERIYA PURANAM[19]

surya namaskar—
embodying the sun

The brilliant sun that shines in every heart

for the heaven's earth and all creatures

What a blessing!

Let it soak my every pore

for the inner splendor it reveals

is a blessing

—RUMI[20]

THE SURYA NAMASKAR MANTRA

Each verse of this mantra corresponds with a movement as illustrated on the next page.

1. *Om Mitraya Namah*
   Salutations to the Friend of All

2. *Om Ravaye Namah*
   Salutations to the Shining One

3. *Om Suryaya Namah*
   Salutations to the Source of Creation

4. *Om Bhanave Namah*
   Salutations to the One Who Illuminates

5. *Om Khagaya Namah*
   Salutations to the One Who Moves through the Sky

6. *Om Pusne Namah*
   Salutations to the Giver of Strength and Nourishment

7. *Om Hiranyagarbhaya Namah*
   Salutations to the Golden Cosmic Womb

8. *Om Maricaye Namah*
   Salutations to the Rays of the Sun

9. *Om Aditaya Namah*
   Salutations to the Infinite Cosmic Mother

10. *Om Savitre Namah*
    Salutations to the Rising Sun

11. *Om Arkaya Namah*
    Salutations to the Source of Life Energy

12. *Om Bhaskaraya Namah*
    Salutations to the One Who Leads to Enlightenment

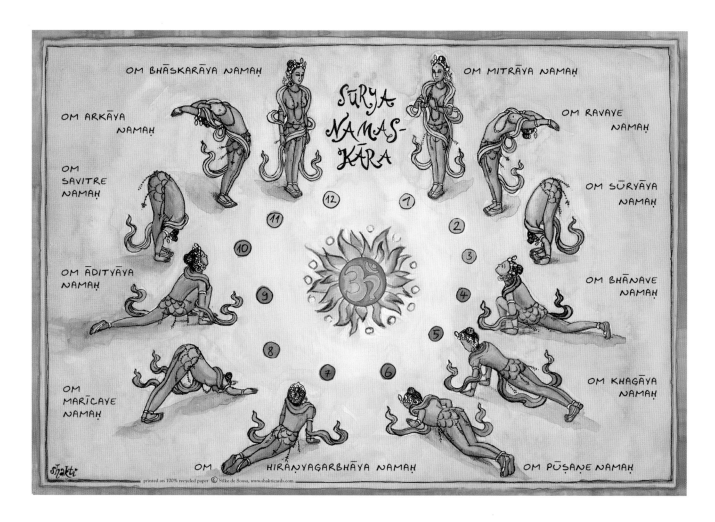

BECOME THE SUN IN THE HEART OF YOUR BODY

Namaskar is a special type of vinyasa, a ritual offering in the form of a synchronized sequence of mudras or asanas. This is a kind of movement alchemy, designed to awaken and transform the mover.

Classical sequences such as *surya* (sun) and *chandra* (moon) *namaskar* are integrated with mantras that correspond to the phases of the sun and moon, to awaken a corresponding inner movement. Namaskar beyond yoga is not yet widely known, yet other "salutation" forms are found in Indian classical dance and martial arts such as *kalarippayatu*.

In Prana Flow–Energetic Vinyasa, the power of namaskar as devotion in motion takes form in more than forty different namaskars connected to fire, water, earth, the heart, and mandalas—circles of wholeness.

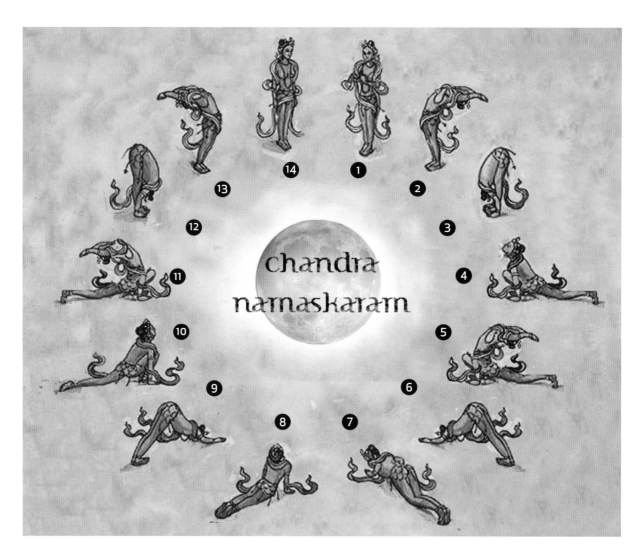

CHANDRA NAMASKAR— EMBODYING THE MOON

Chandra namaskar is the sequence of surya namaskar with the addition of two backbends, for a total of fourteen movements that correspond with the phases of the moon or the *tithis*. The origins of these offerings to the moon are not as well-documented as the sun namaskar, although hymns to the moon and to *soma* are also found in the Vedas. This namaskar carries the restorative nature of the moon and induces slow, inward, *ojas*-generating movement. It is best to cultivate the lunar gaze by circulating these movements while facing the moon, or by visualizing receiving the lunar nectar with every breath. This induces a healing cascade of hormones that you can feel as heart-brain connection. The following mantras correspond with the lunar *tithis*, or phases of the moon, which are connected to the *nityas*, or different aspects of Shakti, the Mother Goddess.

Thirst drove me

to the water where

I drank the moon's reflection.

—RUMI[21]

THE CHANDRA NAMASKAR MANTRA

Each verse of this mantra corresponds with a movement as illustrated on the previous page.

① *Om Kamasvaryal Namah*
  Salutations to she who fulfills all desires

② *Om Bhagamalinyai Namah*
  Salutations to she who wears the garland of prosperity

③ *Om Nitaklinnayai Namah*
  Salutations to she who is ever compassionate

④ *Om Bherundayai Namah*
  Salutations to she who is fierce

⑤ *Om Vahnivasinyai Namah*
  Salutations to she who resides in fire

⑥ *Om Vajreshvaryai Namah*
  Salutations to she whose diamond-like vajra essence is indestructible power

⑦ *Om Shiva Dutyai Namah*
  Salutations to she whose messenger is Shiva

⑧ *Om Tvaritayai Namah*
  Salutations to she who is swift

⑨ *Om Kulasundaryai Namah*
  Salutations to she whose beauty and virtue is the essence of the *kula* family and community

⑩ *Om Nityayai Namah*
  Salutations to she who is eternal

⑪ *Om Nilapatakinyai Namah*
  Salutations to she who is adorned with a blue flag of infinite mystery

⑫ *Om Vijayayai Namah*
  Salutations to she who is ever victorious

⑬ *Om Sarvamangalayai Namah*
  Salutations to she who is always auspicious

⑭ *Om Jvalamalinyai Namah*
  Salutations to she whose essence is the fire

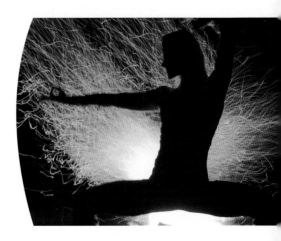

yoga
alchemy

Energetic Vinyasa and the Flow of Rasa

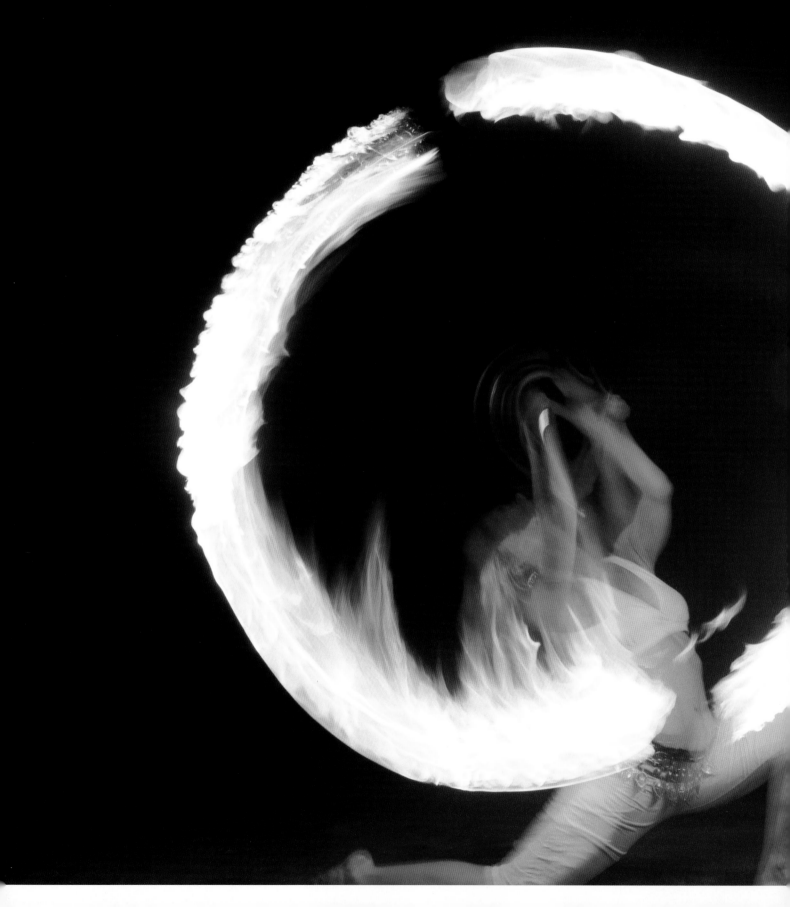

Life is change. Learn to surf.

—SWAMI SATCHITANANDA

Throughout the last chapter, we tended our inner fire
through practices from outward movement (solar)
to inward movement (lunar), including surya and
chandra namaskar, the Sun and Moon Salutations.
In the process of recovering our inherent rhythms
from mechanized ways of "doing yoga," we applied
energetic vinyasa as a way of sequencing to our inherent flow of life force (prana). Too often in the West,
we override our natural state by rigidly practicing a
set sequence or a specific workout without regard
to our actual energy or the rhythm of the day, week,
moon, or season. Moving with the tide of both our
natural energy flow and the macrocosmic cycle is
like tacking your sail to the wind. We have natural
momentum available to us, whether from the lunar,
meditative quality of the waning moon or a Friday
afternoon or winter time, or from the solar, rising
energy of the full moon or spring.

THE EVOLUTION OF ENERGETIC VINYASA— PRANA FLOW NAMASKARS

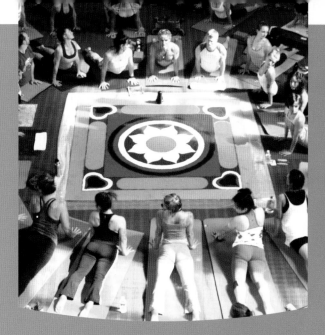

After ten years of Sun Salutations in my body, something began to shift and a different calling started to emerge. I was hesitant at first to move beyond the classical forms I had learned, but I had a deep desire to embody the unique quality of each day, whether through spontaneous sahaja movements of the rising moon or by dropping low to the earth with the falling leaves of autumn.

The Prana Flow Namaskar Mandala, which I have developed over twenty years of practice, offers a framework for approaching the shifts that occur through the wheel of the year and the solar-lunar cycle. (A full description of the mandala is beyond the scope of this book, but I offer it on the book's website, tendingtheheartfire.com, as an additional practice resource.) Here the sixty-four namaskars are arranged around the seasons as well as the elements. It begins at the top of the mandala with the new year and flows through the seasons, connected to the *doshas* (inner wheel of *vata-pitta-kapha*) and the rasas (*vira, sringara, shanti*). These are general guidelines that follow the movement: the solar wheel of increasing light from January through June (the solar, right side of the mandala) and the waning light from June through December (the lunar, left side of the mandala). The namaskars move up the centerline in the flow of the chakras, starting at the bottom with the foundational earth

or *bhumi namaskar* and up through the elements to the most subtle namaskars at the top, connected to our highest devotion. These represent the *deva-devi* namaskars, in which all of our movements are offered to the Source.

It has been my great pleasure in my practice and teachings to see the benefits of the "energetic diversity" reflected in the mandala. I have seen type triple-A, highly driven solar students integrate their fluid nature with great joy. The slow-moving, peaceful movements on the mandala provide tremendous support during the high stress of the holiday season in December. The solar stimulation of the fire namaskars helps stoke the inner fire when it is dim or going out. Firekeeping through the namaskars gives us the ability to be "movement alchemists"—a way of cultivating rasa through changing rhythms and qualities of being. In creating the Prana Flow–Energetic Vinyasa system, my aim has been to empower yoga practitioners to be "agents of change" by respecting, attuning to, and moving with their life force.

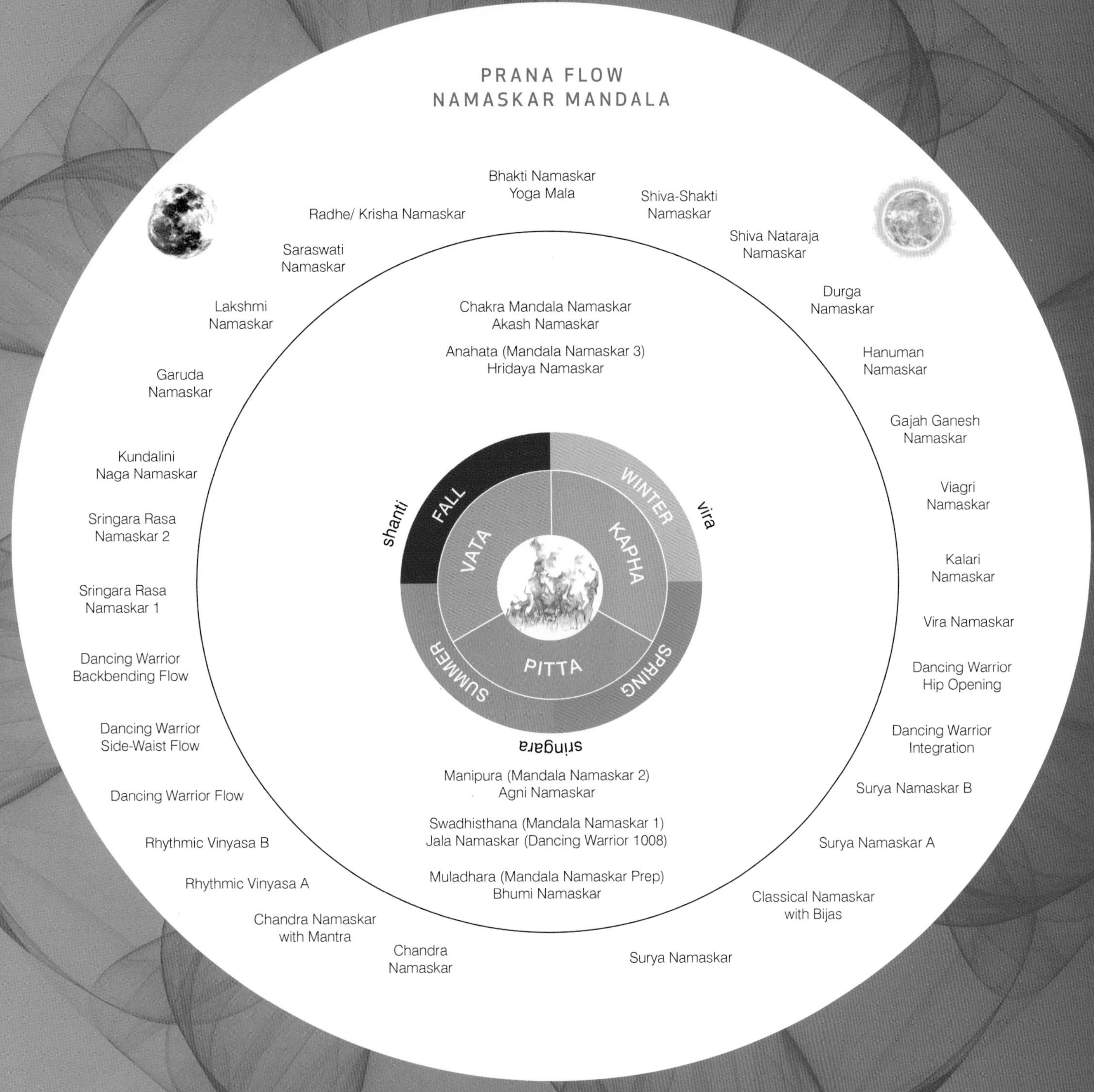

PRANA FLOW
NAMASKAR MANDALA

Bhakti Namaskar
Yoga Mala

Shiva-Shakti
Namaskar

Radhe/ Krisha Namaskar

Shiva Nataraja
Namaskar

Saraswati
Namaskar

Durga
Namaskar

Lakshmi
Namaskar

Chakra Mandala Namaskar
Akash Namaskar

Hanuman
Namaskar

Anahata (Mandala Namaskar 3)
Hridaya Namaskar

Garuda
Namaskar

Gajah Ganesh
Namaskar

Kundalini
Naga Namaskar

shanti

FALL

WINTER

vira

Viagri
Namaskar

VATA

KAPHA

Sringara Rasa
Namaskar 2

Kalari
Namaskar

Sringara Rasa
Namaskar 1

Vira Namaskar

SUMMER

PITTA

SPRING

Dancing Warrior
Backbending Flow

Dancing Warrior
Hip Opening

sringara

Dancing Warrior
Side-Waist Flow

Dancing Warrior
Integration

Manipura (Mandala Namaskar 2)
Agni Namaskar

Dancing Warrior Flow

Surya Namaskar B

Swadhisthana (Mandala Namaskar 1)
Jala Namaskar (Dancing Warrior 1008)

Rhythmic Vinyasa B

Surya Namaskar A

Muladhara (Mandala Namaskar Prep)
Bhumi Namaskar

Rhythmic Vinyasa A

Classical Namaskar
with Bijas

Chandra Namaskar
with Mantra

Chandra
Namaskar

Surya Namaskar

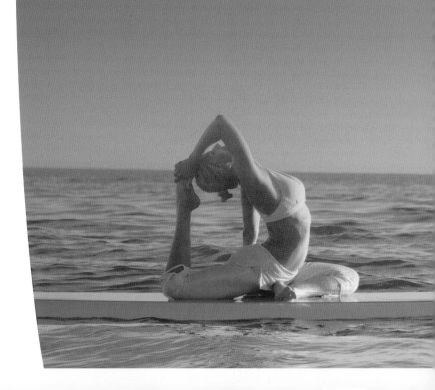

CLASSICAL SEQUENCES

such as surya (sun) and chandra (moon) *namaskar* are integrated with mantras that correspond to the phases of the sun and moon to awaken a corresponding inner movement. Namaskar beyond yoga is not yet widely known, yet other "salutation" forms are found in Indian classical dance and martial arts such as kalarippayatu.

In Prana Flow–Energetic Vinyasa, the power of namaskar as devotion in motion takes form in more than forty different namaskars connected to fire, water, earth, the heart, and mandalas—circles of wholeness.

My heart is pulsing with passion,
like waves on an ocean.

I'm at home, wherever I am …
I can see with closed eyes the beauty that dances.

Behind the veils intoxicated with love,
I too dance the rhythm of this moving world.

—RUMI[1]

This Prana Flow Mandala Namaskar is but one of forty evolutionary namaskars that have emerged from my body and teachings from the source Sun and Moon Salutations. This namaskar embodies flowing qualities (lasya) supported by grounding strength (tandava), balancing the sun and the moon within. The website for this book, tendingtheheartfire.com, has the full flowing version, which you can follow.

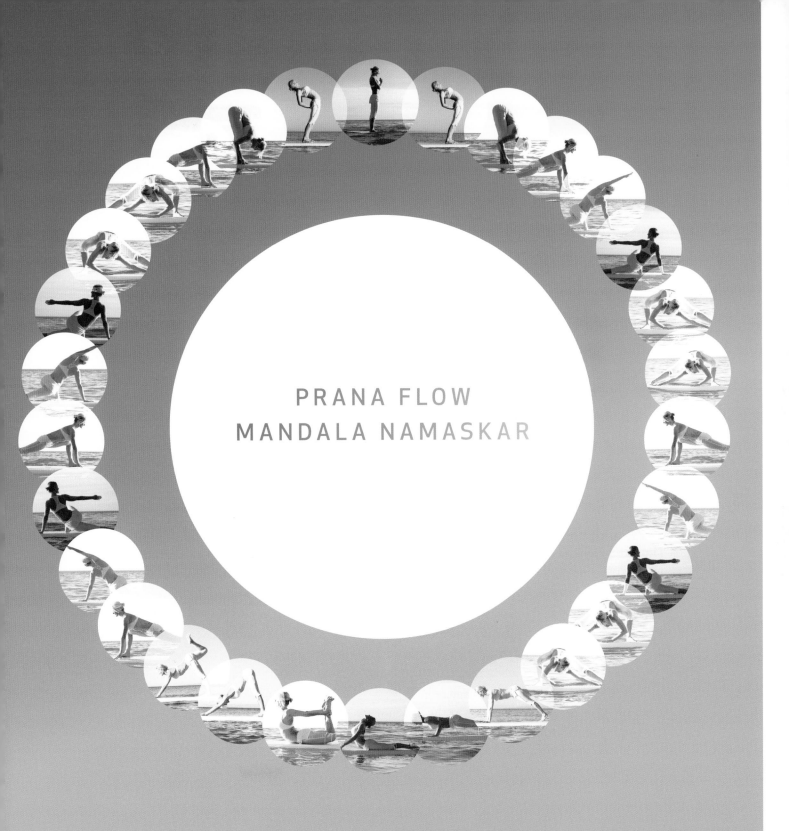

PRANA FLOW
MANDALA NAMASKAR

tending the fire—observing the variables of energetic vinyasa

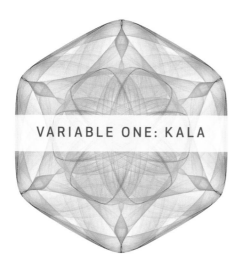

VARIABLE ONE: KALA

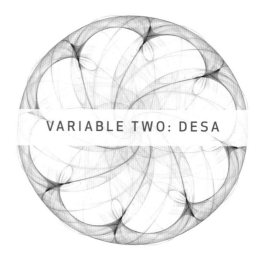

VARIABLE TWO: DESA

Time and rhythm have a profound effect on our energy. The time of the day, week, lunar cycle, and seasonal cycle all strongly influence our practice needs. In general, the rasas vira, shanti, and sringara are correlated to the sun (Vira Rasa, or the activated inner state of the warrior), the moon (Shanti Rasa, or the inner meditative transforming calm), and the interplay of the sun and moon (Sringara Rasa, or the sensual union of the masculine and feminine within).

Desa means "place, home," and has to do with both the ecology and the environment in which you are living or traveling. In hotter or dryer environments, you have to be careful of too much fire so as not to overheat or overstimulate *pitta* or *vata*. In cooler climates, the fire has to be carefully cultivated so that your vital energy does not become too dim. The power of Desa is ultimately within your heart, which leads to the next variable: Bhava-Rasa or Bhavana.

There are four basic variables that guide an energetic vinyasa practice: **Kala** (time and rhythm), **Desa** (place), **Bhava-Rasa** or **Bhavana** (inner state), and **Dosha** (constitution). These principles are fundamental to what I think of as *movement alchemy*.

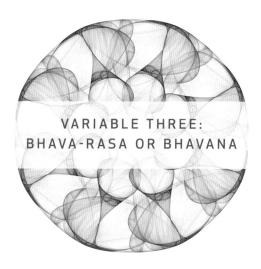

VARIABLE THREE: BHAVA-RASA OR BHAVANA

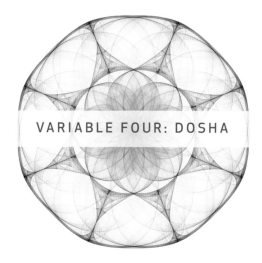

VARIABLE FOUR: DOSHA

Bhavana, your feeling-state, has a profound effect upon your embodiment. Stress and dissonant emotions negatively impact our functioning and well-being, while coherent emotions support these. Coherent inner states, from the lunar calm of loving gratitude to the solar states of passion and enthusiasm, create optimal flow. Focusing on *bhava* within your practice is a beautiful way to balance your inner and outer world through movement.

In ayurveda, the cycle of the seasons mirrors changes in the doshas, the bodily humors of ayurveda: *vata, pitta,* and *kapha.* These need to be balanced in different ways at different times through more solar or lunar energies as well as the rasas. We can balance and enhance our constitution by changing our practice, both seasonally and in accordance with what is arising in our body.

rasa vinyasa—movement alchemy

Rasa is a divine emotional state.
It is eternal, indivisible, and
inconceivable essence of the
supreme transcendental bliss.
It is a state of ecstasy which a
devotee experiences in the
height of his devotion for God.

—SWAMI SIVANANDA[2]

*Rasa has many beautiful, interrelated meanings,
from "nectar" to "taste" to "essence" to "alchemy"
to an all-permeating state of being.*

Rasa vinyasa is a process of movement alchemy in which we can positively integrate our inner state as a living art.

In addition to its other meanings, the word *rasa* is synonymous with soma, *amrita*, and ojas—and in particular the heart. Hridaya Rasa is the essence of the heart, the very essential *para ojas* that resides in the heart from birth. Hridaya Rasa, the highest teachings of yoga tell us, leads to the experience of "one taste" or Eka Rasa—the healing internal flow that can be cultivated through yoga and the arts.

In substances in the body or in food, rasa is the quality of vitality. Restoring your essence is related to ojas in the body and soma in the subtle body. There is also a current that connects soma, rasa, and ojas in relation to the spiritual and emotional states of beauty, joy, love, and sublime ecstasy. Bharata, the author of the Natyasastra, classifies rasa into eight groups: erotic love (*sringara*), heroic (*vira*), marvelous (*abdhuta*), compassionate (*karuna*), comic (*hasya*), terrible, disgusting (*bhibasta*), and furious (*raudra*).

To this the tantric sage Abhinavagupta adds a ninth rasa, *shanti* (the tranquility and bliss of enlightened awareness). He teaches that any one of the eight rasas, all of which carry a degree of intensity, can be a trigger for liberation from suffering, as long as we do not try to reject or cling to any particular rasa that may arise.

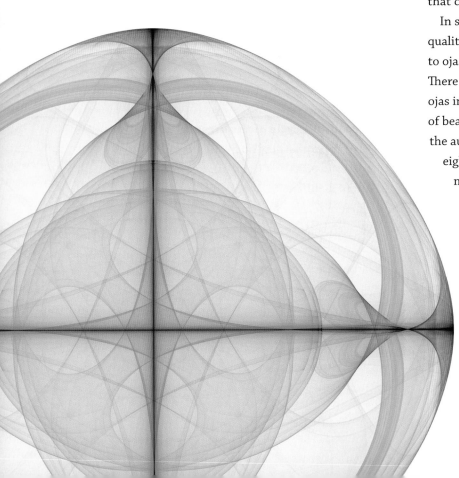

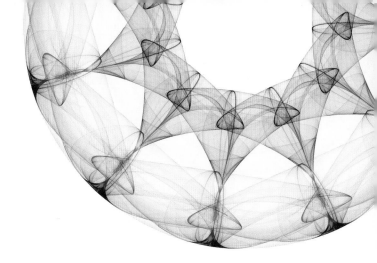

Rather, we can work with the alchemy of the heart with any variation of emotions arising as a particular pulsation of pure shakti (emotional energy), to be honored—that is to say authentically experienced, without any repression or pushing away—as it arises. The intensity of the rasa may then be alchemically transformed through the power of the heart's capacity to transform dissonant emotions. Our feeling-state (bhava) is not an obstacle to yoga but is instead an access point to our heart's presence and a way of working with the authentic truth of who we are in every moment.

Just as an artist learns how to attune him- or herself to the heart energy that is present and access that flow to generate a note, a movement, or a brushstroke, our yoga practice as movement alchemy becomes the art that transforms "thinking mind" into "feeling mind." Through bhava (generation of feeling awareness) and through rasa, the essence—the juice—of life is regenerated.

First try to discover the emotions.
Having embraced them and made love,
You will find the Jewel of Love.
—BAUL SONG[4]

The place of pure wisdom can be accessed through an intense flow of a particular emotion (rasa) arising from within. One who presents a pure-hearted offering with focused attention to a particular rasa will experience the transformation of that rasa into the Supreme, universal consciousness of one's true Self.
—SHRI ABHINAVAGUPTA,
FROM HIS TANTRALOKA (LIGHT ON TANTRA)[3]

The following exploration is based on my practice and the development of offering Rasa Vinyasa—Movement Alchemy, a practical process to balance and enhance the emotions arising to enter into deeper states of flow in life and within yoga. In Rasa Vinyasa we focus on the three primary rasas utilized in Indian classical arts: Vira (solar energy), Shanti (lunar energy), and Sringara (the alchemical flow of love) as a way to affect the flow of our life-journey through the power of our movement practice, which includes a prana rasa vinyasa, movement meditations, namaskars, mudras, wave sequences of yogasanas, mantra, and internal meditation, which are featured in Part Two. The online practice companion to the book integrates this approach to living alchemy.

energetic rasa vinyasa— three primary rasas

As you learn to circulate the appropriate rasas, the juice of your life force revitalizes. You become a reflection of the full spectrum of nature.

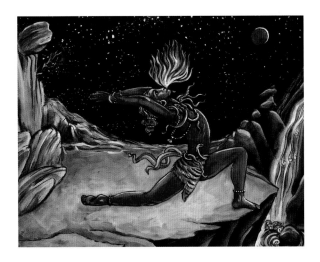

VIRA RASA— ACTIVATING SOLAR POTENCY

Vira Rasa is the natural invocation of the rising energy of nature, which can be felt at any time when change is being ignited as a force of growth, evolution, and vital energy. Derived from the root meaning of the word *vira* as "hero," vira is the embodied state of inner and outer strength, potency, courage, and verve. Vira Rasa is related to the yogic process of tapas—unwavering commitment and dedication. It is the activation of solar energy to cultivate the juice of your life (ojas)—not, as ayurveda cautions, to burn ojas up.

Tending Vira Rasa: Igniting the Fire

Kala/Tala (time and rhythm): Optimal times include the initiation of any cycles as well as the peak waxing energy, morning or before sunset, new moon through full moon, Tuesdays (the day for Mars), or any day of the week when you are naturally energized or when you need to awaken a dim fire. The rhythm of Vira Rasa is activating and steady, supporting the ability to build energy and ecstatic intensity.

Desa (place and ecology): Environments of high prana that are naturally energizing.

Bhava (somatic mood): Warm, engaging, energizing, awakened, naked feeling-states that are often beyond one-word descriptions. These feeling-states have the clear, passionate, present, noble, wisdom-in-action, and expansive heart qualities that inspire us at a deep ancestral and spiritual level. Vira states enable us to face our own shadow tendencies with truth, courage, and the heart of a warrior, unafraid of the dark, contracted, difficult spaces in life.

Dosha (constitution): Vira Rasa is a natural mode of being for pitta- or fire-predominant types, but it can cause excess heat, agitation, and burning of one's life-energy if practiced under stress or when one is tired. Vira Rasa is excellent for the kapha constitution to generate energy and stimulate the fire element in one's body and life.

Yoga Practice: Dynamic solar namaskars; Agni Kriya; shaking movement meditation; sequences involving concentration, alignment, and breath. Linear asanas with strong lines such as the warrior family (*virabhadrasana*), arm balances, standing balance poses, and core cultivation all activate Vira Rasa. *Pranayama: kapalabhati, bhastrika,* and *ujjayi pranayama* with retentions. Solar meditations.

Living Vira Rasa: Vira Rasa stokes the fires to help us overcome any obstacle, challenge, or regressive habit by encouraging the embodiment of courage, stamina, and steadiness within our daily lives.

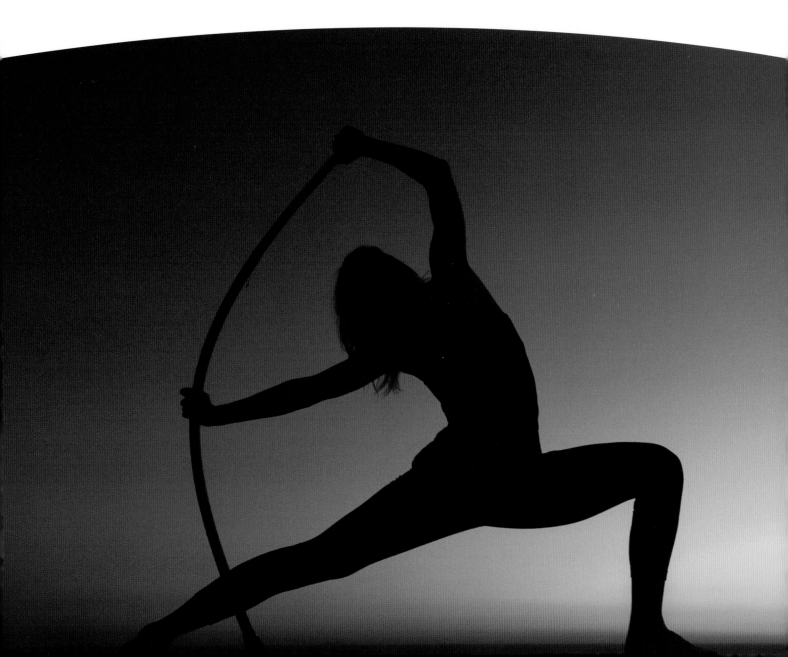

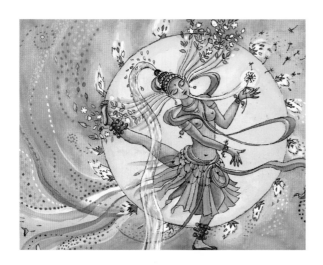

SRINGARA RASA— THE WAY LOVE MOVES

Sringara Rasa is the rhythm and way of moving as love. We find it in the spontaneous backbend that arises when we taste something sublime; when we fling open our arms in response to a beautiful sight in nature; when we hear a lovely piece of music and close our eyes and smile; when we make the humming sound *mmmm* in the pleasure of a delicious taste or in lovemaking, in feline purring and the buzz of the bee's pollinating dance. These naturally arising movements of sringara trigger a response in heart rhythm-brainwave flow that stimulates the slower heart-rate rhythms and the flow of hormones of love—oxytocin, seratonin, dopamine, and endorphins. If you are not feeling loving, try moving as love, which has an instinctually fluid, connected quality that is part of the art of Sringara Rasa, expressed in curving movements and music with notes and melodies that bend and sway.

It is impossible to be rigid and express love at the same time. Sringara Rasa is the cultivation in the heart of the love union of male and female. Sringara Rasa is fire and water, sun and moon, passion and peace. It is a cultivation of the heart and sensuality of yoga that helps us to feel and generate loving energy toward ourselves, others, and ultimately the Divine. If you too often feel dry, brittle, bitter, or lacking in heart energy, learning to cultivate Sringara Rasa in your body and life is like discovering a secret well that flows inside you and can never run dry.

Love moves in natural sways.
The taste melts, the spine
arches, the heart stirs —
the way love moves in
spontaneous freedom.
We can move as love to
trigger the alchemy.
When the heart regions
open and love's sway
begins, the heart nectar
pours through the body.

Tending Sringara Rasa

Kala/Tala (time and rhythm): It's best to practice Sringara Rasa before we have become hardened, mechanical, or lacking in feeling or connectedness with our own body or with others. It can also be practiced to shift the energy when we are already experiencing those states. Sringara Rasa is suitable for all times of practice and all seasons, particularly to cultivate bhakti during holidays of love such as Valentine's Day, before lovemaking, or for any cycle where you are intentionally stoking the love fire. The rhythm of Sringara Rasa is a melodic, meandering, smooth, passionate, building dynamic leading to a peak orgasmic release and then integration/communion into bliss. This rhythm is found in all forms of art, from music to dance and drama, as it is the rhythm of the climax of creation that makes Sringara Rasa so compelling.

Desa (place and ecology): All places, particularly rasa-filled natural environments by the ocean or in tropical regions where nature's sway and abundance relax your whole being into the eros of nature.

Bhava (somatic mood): Sensual receptivity, seeing/feeling/hearing/tasting the Beloved in the diversity of life and within one's being.

Yoga Practice: All movements that are circular, wavelike, and fluid mirror the sway of love that Sringara Rasa invokes most, typified in the heart-liberating flow of backbends in *yogasanas*. All meditations, mantras, mudras, and chanting within asana (lengthens exhale, awakens the vibration in the heart center), as well as *viloma* and *anuloma pranayama* (drinking and savoring the breath in stages).

Dosha (constitution): Sringara Rasa is excellent for all doshas, particularly pitta and vata types who can easily sacrifice love, enjoyment, and fluid flow to the physical agenda of achieving. Sringara Rasa is nourishing and healing for any form of stress.

Living Sringara Rasa: Open to the experience of life in its sensual fullness. Touch, taste, see, and hear the world, and experience each breath as a form of the Beloved. Notice how your movement and voice change and become smoother and more elegant and regenerative for yourself and others.

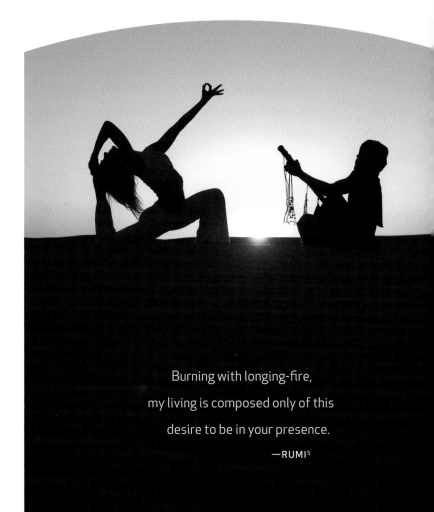

Burning with longing-fire,
my living is composed only of this
desire to be in your presence.

—RUMI[5]

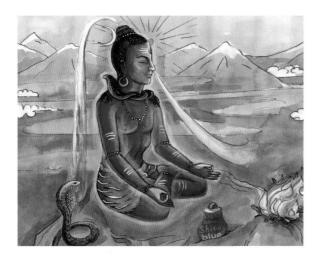

SHANTI RASA—BEING PEACE

Shanti Rasa is the embodiment of deep peace. The lotus rising from the mud is the timeless yogic symbol of Shanti Rasa, for peace is not dependent on cloudy or clear water, or external circumstances, but a deep connection to eternal essence within. The rhythm of Shanti Rasa is inwardly connected, even if outer rhythms are turbulent or dissonant. For most people, cultivating Shanti Rasa in movement involves slowing down and allowing their movements to become very simple and yet powerful, often moving close to the earth, as with the prostrations that we learned in Chapter Four. For this reason, Shanti Rasa is closely connected to lunar *sadhana* and is regenerative in nature, like fertile earth nurturing the seed. Shanti Rasa is good to cultivate when you feel depleted, while traveling, or whenever you feel ungrounded. Shanti is the state of living, breathing peace.

Tending Shanti Rasa

Kala/Tala (time and rhythm): Shanti Rasa is best to circulate when you are feeling stress or too much fire; it is suitable for all times and seasons, but particularly early morning, early afternoon (siesta time), evening before bed, and waning energy (full moon through new moon). Shanti Rasa is important during the summer months of high heat as well as late fall, particularly the last six weeks of the year between October 31 and December 21 during the vulnerable seasonal transition. Keeping a slow and balanced rhythm that is steady, smooth, spacious, and without extremes is the key to being in peace.

Desa (place and ecology): Moving in peace is essential in quiet natural settings to allow you to absorb the subtle energy or prana of nature. It is also good to do in places of high stimulation such as New York City or Hong Kong.

Bhava (somatic mood): Calm, *sama* (evenness), equilibrium, acceptance, karuna (compassion), *santosha* (contentment).

Yoga Practice: In applying Shanti Rasa to vinyasa, slow and even movements are best. In asanas, all forward bends, hip openers, inversions, and any asanas approached with equanimity and a "cooling" bhava are movement medicine. Pranayamas such as *nadi shodhana, sama vritti ujjayi pranayama* (even inhale and exhale), and ujjayi pranayama with an emphasis on increasing exhale (twice as long as the inhale) are also tremendous movement tonics for healing any stress or dissonance in your heart field.

Dosha (constitution): Shanti Rasa is excellent for all doshas, especially when practiced in the early morning or evening when the solar or vira energy of the day has been satiated. Pitta and vata types will often resist the slower mode of Shanti Rasa that emphasizes being over doing, so it is important to choose the right timing to cultivate Shanti Rasa, including when signs of excessive or wavering fire connected with pitta and vata doshas are present. Shanti Rasa is the lunar quality that balances and calms the inner fire.

Living Shanti Rasa: Slow down and feel the release of any pressure as you find the rhythm of nature, the ocean tide within the rising and falling of the "Ten Thousand Things" as it is described in the Taoist text, the Tao Te Ching. Cultivate an authentic value of inner balance, equilibrium, wisdom, and serenity that is the fruit of living yoga.

Om Shanti Shanti Shanti

ॐ शान्तिः शान्तिः शान्तिः

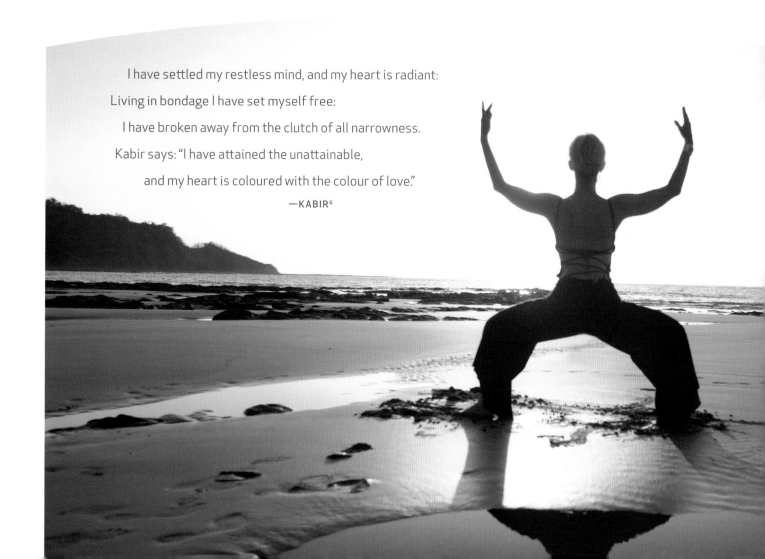

I have settled my restless mind, and my heart is radiant:

Living in bondage I have set myself free:

I have broken away from the clutch of all narrowness.

Kabir says: "I have attained the unattainable,

and my heart is coloured with the colour of love."

—KABIR[6]

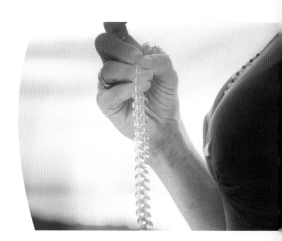

heart fire meditations and life practices

If you meditate in your heart,

you will then melt into supreme consciousness.

— VIJNANA BHAIRAVA TANTRA

115

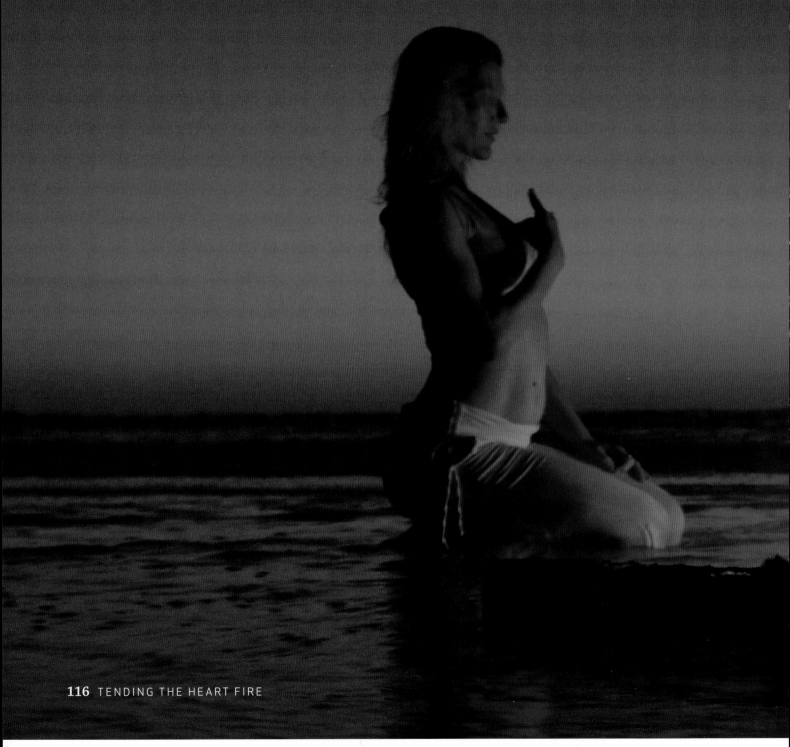

gazing at the inner fire—
dristi and *dharana*

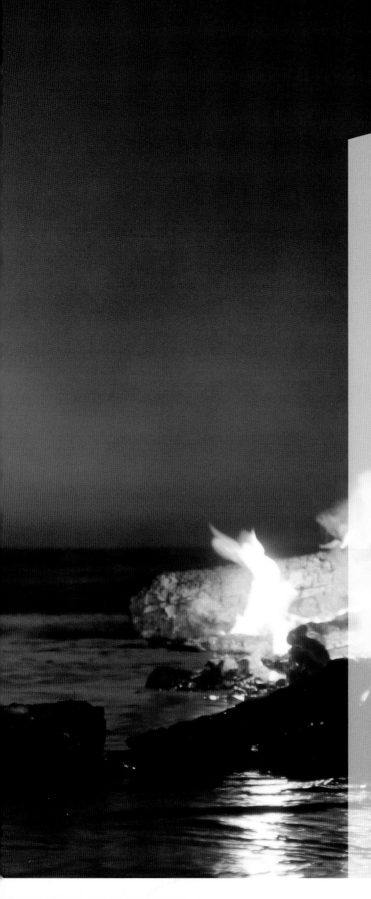

OUR EYES ARE NATURALLY DRAW TO THE CENTER OF A FIRE,

and we experience an inward shift. The same is true when we gaze at the sun during twilight hours. One of the oldest formal instructions in the world's meditative traditions is to steady your eyes and feel the sacred presence. In this way we can behold the fire of consciousness. Once our gaze settles, we enter states of awe, reflection, and adoration. We relax and become centered in contemplation, creating a sacred space for the spontaneous flow of insight, for our own creative and spiritual unfolding. This is the power of dristi: the inner gaze, or seeing with the inner eye for understanding. Even as infants, we gaze at the sun, the moon, the sky, at one another, at the world in motion, and we enter a quiet inner space.

The inner gaze emerges from the heart and can stream anywhere and everywhere within the body. The *hridaya bindu* meditation is a form of dristi that begins with re-envisioning the body as a yantra—or essential form—that originates from a central energetic point: a *bindu,* or a seed vibration. The bindu represents the vibrating origins of a form that in the yogic body is connected with the heart center.

Strengthening the natural meditative gaze through ritual devotion becomes the "technique" of gazing. It is important not to lose the naturalness or to introduce any tension through effort. Simply gaze, as we innately know how to do. When we add the spark of our feeling (bhava), our gaze effortlessly activates our Heart Fire energy like a spark creates flame.

awakening the heart bhava through the gaze

The nature and essence of bhava are pure consciousness. Bhava ushers in *prema*, or love, just as the rays usher in the rising sun, and melts the heart.

— SWAMI SIVANANDA[1]

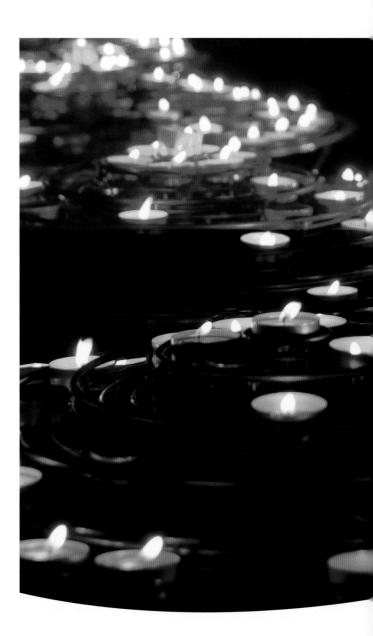

As our gaze brings us into a deeper state of presence, we become aware of our own bhava, a rich inner state of heart feeling. From the root word *bhu,* or "to be," bhava is the ground of being of the heart, just as *bhumi* is Sanskrit for "ground" or "earth." Bhava can also be translated as a verb, *bhavana,* a method of contemplation through the heart.

Dristi offers direct access to this feeling-state. As soon as our eyes become steady, a natural entrainment of the breath, heartbeat, and brainwaves takes place. We become more aware of what we are experiencing beneath the surface. This state of entrainment facilitates a natural contemplative quality that is associated with meditation. Contemplation, presence, insight, feeling, devotion, emotional stirrings, dissolution, and heart-based realization all arise out of bhava.

meditations

Here are a few dristi meditations that move us into the bindu of the heart and the feeling-state of bhava.

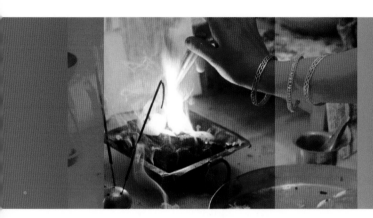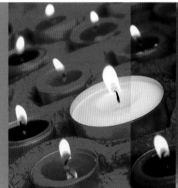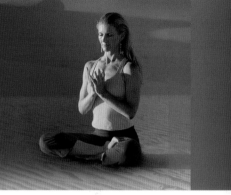

GAZING AT THE FIRE—TRATAKA

Fire-gazing may be the oldest meditation, a steady resting of the eyes upon the brilliance of flame. *Trataka* is the yogic version of this practice, in which we consciously gaze at a fire and internalize the gaze to realize the link between our inner power and the outer power of fire. Through trataka, the inner eye is awakened.

To begin, light a candle, an oil lamp, or a little fire in the hearth, accompanied by a prayer or an intention. With relaxed focus, feel your gaze settling upon the fire.

Let yourself remain relaxed and comfortable, naturally attentive, with minimal blinking, ignoring any visual distractions.

As you steady your gaze, you'll notice a meditative state arising from within. Slowly close your eyes and visualize this inner flame in your heart. Be with the sensations of your energetic heart and the power of your gaze to direct the light of your awareness.

HEART GAZE—HRIDAYA DRISTI

Keeping your outer gaze upon the fire, begin to awaken the *hridaya dristi* (inner gaze upon the Heart Fire). You can kindle and cultivate a continuous connection to your inner Heart Fire through repeated experience and practice of this inner heart gaze.

Begin by relaxing the backs of your eyes. Feel a quality of streaming your awareness in a downward cascade toward your heart center. There will be an immediate shift toward your "feeling mind." This is because when your brainwaves are vibrating at high frequencies, stimulated by the usual plethora of thoughts traveling through the mind, your somatic experience is one of excess energy. This inner gaze instantaneously shifts your awareness through the heart field; your gaze ignites it and allows it to come to prominence in your inner state.

With your dristi, feel or visualize the power of your Heart Fire. This is not a time to analyze it, but to nourish the inner fire through the power of dharana, a meditative focus that kindles devotion.

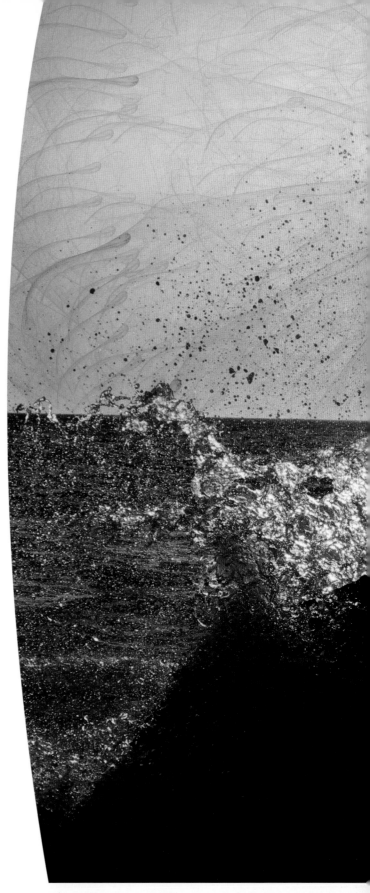

solar heart fire meditations

When people get around a central fire or gaze at the sunrise or sunset, they enter into a state of reflection and presence—a natural meditation. We have not forgotten. The great fireball in the sky still captures our imagination; the sunrise and sunset still envelop us in awe.

SUN GAZING—SURYA DRISTI

Gazing at the sun during sunrise or sunset (*surya dristi*) is an ancestral practice that has the effect of synchronizing our biorhythms with the rhythms of the cosmos, the radiance in our heart with that of the sun. The soft light at these sacred junctures allows our eyes to take in the full spectrum of light frequencies that the pineal gland requires for proper functioning.

The sun is the fire altar of our planetary life. As you gaze at it as it rises or sets, feel the rays reaching you from ninety-three million miles away and recognize that this is the source that generates and regenerates all life. Sun-gazing is a meditation in itself that is practiced within yoga and around the world. As your eyes drink in the beauty of the moment, all other thought waves naturally rest. This is the state of namaskar, or bowing, to the extraordinary source of fire around which our lives literally revolve.

SOLAR BHAVANA—FEELING THE SUN

Feel your own radiant, life-giving energy, generosity, and all of the healing emotions that arise through that embodiment of the sun (the solar *bhavana*: joy, enthusiasm, connectedness, confidence, creative potency, and sustaining power.

COSMIC BREATH—
CIRCULATING THE INNER SUN

As you saw earlier in the book, the cycle of the breath is envisioned as the union of the sun and the moon, soma and prana, within the fire of the heart connected to the core tantric practice of *ucchara*. Each breath can also be visualized as the full cycle of either the sun or moon. The inner *nyasa*, or circulation of awareness, comes and goes on the in-breath and out-breath.

As you're gazing upon the sun, you can draw solar prana into your heart with the breath. As you inhale, feel that radiance drawing into your body through the corresponding sandhyas, or sacred junctures:

> **Inhale the solar light** from the crown of the head to your third eye.

> **From the third-eye center** to the palate of the mouth.

> **From the palate of the mouth** to your throat center.

> **From your throat center** through to your heart center.

> **Bow your chin toward your heart** and pause in *kumbhaka* (retaining the inhale without straining) and feel the space outside of time. Offer prayers and mantras within that space as offerings to the inner Heart Fire.

Om Ravi-Prakhyayai Namah

I bow to the One who shines with the special brilliance of the sun.[2]

You have the option to circulate the mantra *Om* or the solar mantra *Om Hum Suraye Namaha*. As you exhale, feel the solar breath return from the heart center back to the crown. Continue to breathe the light of the sun through the cycle of your breath, adding a mantra if you wish. You can enjoy this for several rounds, then rest in meditation.

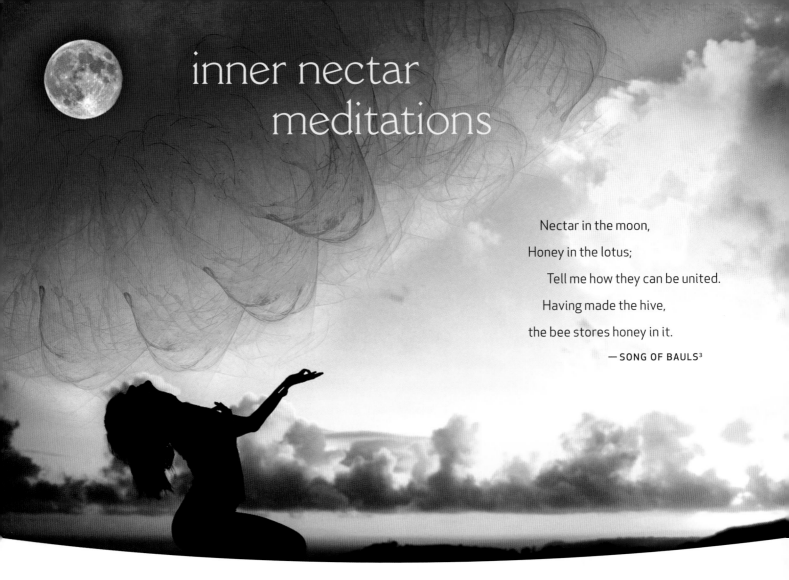

inner nectar meditations

Nectar in the moon,

Honey in the lotus;

Tell me how they can be united.

Having made the hive,

the bee stores honey in it.

— SONG OF BAULS[3]

LUNAR GAZING—SOMA DRISTI

Behold how the moon-beams of that

Hidden One shine in you. —KABIR[4]

Gazing at the moon (*soma dristi*) is a sacred practice that harmonizes your body and heart with meditative energy. It also offers the opportunity to see the gradual changes in your day-to-day energy reflected in the moon's journey from new to full and back again.

You can cultivate this practice through all the seasons, sleeping outdoors in the summer (taking a moon bath) or bundling up and enjoying a harvest or winter moon for a few minutes—or longer—by the fire. You can offer the mantras of the Goddess (listed in chandra namaskar on page 95) that are associated with each phase of the moon, or simply soak up the healing radiance of the gentle rays as the plant world does.

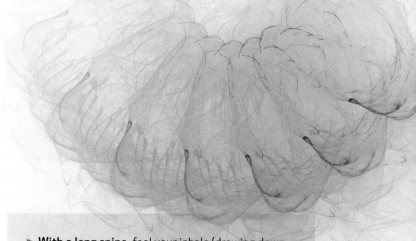

LUNAR BHAVANA— DRINKING THE MOON

Cultivating lunar bhavana awakens within the heart love for the subtle mystery of our being. The essential quality of the lunar bhavana is a shift toward receptivity, allowing the quiet power of relaxation, fluidity, and grace to circulate through the bloodstream. This is the yogic metaphor of the "nectar of the moon." You can nurture the lunar bhavana by contacting and amplifying any healing quality.

Whether you are gazing at the actual moon or visualizing the moon, draw the inhale from that reflective light down through the crown of the head through the backs of the eyes, as if drinking a supreme elixir, amrita, a mystical experience of the sublime nectar of the self.

COSMIC BREATH—CIRCULATING THE NECTAR OF THE MOON

The inhale is the cooling part of the breath cycle associated with imbibing the lunar nectar, the regenerative energy of the moon. The journey of the inhale begins with the new moon entering at the crown of the head, then waxing to full moon in the heart with the greatest concentration of lunar energy at the top of the inhale (*kumbhaka*). Then as you exhale, the journey reverses from full moon to new, and from the heart to the crown of the head. This waning energy gives us the opportunity to let go with every exhale. Open your heart as you embody this journey by cultivating your hridaya dristi, or heart gaze.

> **With a long spine,** feel your inhale (drawing down the moon) by visualizing a stream of lunar nectar flowing from the lotus at the crown of the head. As you gaze at the moon, draw your inhale from the crown to the heart as the expression of increasing light. This is a time to nourish whatever has been coming into being inside you.

> **Inhale from the crown of the head,** slowly, down into the heart center,

> **From the crown of the head** (new moon) to your third-eye center (quarter moon),

> **From the third-eye center** to the palate of the mouth (half moon),

> **From the palate of the mouth** to your throat center (three-quarter moon),

> **From the throat center** through to your heart center (full moon).

> **You can pause now in kumbhaka,** retaining the breath, and circulate a mantra where the sun, moon, and fire of the heart align with the crown of the head.

> **As you exhale,** slowly release the breath, allowing it to pass through the throat, palate, third-eye center, and crown of the head as if exhaling the waning moon.

> **Circulate one, two, three, or 108 rounds.** Complete the process by resting in natural meditation.

heart mantra—
sound of the sacred

The universal practice of mantra evolved from the spontaneous chanting and singing that began around the fire. These expressions became refined as the mantras of firekeeping, or *homa* in the Vedic tradition. The vibrations of mantra are seen as the actual subtle-body form of the divine.

We can now see these subtle-body vibrations, using an instrument called a cymascope, as the geometric patterns formed by sound vibration. Tuning ourselves to sacred vibration by chanting mantras has profound effects, unifying our inner rhythms of heart-brain flow.

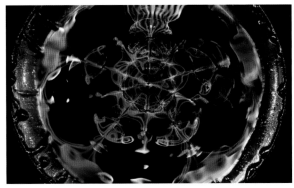

A cymatic image of a 34Hz Triangle wave in alcohol.

The universal mantra sound of *Om* is not only found in yoga; it also appears throughout spiritual cultures in differing yet recognizable forms: *Awen* in Celtic culture, *Amen* in Christian culture, *Shalom* in Jewish culture, *Allah* in Sufism.

Many people relate to the One in formless ways, such as the mantra of the breath or as light invoking light. Connecting mantra to form is a natural process of feeling a connection through differing rays of the One. Always honor your personal spiritual beliefs here; the mystic heart feels an affinity for all the world's spiritual traditions.

Sva Diksha mantras are universal mantras that can be chanted from one's heart feeling. Sva Diksha mantras are infused with the power of the guru or teacher who is empowering the vibration of the mantra with the Shakti or energy of his or her realization. Although many of these mantras—such as the Sri Vidya mantra *sodaskshi,* or sixteen-syllable mantra—are available on the Internet, the Sva Diksha mantras are part of an internal process that requires years of guided practice and many *purascharana,* or one thousand *malas* (prayer beads) of mantras, as part of the gradual awakening.

Om Sarva-Mantra Svarupinyai Namah
I bow to the essence of all mantras.[5]

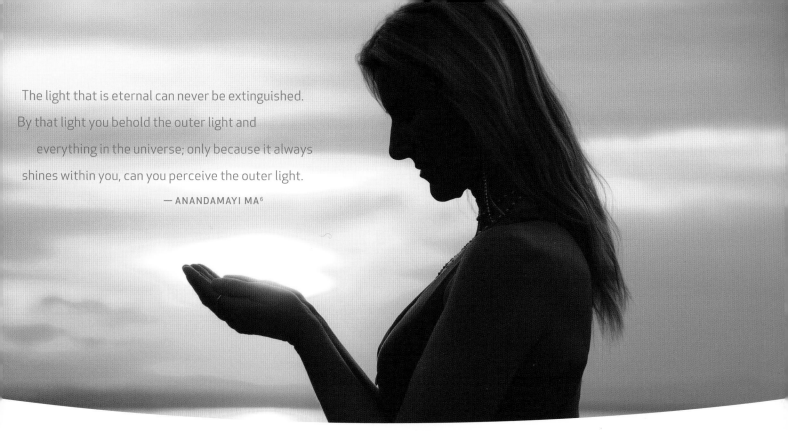

The light that is eternal can never be extinguished.
By that light you behold the outer light and
everything in the universe; only because it always
shines within you, can you perceive the outer light.

— ANANDAMAYI MA[6]

ISHTA DEVATA—YOUR PERSONAL CONNECTION TO THE SOURCE

Your *ishta devata* is your personal connection (*ishta*) to a shining source (*deva*), the intimate experience of connection to life, the source we call upon when we are at our greatest need or enraptured in our highest joy. This is the intimate space of our heart's devotion, the heart of our prayer.

Some people sense their ishta devata in the anthropomorphic form of a god or goddess or *saguna,* as in *sa* ("with") *guna* ("form"). Others have the non-anthropomorphic experience of the source as light, the fire of consciousness, or flame of love, which is referred to as *ni* ("without") *guna* ("form"). The yogic traditions emerged in India within the soil of devotion, as the mantras (nama, or sound signature within a name or seed sound) and form (*rupa*) of the One are considered to be as innumerable as rays of the sun or pathways up the mountain. The primary pathways are often described as three: the Shakta path, for those who connect to the divine through the Great Mother Devi; the Vishnav path, for those who follow the way of love through Vishnu; and the Shaivite path, for those who invoke the supreme reality as Shiva. For still others, the divine One is the union of the divine masculine and feminine.

Mantra and the healing power of sacred sound offer pathways for experiencing the divine current. Those represented here are but a few of the primary ishta devatas within yoga and other world traditions. *Mantra japa,* or the circulation of sacred sound, is a universal expression that can be traced back to our lifted voices around the fire.

Om Hridayayai Namah

I bow to the One who is the essence of the heart.

Student, tell me, what is God?

The breath inside the breath.

— KABIR[7]

the pulse of life—heart, breath, and mantra meditations

hamsa—natural breath mantra

Air is exhaled with the sound SA

and inhaled with the sound HAM.

The reciting of the mantra HAMSA

is continuous.

— VIJNANA BHAIRAVA TANTRA[8]

All beings are being breathed by a natural mantra, *hamsa,* 21,600 times a day—bringing the opportunity with each inhale and exhale to realize the inner meaning that is carried on the sound of the breath. As you inhale, you can hear the spontaneous mantra *ham,* which in Sanskrit means "I am." As you exhale, you can hear the mantra *sa.* Hamsa can be felt in a calm flow that embodies the unifying meaning of the mantra, the miraculous breath breathing us all—"all that is." Circulating a mantra upon the breath is the most natural of mantras, a rhythm that ceaselessly courses through our being.

As you inhale and exhale, listen intently to the ocean sound of your breath. You can experience this naturally as it comes, or through the technique of *ujjayi* breathing. As you circulate the cosmic breath, you can circulate the sacred sound of mantra along the pathways of the body.

UJJAYI BREATHING—
OCEAN RHYTHM OF THE BREATH

Ujjayi, or "victorious breath," is the drawing of the breath along the back of the throat in a receptive flow without tension. It sounds like the echo of the sea heard in a shell. The ujjayi breath is a continuous, streaming tide that links your heart and breath rhythms through slowing down into the sound of deep time—the eternal waves that have been pulsing for billions of years. Throughout the day, during pranayama or movement meditations, keep opening to the flow of breath as the flow of consciousness—the mystery of the breath that becomes the basis for this and all of the other breath mantras that follow.

BRAHMARI BREATH—
MAKING HONEY IN THE HEART,
A PRIMAL OR UNIVERSAL SOUND

Brahmari breath is a simple yet profound breath mantra that connects you to the humming sound of bees. It can be visualized as making honey in the heart with the *hummmm* of creation. It is as simple as inhaling and then sounding the *hummmm* of a bee with a droning, or an *mmmm* plus *ngggg,* sound. This is the ending sound of *Om*—the sound of a hive in natural mantra. In the Tantras, our consciousness is likened to a little bee by the name of Uhli: Uhli, the little "soul bee." The little bee of consciousness hums to create the nectar in the heart.

Breath is the mantra . . .

the highest place of pilgrimage.

— VIJNANA BHAIRAVA TANTRA[9]

heart mantra meditations

DUM DUM—MOTHER OF SOUND

Bring your hands to feel your pulse at your carotid artery (just below your jawbone). Feel the sonic sensation of "hearing your pulse"—a unique capacity we have to hear what we feel. Internally or aloud, chant *dum dum* with each pulse. *Dum* is the *bija* mantra connected to the Great Mother, the sound to which our hearts synchronized as we were sonically permeated with our mother's heart rhythm. Dum can be seen as our first Sva Diksha, or naturally initiated mantra, connecting us to the extraordinary womb retreat where our first yoga movements, which assisted in growing our body, also unfolded. Go deeply into the *dum* mantra. Feel your heart connection to the mother of sound—Matrika Shakti—from which all mantras emerge. You can also combine *Om* with the mother mantra of *Om Dum Durgaye Namaha.* Feel the deep resonance within and the shimmering that increases in your body with the rounds of mantra.

SOUNDING OF OM

Offer the *pranava Om* as an invocation, as a continuous part of your meditation, or with the ucchara, or raising of the mantra practice, below. Offering *Om* in the full cycle of *a-u-m* is the essence of vinyasa, as the sound of creation (*a*) emerges from the heart, is sustained at the peak (*u*) in the palate of the mouth, and dissolves in the *hummmm* with a drone sound of *ngggg* at the lips and skull center. Feel how sounding

O Bhairavi, sing OM, the mantra of the love union of Shiva and Shakti, slowly and consciously. Enter the sound and when it fades away, slip into freedom of being.

— VIJNANA BHAIRAVA TANTRA[10]

Om naturally increases the flow of your exhale—a way of purifying excess thinking and bringing more relaxation and resting to the heart.

BODY MANTRA

Circulate the natural mantra of the breath for several rounds until you feel the calling for a more specific mantra that you can circulate with your breath along your body as an offering to your Heart Fire. You can offer universal mantras such as *Om Namah Shivaya* or mantras of your own spiritual tradition—"Shalom," "Amen."

Or as you inhale, you can repeat several rounds of a universal mantra, such as *Namah Shivaya,* drawing the mantra as one long flow—*Naaaammmmah Shivaaayyyaaa*—or as a continuous, rhythmic flow with your breath. Visualize the mantra as being offered to your Heart Fire, inwardly chanting a few more rounds of *Namah Shivaya, Namah Shivaya.* Then exhale and continue chanting the mantra along with the flow of the exhale. Feel the mantra resonating within you.

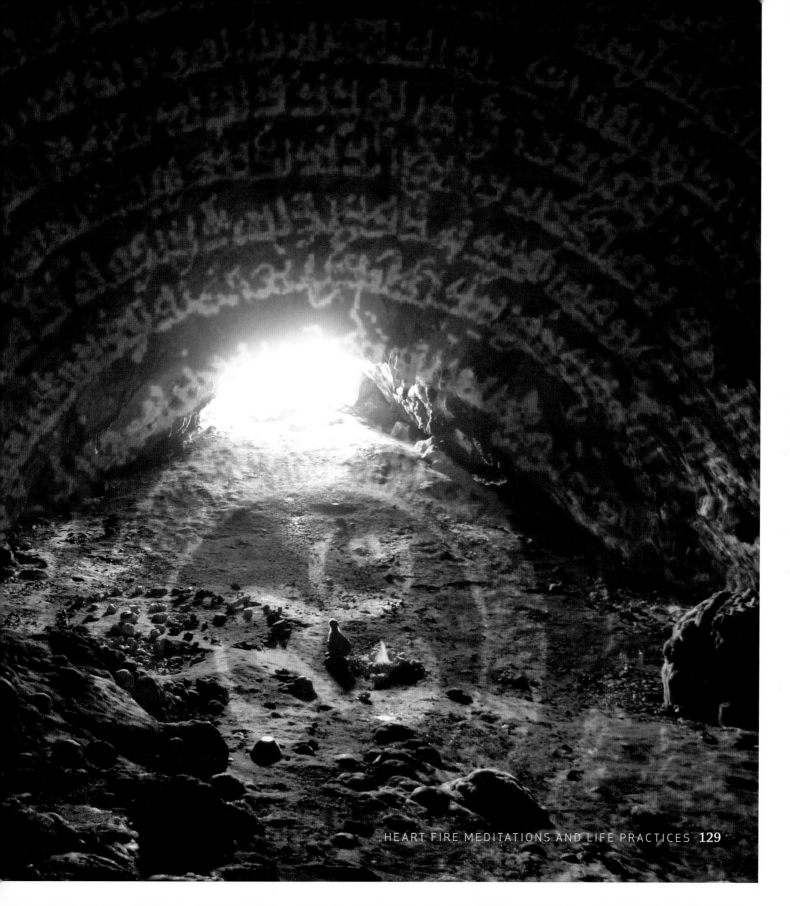

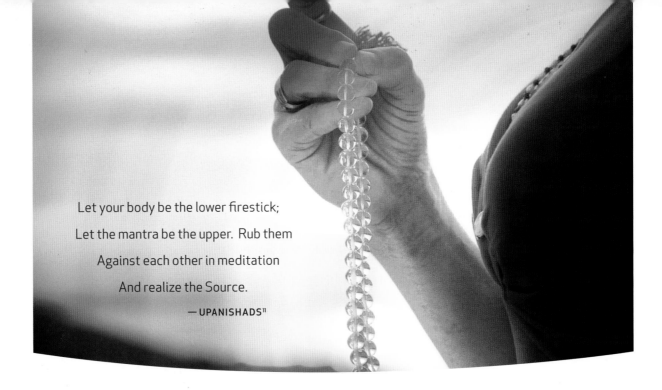

Let your body be the lower firestick;

Let the mantra be the upper. Rub them

Against each other in meditation

And realize the Source.

—UPANISHADS[11]

MANTRA JAPA

The daily circulation mantra (*mantra japa*) is beautifully cultivated using a string of 108 mala beads. Each mantra coincides with the movement of a bead with the thumb as the mala is slowly turned, held at your heart or in your lap. One round is from the "guru bead" (held by a large bead or tassle) to the guru bead again.

You can offer mantra to your heart, as in the ucchara practice below, while turning your mala by counting with your fingers, or by using a "body mala" practice I have developed, in which you circulate three rounds of mantra in each of the six chakras, from the root chakra (*muladhara*), creative center (*swadhisthana*), navel center (*manipura*), heart center (anahata), throat center (*vissudhara*), and vision center (*ajna*), making eighteen rounds. Do this six times to equal 108. This transformative cycle creates a ritual space in which to be transformed by the sacred current of sound. You can offer Sva Diksha (self-initiated mantras), universal mantras, or the sounds that your teacher has whispered to you. Feel the accompanying transformation in your energetic body, which is viewed at its source as mantra.

NADI SHODHANA WITH MANTRA

Nadi shodhana is an essential practice for balancing sun and moon in the body, the sympathetic and parasympathetic parts of the nervous system that regulate the balance of the hemispheres of the brain: active and receptive. Nadi shodhana is the core pranayama householders can practice to reflect upon the state of their nervous system.

Be aware, as you begin this practice, of any grasping, pushing, or expectation, or rushing to complete it: these are all signs of excess solar energy in your system. This pranayama always begins with the left nostril, or lunar channel, so as to start in a relaxed state. There are several different approaches from

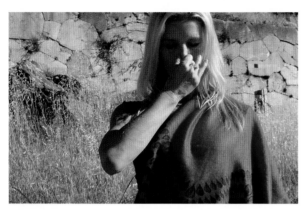
Nadi shodhana

different schools of yoga, as well as practices that involve advanced ratios of left-to-right breathing. My approach with nadi shodana, as with all pranayamas, is to breathe with devotion for a long time before adding any breath retention. Mantra can be your rhythm.

As you inhale through your left nostril, close your right nostril and slowly drink in your breath, listening to the ocean sound or offering mantra as you inhale. Pause at the top with your chin slightly bowed to the heart (*jaladhara bandha*), and rest in the silence or offer mantra to your heart. Close the left nostril and slowly exhale through the right nostril with the sound of the breath or mantra. Pause again in the stillness of complete emptiness, purifying your nervous system of all grasping. Before any strain, slowly inhale through the right nostril, with or without mantra. Pause at the top in silence or in mantra as if embraced by the breath. Exhale—close your right nostril and slowly release your breath as if setting down a sleeping baby, with silence or mantra. Circulate left to right and right to left for a minimum of three cycles or more. Enjoy the balance of the solar and lunar current.

KAPALABHATI AND BHASTRIKA— SOLAR PRANAYAMAS WITH SOLAR BIJA HRAM

These solar pranayamas are heating and purifying, cleaning out old air and thoughts. They should be respected and never practiced with strain, during a lunar state such as a woman's moon cycle, or when a heating condition such as ulcers or hypertension is present.

Enjoy a short inhale and then pump your breath with your belly as if stoking a fire. This is known as *kapalabhati* or "skull" (*kapala*) "shining" (*bhati*) breath, and can be circulated for one to five minutes for several cycles without strain. You can combine this with solar mudras or the solar bija mantra *Hram* for activating prana and mantra. *Bhastrika,* or "bellows breath," is a slower rhythm and includes an even drawing in and out as the exhale is pumped out with the belly and the lungs fill with the inhale. The rhythm is slow and percussive, purifying but calming. Offer for one to five minutes with pure breath or add a solar mantra. Enjoy the clear channel of the breath.

SITALI PRANAYAMA WITH SHANTI MANTRA

The cooling *sitali pranayama* is experienced by curling your tongue to form a "straw" from which to inhale the cooling lunar breath, and by exhaling through the mouth. As you inhale, meditate upon the moon and the quality of peace, as offered in the mantra *Shanti, Shanti, Shanti,* whispered internally upon the breath to create a more calming bhavana when you are experiencing excess fire in your practice or life.

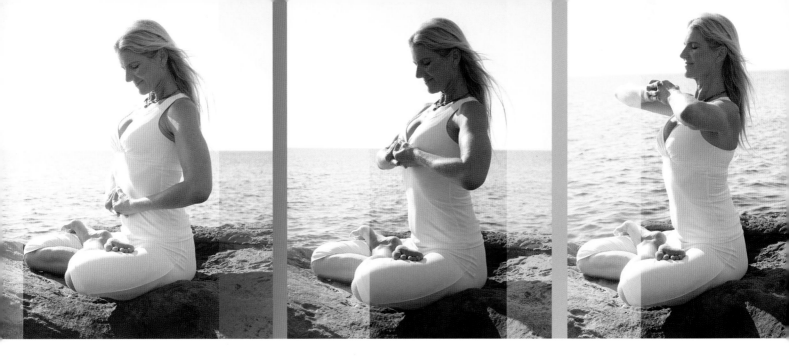

UCCHARA WITH INNER SANDHYAS—COSMIC BREATH MEDITATION

This is a wonderful mudra vinyasa for harmonizing the solar and lunar currents inside the heart, based in the earliest tantric traditions. The first phase of this meditation, which in essence means "rising (*u*) as in *udana* movement (*chara*)," is taught within our teacher-training community by tantric scholar Christopher Tompkins.

> **Relax into a state of presence** and feel your inner heart gaze.

> **Begin the ucchara** by lifting your hands together over your crown in *jaya mudra*.

> **As you inhale,** receive the lunar breath by tracing the pathway from the crown to the heart, slowly drawing your hands through *prana mudra* in a downward circle that meets with your hands connected in chin mudra (index and thumb touching and connected with fingers overlapping at your navel).

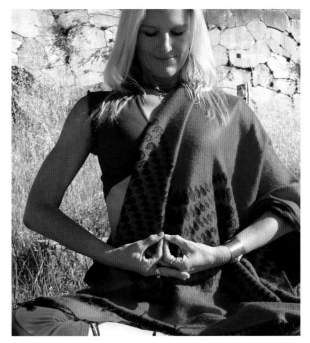

Chin mudra

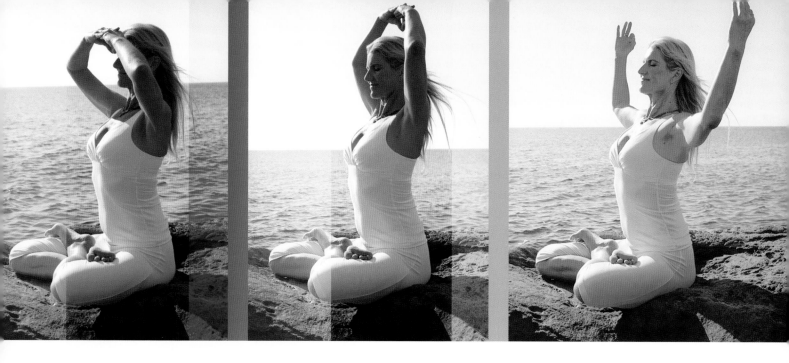

> **Bow your head and pause** in your own natural kumbhaka, or breath retention, between three and fifteen beats of the heart.

> **While in kumbhaka,** make a fire offering of a seed mantra such as *Om* or *Hum* or *Hrim* with natural devotion and ease. Connect to the central channel of your spine, visualizing the agni (fire) from your navel generating heat to forge the alchemical union of the solar and lunar breath within your Heart Fire, now joined in the sacred pause between in-breath and out-breath.

> **Feel your connection** to the universal pulse, the feeling within your heart, your heart guru. Visualize the Heart Fire. Merge with the deep vibration you can feel within the heart's pulse.

> **As you exhale,** feel the purifying solar breath carrying a seed sound mantra such as *aaa* (in the throat), *eee* (in the palate), *mmm* (in the third eye), and *nggg* (in the third eye and crown) in the original meaning of *ucchara* as "raising the mantra" from the heart to the crown.

> **While chanting,** draw your hands upward from your heart along the same path and then sweep your arms open into prana mudra. Keep your hands even with your eyes and ears, and feel the fullness of the peak expression of sound. Now inhale and bring the arms down along your sides, bringing your hands together at the navel to begin the cycle again for at least three rounds.

You can enjoy this meditation with mantra and mudra for a minimum of three breaths or cycle it for nine cycles or more in mantra japa.

mudra dhynam—
heart mudra meditations

In all of my practice and teaching I have found mudras of the body, hands, and the movement of mudras as mudra vinyasas to be the most effective form of awakening heart consciousness. They can be done at any time, any place and for everybody from children full of life to those great souls who are on their death beds. The power of touch and the shape of the mudra inherently contain profound shifts of being—a shift toward listening when there is static. A spark to awaken a dim flame when we need to rise up.

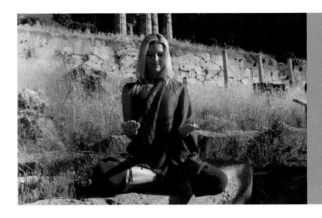

ABOUT HEART MUDRA PRACTICE

I hope that you will experience at least one of these mudras—if not all—even if they look very simple. For all mudras begin by invoking the freedom and ease of the body and breath. Open your eyes and gaze into your heart. For every mudra, I have offered a mantra and/or a *aham bhavana* (feeling state) that can be circulated effortlessly within the mudra—or you can rest in pure presence. Aham Bhavana is a process of generating healing states that can be circulated in mudra. Aham or "I am" is the deep sense of self within Self. AHAM is created by "ah" Shakti and "mmm" Shiva in union to create all the souls of all creation. I always invoke the time in a mudra as "108 moments" for roughly two minutes of practice, or 1,008 moments for an almost twenty-minute practice. You can rest in mudra or include mantra japa with mudra meditation or begin or end a vinyasa practice. Enjoy the transforming power of heart mudra.

HASTA MUDRA

Bring your hands in front of you, palms facing up. Feel the very center of your palms, referred to as *tala hridaya,* as a place of great receptivity.

Feel your hands like two open vessels, emptying the mind of static. As you rest in this mudra, you will begin to feel yourself shift into listening to your heart center. This is a wonderful way to begin a mudra sadhana and to energize the hands with hearty energy.

Om Karuna Rasa
Sagarayai Namah
> I bow to the One who is the
> Ocean of Compassion

Aham Karuna
> I am the essence of Compassion

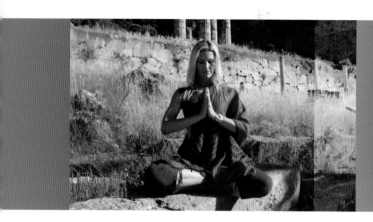
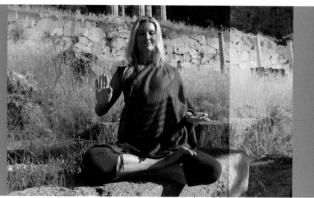

ANJALI MUDRA— HEART OFFERING MUDRA

To practice *anjali mudra,* place your hands before you, palms up, as in hasta mudra, on the previous page. Feel the solar current in your right hand and the lunar current in your left.

Now experience the central energy channel that runs along your spine (*sushumna*) and your heart, representing the place of union between the two energies expressed through your hands.

Om Premaye Namah
  I bow to the One who
  is the essence of Love

Aham Prema
  I am the essence of Love

ABHAYA MUDRA— FEARLESS BLESSING MUDRA

Abhaya has two simultaneous meanings: "have no fear" and "blessing mudra." This is often the mudra that gurus and elders offer. Bring your left hand to rest on your heart, allowing your right hand to face outward, at heart level, in *abhaya mudra.* Feel transformed by this process of resting in the place of no fear and the blessing that can stream from the heart.

Om Shantayai Namah
  I bow to the One who is
  the embodiment of Peace

Aham Mangalam
  I am Auspiciousness

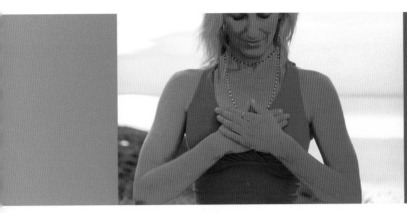
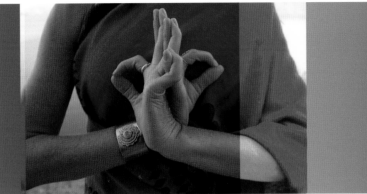

SVASTIKA MUDRA—AUSPICIOUS MUDRA FOR THE HEART

The simple mudra of crossing your hands over your chest—*svastika mudra*—has the same effect as anjali mudra but often with the quality of reverence and intimacy. The arms combine the quality of embracing yourself (*sva*) with the quality of auspiciousness, the feeling of life in its regenerative blessing. Rest here as part of your meditation or anytime during the day when you need to come home within your Self.

Om Svasthayai Namah
　I bow to the One who abides
　in their own nature
Aham Svabhavah
　I am the essence of the Self

ABHAYA HRIDAYA MUDRA—COURAGEOUS HEART MUDRA

To practice *abhaya hridaya mudra,* cross your hands in front of your chest with the backs of your hands touching, right hand closest to your heart. Interlink your little, ring, and middle fingers and then join the tips of your index finger and thumb with both hands to form two circular rings. With your hands in front of your heart, release any fear or doubt by feeling the awakened presence emanating from your heart.

Om Viryaye Namah
　I bow to the One who is
　the essence of Vira
Aham Viryam
　I am potency and
　courage beyond fear

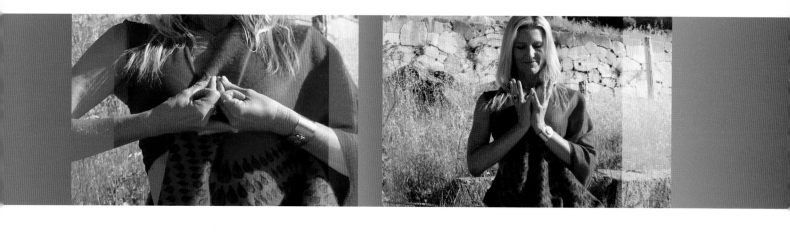

HRIDAYA MUDRA—HEART CONSCIOUSNESS MUDRA

With each hand create the same mudra: coil your index finger to the base of your thumb while connecting your thumb to the tips of your middle and ring finger. Now extend your little finger and feel the calming, heart-generating bhava as you move your hands to rest upon your thighs.

Om Hridayayai Namah
I bow to the heart
conciousness

Aham Hridayam
I am the essence of the heart

HRIDAYA PADMA MUDRA—HEART LOTUS MUDRA

To practice *hridaya padma mudra,* bring your hands to your heart in the shape of a lotus bud. Experience the generation of bhava—regenerative emotions such as compassion and gratitude—like fragrance rising from a lotus bud. With each inhale you offer to your Heart Fire, silently repeat the quality that is arising: shanti (peace), *prema* (love), *santosha* (contentment). As you rest in these healing qualities, offer up any dissonant thought waves, subconsciously held tensions, or contracted emotions into the fire of your heart. Make a final prayer or dedication and then bring your hands gently overhead and let them move down your body in a cascade of renewal.

Om Om Hridayasthayai Namah
I bow to the One who resides
in the heart.

Aham Amritam
I am the essence of the
heart nectar

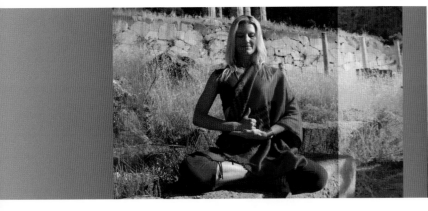
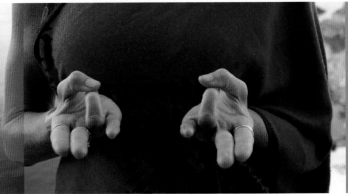

SHIVA-LINGAM MUDRA—UNION OF DIVINE MASCULINE AND FEMININE

Shiva-lingam mudra is the embodiment of the union of masculine and feminine at the heart of creation. It balances the *ida* and *pingala* nadis, the active and receptive energy channels running along your spine. As you inhale, draw your left hand just below your navel and place it at swadhisthana chakra, related to the yoni, the moon in the female body, or the seed center in the male body.

With your right hand, bring your fingertips together in a fist with your thumb extending upward. This hand represents the lingam, or male principle of ascending energy. Place your right hand over your open left palm at your navel center. Breathe here, maintaining your inner heart dristi and slow, rhythmic breath while experiencing your whole body entering the state of union. You can visualize your entire spine as the lingam and the base of your body as the yoni, or you can visualize the *shiva lingam* inside the inner sanctum of your heart.

Feel any tension, feelings of separation, or inner conflict between polarities within you—such as intellectual activity versus feeling/dissolving. Allow your experience of shiva-lingam mudra to be fresh and new every time.

Om Namah Shivaya
 I am the essence of Consciousness

SURYA MUDRA— SOLAR RADIANCE MUDRA

Now experience the activating energy of the sun in a simple hasta (hand mudra). For *surya mudra* with one hand or two, in seated meditation or at any time, cover the nail of the ring finger with your thumb while extending the remaining fingers like rays of the sun. Place your hands on your thighs or at the level of your heart. Relax and feel the subtle difference of the activation of pingala nadi, or the outward-moving solar current, to generate energy, confidence, and presence.

Om Suryaye Namah
 I bow to the energy of the Sun
Aham Surya
 I am the essence of the Sun

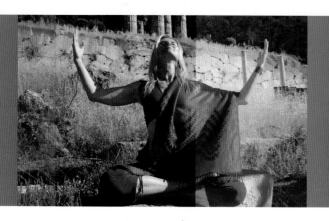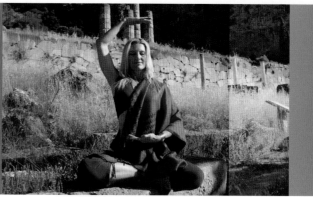

SURYA PRANA MUDRA—
VITAL ENERGY MUDRA

In a comfortable position,

hands open at shoulder level,

an area of radiant spatiality gradually

pervades the armpits, ravishes the

heart, and brings about profound peace.

— VIJNANA BHAIRAVA TANTRA[13]

To practice the radiant *surya prana mudra,* extend your arms from the heart to the level of the eyes and ears with your palms facing inward as if to form a chalice for receiving energy. At the same time, radiate energy from your heart, just as the sun simultaneously draws energy in to then create its omnidirectional rays. Feel the empowering qualities that the solar current activates within your heart. This mudra is a healing tonic for any weak fire or contracted emotional state.

Om Hram Suryaye Namah
I bow to the radiance of the Sun

Aham Prana
I am the Vital Prana of the Sun

SOMA MUDRA—
LUNAR NECTAR MUDRA

To practice *soma mudra,* bring your hands to your heart to generate your connection to your heart energy. Slowly draw your open right palm over your head or upon your crown and bring your left hand to rest upon the heart or extend outward as a gesture of offering. Touch the crown of your head for a moment to feel the energy of a blessing that you have received since you were born—a streaming of pure benevolence. Feel how the hand at the crown of the head activates the inner entrainment of brainwaves with heart rhythm. Relax and become completely receptive as you feel a shift toward regeneration. The lunar nectar flows down from the inner moon at the crown of the head and down the inner brain, palate, and throat, and then pours into the heart. This is the stream of soma that stimulates the healing hormonal flow of serotonin and oxytocin and a healthy cerebrospinal pulse. In this mudra, draw the lunar nectar down on the inhale and receive it with your left hand at your heart center.

Om Somayayai Namah
I bow to the essence of Soma

Aham Soma
I am the essence of Soma or
regenerating nectar

Om Mani Padme Hum
The Jewel is in the
Lotus of the Heart

heart mandala meditation

This meditation is found within most of the world's spiritual traditions. It extends the circle of love from within your own heart and ripples outward to all beings. It is also based on the practice within Tibetan Buddhist meditation on invoking, receiving, and offering love.

> **Settle into a comfortable seated position** and connect your hands to your heart and your inner gaze to your Heart Fire, feeling the shimmer and heat within. Allow yourself to first open and receive. Imagine manifesting from the center of your heart a being who radiates love and acceptance toward you: a grandparent, your beloved, a teacher, or any great being whose eyes radiate the healing stream of love beyond condition. Imagine this manifested being in front of you, about an arm's length away from you, and elevated slightly above you. (It's helpful to have images centrally placed on your altar of beings who express to you all the qualites of unconditional love, all-embracing compassion, and penetrating wisdom.) Let the power of their unconditional love overcome even the slightest hesitance or disturbing emotion, such as being unworthy to receive such love. Bathe in a love that completely accepts you and knows your heart of hearts.

> **Feel that love energy** as it kindles within and radiates to all of your cells. You can chant a prayer or mantra as you extend out the wish so that the wish is carried on the vibration of sound. Even if your Heart Fire feels like a tiny flame, let that flame be nourished in this stream of love as an offering that fuels your love fire. Spend as much time in this first stage of the meditation receiving love to the depth of your being until you feel completely ready to move on.

> **While continuing to receive love from above,** invoke connections from your own heart—nadi lines that radiate out to your immediate home and household, your beloved, your children, pets, or animal friends. Invoke your parents—wherever they may be—your brothers and sisters, and extended family. You can expand the definition of children to include any beings who activate a nurturing force within you. Visit them one by one and radiate love and good will, visualizing or feeling their presence silently, by offering your own prayer, or by saying: "May (invoke their name) be blessed," or "May (invoke their name) have love and goodwill and experience the blessings of innate happiness." Extend this healing wish to include all by chanting a universal prayer or mantra such as "Om" or "Om Mani Padme Hum." This integrates your body, speech, and mind into the meditation.

> **Continue to create your heart mandala in this way.** Next connect to a teacher who opened your heart. Surround yourself with the light and love of gratitude for his or her love and guidance. In truth, all of the beings you have reached out to are your teachers.

> **Now radiate the Heart Fire to your close friends, extended community, students—** whoever comes into your heart field and to whom you can radiate goodwill.

> **Now include your colleagues and collaborators** or anyone with whom you have a heart bond of respect.

> **Now include "precious jewels": anyone with whom you have conflict.** Without these precious jewels, we may not practice so intensely to keep our Heart Fire alive. Send clear energy outward and work with that nadi line to transmute any regressive qualities, such as bitterness or ill will, that are not useful in a healing process.

> **Now extend out with your heart to any places in nature**—intimate places, a special tree or place by the river, pilgrimage sites, places that are in crisis or war torn, places where there is any suffering. Find any place that moves your heart and radiate goodwill toward it.

> **In the final phase, the visualization dissolves** and returns to the center of your heart mandala as you are never separate from the source of unconditional love. Feel the power of your heart mandala connecting in all directions to your heart field. You can bring your hands to your heart or slowly radiate your arms from your heart to viscerally embody and feel the fullness of your heart field. Stay in this state with presence or prayer for as long as you like, connecting to the vibration of the heart mantra and its universal wish for all beings to be awakened and experience intrinsic happiness. Then, when you feel complete, slowly bring your hands back to your heart. Offer the mantra of peace from your own spiritual tradition or by chanting *Om Shanti, Shanti, Shanti.* Peace, Peace, Peace.

micro-meditations: life practices for tending the heart fire

One of the most important qualities of a practice is whether it is effectively integrated into our daily lives. Tending the Heart Fire is not a cliché or a romanticism but is instead a tangible, practical, instinctual way of transforming the conditioned patterns that limit the flow of love.

Householder yoga embraces the yoga of living and the integral way our view of ourselves and the world affects our embodiment, which then affects our energy exchange with all of life. Firekeeping in daily life dances with our shadow—what is neglected, unconscious, disconnected, and disowned as each person evolves along with cultural shifts and breakthroughs. Embodying and living from the energetic heart is radical and yet completely natural, offering to a fragmented world a rediscovery of and new applications for ancient wisdom and rhythms. This is a living yoga sadhana.

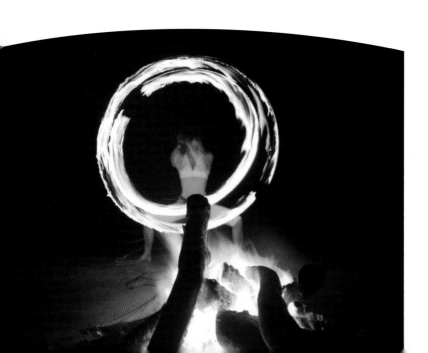

MICRO-MEDITATION— LIVING YOGA IN THE FLOW OF LIFE

Within the lifestyle of householder Tantrica from the eighth century to the present, the flow of meditation was cultivated through dharanas—living contemplations such as 112 meditations with the Vijnana Bhairava Tantra—that transform everyday movements into firekeeping acts of realization.

These micro-practices are part of a natural way of tending the Heart Fire—of generating love, presence, and wisdom—at times fierce and passionate, at other times tender and calm in the midst of all the activity of life.

EMBODYING THE HEART FIRE

> **Listen to your pulse** and perceive the underlying rhythmic message of your state of being radiating to every cell of your body.

> **Feel the wave of your breath** connected to your heart. Rest your awareness in your heart as you move through the day.

> **Bring one hand to your heart** and the other to your forehead and then your belly. Feel your breath bringing your inner rhythms and intelligences into coherence or the state of flow.

> **Be aware of any holding** in your feet, belly, shoulders, jaw, and backs of the eyes, or any place that may block the flow of your connection to the whole.

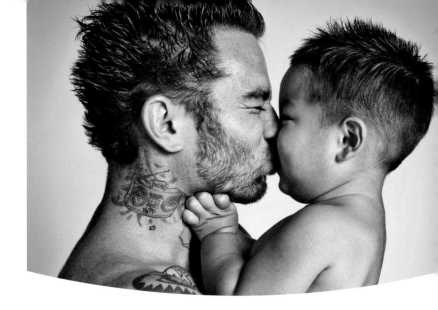

- > **Experience a natural expression of your heart field** extending beyond your body. Visualize the electromagnetic energy of your heart illumined from within like an inner sun, radiant in all directions.

- > **Feel the sensations in your heart region—** a heat, a shimmering, a tiny vibration—as an awareness or a barometer for the quality of your inner heart fire. When you lose your awareness, or when your sensations wane, notice the outcome.

- > **When you are in synch—**when your thoughts and feelings, brainwaves and heart rhythms are in a unified flow, experience how this nonverbal knowing guides you as you move through the world.

HEART BONDING AND THE COLLECTIVE HEART FIELD

- > **Feel your partner's energy field** by holding your hand to his or her heart—physically in the front or back, or just through your perception. Connect subtly through your body sensations until the shimmer becomes a living field that connects you both completely.

- > **Perceive your pulse connected to seven billion human beings,** to countless creatures, to the breathing earth itself.

LIVING IN RHYTHM AND FLOW

Before taking any action, pause for a moment. Feel the alignment of your awareness as your breath connects with your heart, giving it the space to clear tension and express your next moment in a state of flow.

- > **Spend a day in a state of offering,** pausing before every action and offering your awareness to the source of action, an offering to the altar of the heart, allowing the highest flow possible.

- > **Experience the state of flow** as a seamless awareness, a continuous dance, a stream of consciousness, an optimal presence, an oscillating balance navigated by the inter-rhythmic unity of the heartbrain.

- > **Feel the turning of the earth,** the moon, the solar system, the galaxy, and your rhythmic body—all the movements in the cosmic symphony of life.

- > **Spend a day in a state of devotional offering,** pausing in prayer and transforming every action, every breath into an offering.

- > **Pay attention to the cycles within your life from morning to night**—the way you begin a cycle and sustain and complete each vinyasa to create a flow. When the flow is lost, some part of the intelligent cycle—the vinyasa of nature—has been broken.

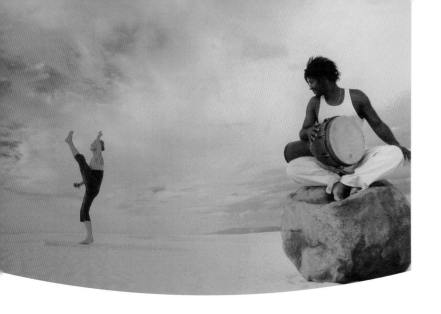

rasa vinyasa in the world

MICRO-PRACTICES FOR SRINGARA RASA

> **Contemplate the love** that every being is born with. All humans are born as lovers.

> **Experience your breath** as your highest slow-dance partner initiating you into the deep movement of your being.

> **Offer a benevolent gaze** that melts the hardened places.

> **Move with your beloved** so that you stay naturally connected in the ordinary and extraordinary flow of life.

> **When you feel your energy of connection waning,** be aware of what may be weakening your bond and try to nourish the fire of love and affection.

> **Touch everything with your hands,** feet, and body in a circular energetic exchange. Feel how the earth vibrates with your feet. Caress the air. Move with space.

> **See the light in all eyes** as a reflection of the Source. Trace the spark, whether dim or blazing, beyond the outer coverings of separation to discover the fire blazing in all.

> **Slow down and savor a drink** as life-giving fluid, a taste as the nectar of life. Experience Shakti as the energy within simple moments of bliss.

> **All music affects our heartbeat.** Enjoy music as a whole-body experience that can bring you into meditation.

> **Take time for self-care,** including getting massage, enjoying life, and nurturing your relationships.

SACRED ACTIVISM

> **Ask yourself what moves you,** what you would give your life for. Find a way to give back for future generations from your heart.

> **Care for the earth, for your food, and for energy sources.** Use natural sources of food, light, and energy and feel the difference in your energetic body.

- **Unplug** and take responsibility for your energy exchange in the world.

- **Whatever your greatest difficulty is,** apply the opposite and find someone to serve. If you feel contraction, offer a generous act. If you have wavering doubt, be a steady hand for someone near. When you feel overwhelmed, put your hands in the earth and serve what is needed right in front of you.

MICRO-PRACTICES FOR VIRA RASA

- **Know in your heart** the courage and stamina of your ancestors: feet that have walked miles, arms that have paddled across seas, a Heart Fire that has weathered every storm.

- **Feel your truth** as the core fire in your heart. Tend this fire with the power of self-integrity.

- **Triumph over mediocrity** with a penetrating presence, an original action, a fearless knowing.

- **Roar with the cosmic sound** of being ignited again.

- **Blaze through self-imposed limitations.** No covering can dispel your luminous light.

- **Have the courage to make changes,** and to reignite a dim fire of a love, a passion. Support something you care about as it starts to waver. Be brave and let go into the fire when it is time to transform and be reborn to a life anew.

MICRO-PRACTICES FOR SHANTI RASA AND MORE

- **Keep your heart at peace** as crazy, disconnected rhythms come your way.

- **Slow-dance to intense rhythms.** Be vibrant inside the dullness. Be steady inside wavering.

- **Be aware when your heart gets too heavy.** Remember the radical smile and open arms of people in the world who have nothing but the lightness of Being (Hasya Rasa), even when the house has burned down.

- **Smile from the natural joy in your heart** (Hasya Rasa) and feel the radiant effect on your energy field.

- **Drop your jaw permanently** in a state of wonder and awe (Abdhuta Rasa) whenever the mind-blowing beauty and perfection of nature in all forms overwhelms you with delight.

- **Awaken compassion** (Karuna Rasa) and feel repressed emotions in yourself or others being given love to release and heal.

MICRO-PRACTICES FOR DIFFICULT TIMES—THE FIRE OF LOVE IN THE DARK

- **Take a gradual step,** breath by breath, toward the next cycle. The sun also rises.

- **Claim a sacred space right where you are.** Go to the refuge of your heart and let go of all mental projections of past, present, and future.

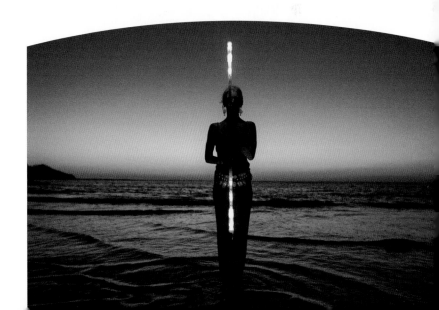

- > **When dissonant rhythms arrive,** listen to your heart and slowly navigate your way through the jungle without fear or anxiety.

- > **When you encounter difficult people,** remember the tree, a saint, or Tibetan monks or nuns in prison, and radiate with an energy field like the sun that can never be dimmed or extinguished.

- > **When life gives you manure,** roll up your sleeves and make fertilizer for something even more powerful to grow.

- > **When life's rhythm is stressful** and accelerated in time, slow down inside and dance with the swift rhythm while staying peaceful inside.

- > **When you feel the contracted way that fear moves,** or the sharp way that agitation moves, or the scattered way that anxiety moves, or the tight way that control moves, move the way love moves.

- > **When all else has failed,** when there is nothing more to do, when you have exhausted every branch, when you feel tired like you want to give up, when the world is overwhelming, go into a prostration or a whole-body mudra. Then listen and receive fully at the heart of prayer.

- > **Dance with your Shadow** as a tender human; clean your wounds with compassion; embrace the hardest, most neglected places within yourself with a lava flow of love that dwarfs the tiny ash of the smallest self.

- > **The "real world"** is just a covering on top of the mystery. As you gaze at a sunrise or sunset, experience a connection in deep time that will dissolve every deadline, every obstacle into the dust of a billion years, a billion stars, a billion forms of light.

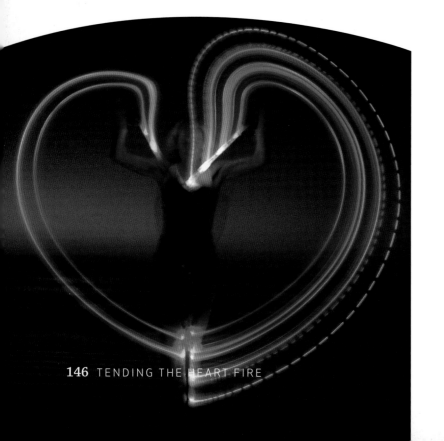

146 TENDING THE HEART FIRE

As you've discovered in this book, firekeeping is our universal practice lineage. Long before any formal meditation, our simple gaze upon the fire led human beings to a natural state of presence and connectedness—an attunement that has been retained in our cellular memory for some two million years. We must remember, within the fragmentation and distractions of modern life, that this connectedness is innate, natural, and yet a process that must be tended and cultivated. When we are living in flow, we can tend our inner fire of consciousness all day long and through all rhythms and life activity.

living in rhythm

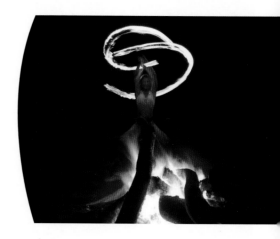

tending the
fire of creation

Ayurveda and Inner Firekeeping

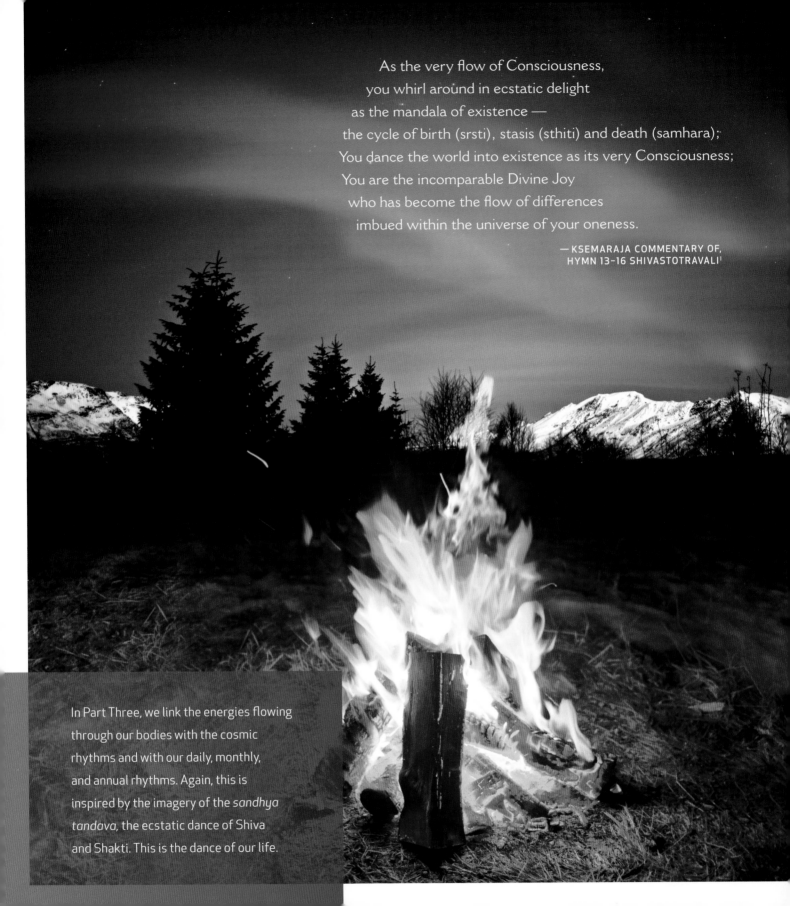

As the very flow of Consciousness,
you whirl around in ecstatic delight
as the mandala of existence —
the cycle of birth (srsti), stasis (sthiti) and death (samhara);
You dance the world into existence as its very Consciousness;
You are the incomparable Divine Joy
who has become the flow of differences
imbued within the universe of your oneness.

— KSEMARAJA COMMENTARY OF,
HYMN 13–16 SHIVASTOTRAVALI[1]

In Part Three, we link the energies flowing through our bodies with the cosmic rhythms and with our daily, monthly, and annual rhythms. Again, this is inspired by the imagery of the *sandhya tandava*, the ecstatic dance of Shiva and Shakti. This is the dance of our life.

sandhya— sacred junctures of time

Yoga can be thought of as a process of moving beyond the continuum of time—the span from past to future—and dropping into the moment. It is only here that we can savor the pure rhythm of the pulse of life without distraction. Our lives unfold moment by moment according to their own flow, yet some are highly potent moments known in yoga as *sandhyas*—a sacred juncture of transition and transformation. We experience these outside of time, and we will go deeper into their meaning for daily life in this chapter.

In the body, sandhyas are found at its junctures. These are the joints, the intersections of bone and ligament that form pivot points and allow us to move. They are the nexuses of subtle-body energy: the chakras. Having spent much time learning about the heart chakra in Part Two, we now know that this particularly powerful energetic nexus governs our lungs, circulatory system, emotions, intelligence, and the radiant electromagnetic field that connects us to other people and the entire sentient world.

Moving outward from the body, sandyas are also found on the earth: at the sacred unions of river and valley and at other geographic junctures. On an even larger level, sandhyas are nexus points in the continuum of time and in the changing flow of sun, moon, and cosmos. We have the opportunity to align ourselves with these heightened points of transition in time, where we can listen deeply to the momentum of forces greater than our individual self—sunrises and sunsets, new and full moons—for a deeper attunement to the cosmic cycles themselves.

Our ancestors understood the incredible energy and sense of harmony that came about when they honored the natural world's sandhyas; this is why the vast majority of holidays (holy days) coalesce around solar and lunar sandhyas.

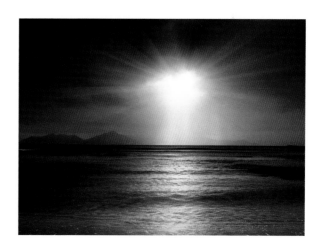

shiva's dance—the rhythm of the heart as the creation of the cosmos

From the pulse of our heart to the pulse of the moment in which it beats, all rises from the *spanda*—the pulsation of consciousness that throbs from the source rhythm of Shiva's own heart consciousness, as symbolized by his *damaru,* or two-sided drum. The sandhya tandava is not just a moment of intimacy between the great lovers Shiva and Shakti (two as One); it is an essential cosmic act creating the movement of this world, from the vibration of the atom to the galaxy's swirl.

The sandhya tandava is the source of the five principal manifestations of eternal energy, or *panchakritya:*

SRISTI—THE CREATIVE POWER

The first manifestation, *sristi*, is the creative energy of consciousness symbolized as the damaru that brings forth the rhythms of creation, dissolution, and creation again. The shape of the damaru includes symbols of male generativity (the lingam) and female generativity (the yoni). The point where these symbols meet is where creation begins; when they separate, destruction ensues.

The damaru is the consummate symbol of the ceaseless rhythm of time within the vinyasas of life. These exist as the pulse of the heart, inhalation and exhalation, sunrise and sunset, and the waxing and waning polarity that underlies all of creation.

STHITI—THE SUSTAINING POWER

Sthiti is the sustaining power of the dance of life that preserves and supports all aspects of creation. This is the miraculous power of resilience, the ceaselessness of the heartbeat that flows from Shiva's drum. The gesture of abhaya mudra, translated both as "have no fear" and "blessing the way before you," expresses Shiva's effortless movement as he dissolves obstacles during his dance with a single stamp of his foot.

SAMHARA—THE POWER OF DISSOLUTION

Samhara is dissolution or absorption, and it is symbolized by the fire in Shiva's hand. Fire is the transforming spirit that ignites, transforms, and dissolves, creating ashes to form soil for new life to emerge.

TIROBHAVA—THE POWER OF MYSTERY

Tirobhava is the power of consciousness to conceal the divine within any form or action. It is represented by Shiva's powerful right foot dancing upon the "dwarf of ignorance," our limited awareness.

ANUGRAHA—THE POWER OF GRACE

Anugraha is the grace of liberation represented by Shiva's left foot and lower left hand, held in *gajahasta* (elephant's trunk) *mudra*. This symbolizes the path of liberation.

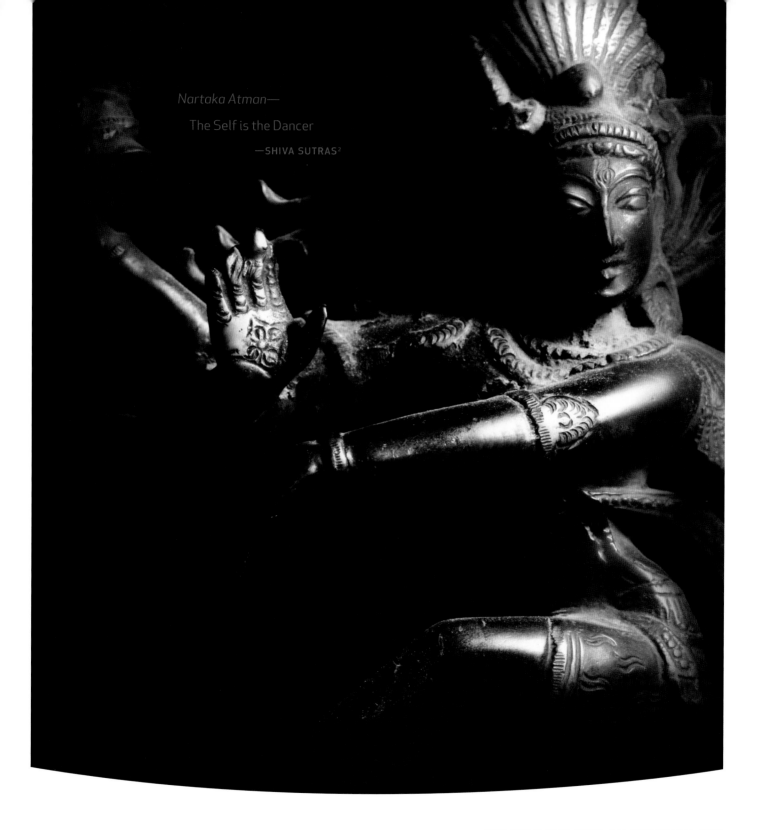

Nartaka Atman—

The Self is the Dancer

—SHIVA SUTRAS[2]

the rhythms of creation—
the planets, elements, and ayurvedic doshas

The sounding of Shiva's damaru creates time and rhythm in the unfolding of creation. Five beats evoke a five-syllable mantra, *Namah Shivaya*, with each sound creating a different element.

> In your body is Mount Meru
>
> the rivers are there too,
>
> the seas, the mountains, the plains,
>
> and the Gods of the fields . . .
>
> The stars are there, and the planets,
>
> and the sun together with the moon;
>
> there too are the two cosmic forces:
>
> that which destroys, that which creates;
>
> and all the elements: ether,
>
> air and fire, water and earth.
>
> Yes, in your body are all things
>
> that exist in the three worlds,
>
> all performing their prescribed functions
>
> around Mount Meru;
>
> he alone who knows this
>
> is held to be a true yogi.
>
> —SIVA SAMHITA[3]

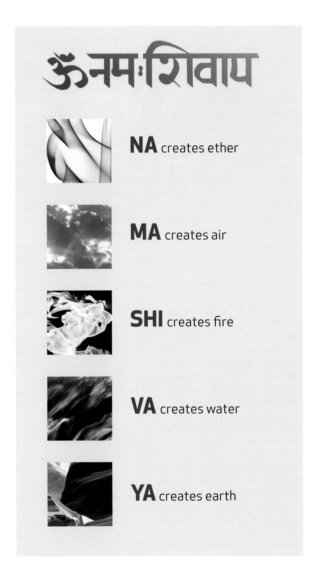

ॐनमःशिवाय

NA creates ether

MA creates air

SHI creates fire

VA creates water

YA creates earth

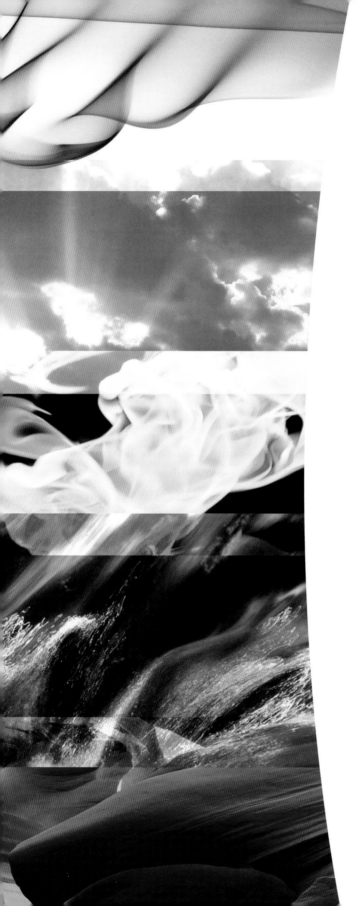

EMBODYING THE FIVE ELEMENTS

Ether *(akash)* is the pure space that first manifests from consciousness. Space is not considered inert but is instead filled with vibrating particles that change, depending on the observer's point of view, from energy to matter and matter to energy in less than a billionth of a second.

When ether condenses, atoms and molecules are formed, such as hydrogen, oxygen, and many other gases. These are all part of the **air** principle, which is movement, or vata.

When movement intensifies, heat emerges as **fire** *(agni)*. Fire is the principle of metabolism in life forms and heat in the non-sentient.

From fire, the **water** principle *(apas* or *jala)* is born, just as when hydrogen (an element of the air principle) burns and water is produced. Intense heat melts many metals, transforming matter into a fluid state.

From water, the **earth** principle *(prithvi)* evolves, representing the solid state of matter characterized by form and structure.

Our body, mind, and spirit are also made up of these five elements at both the gross and subtle-body levels, including the chakras. Our five sense organs—ears, skin, eyes, tongue, and nose—and their underlying qualities—sound, touch, vision, taste, and smell—are governed by the subtle principles of the five elements. Sound is governed by space, touch by air, vision by fire, taste by water, and smell by earth.[4]

The Source of Love is above name and form. He/she is present in all and transcends all...the source of space, air, fire, and water and the earth that holds us all. Fire is his head, sun and moon his eyes... the air his breath, the universe his heart... The Lord of Love is the innermost Self of all.

—UPANISHADS[5]

ayurvedic firekeeping— *swastuvritta*—being in the flow of nature

Within ayurveda, the five elements brought forth by Shiva's drum are found in the three principles of vata, pitta, and kapha that govern all the activities of our embodiment. These are called doshas, or bodily humors that create our constitution (*prakriti*) and also can become imbalanced through our lifestyle (*vikriti*). Vata—combining air and space— is the force behind all movements, such as breathing, circulation, and the elimination of waste from the body. Kapha—combining earth and water—is the binding principle and provides the building substance in the body. Pitta is the fire and water element that governs all metabolic, transformative activities. This combination of the elements into the primary forces of vata, pitta, and kapha become the ayurvedic *prakriti-vikriti* model in which each person is born with a constitution combining the forces, with one or two that are predominant. This natal constitution can become imbalanced (vikriti) as one ages and as a result of other changes in life: stresses, challenges, and even powerful positive change.

Most imbalances that we experience are a result of going against the flow of nature known as *prajna* ("wisdom") *parada* ("to go against") in the psychological (mental and emotional) or somatic realms. Applying the ayurvedic understanding of householder life, we strive to be a *swastha*, a person who is aligned with their sva (or self) nature and who tends these varied levels of health, well-being, and evolution by attuning him- or herself to optimal flow.

Ayurveda views human beings as psychosomatic-spiritual entities in which the interplay between thought impressions, emotions, body experiences, life actions, and macrocosmic forces are understood through a rhythmic lens. Ayurveda seeks to harmonize the many elemental rhythms of our life—the dynamic with the stabilizing, and so forth—so that we can tend the overall fire of our life force and align ourselves with our heart's pulse, literally. Listening to one's heart rhythm is both a high-level diagnostic tool in ayurveda and the central metaphor of being in *swastha vritta*. Shiva's sandhya tandava, which creates the doshas, also creates the sacred rhythm that affects the flow of our daily (*dinacharya*) and seasonal (*rtucharya*) life.

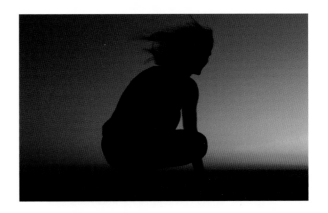

VATA

The word *vata* is derived from the verb *va* which means movement. Vata is air or wind responsible for all movements. Vata is that which moves and acts as a vehicle. Vayu is another name for vata as the energy of circulation.

ELEMENTS space and air

GUNAS mobile, light, dry, cold, rough, subtle, clear

RASA (TASTE) astringent and bitter; balance with sweet, salty, and sour

SEASON fall and early winter

ASSOCIATION WITH BODY colon, joint, heart/brain connection, thighs, bones, ears

ACTION IN THE BODY all movement, muscle and ligament strength, nervous system impulses, all actions in the body, movement of awareness, perceptions and thoughts, respiration, circulation, sensory perception, memory and speech, creativity, introspection

PHYSICAL ATTRIBUTES dry skin, joints, eyes, low weight, thin bones and body frame, angular chin, irregular teeth, sunken chest/underdeveloped breasts, uneven shape to nose

MENTAL ATTRIBUTES creative, fast speech and mannerisms, fear, anxiety, uncertainty, short-term memory, quick intellect, fast to respond

ACTION, INTENTION, AND RHYTHM variability, mobility, adaptable, circulation, flexibility, complete one action at a time

PACIFY slowly, steady, moving with awareness, focus

SIGNS OF IMBALANCE emaciation, hernia, abdominal distention, constipation, dry skin, numbness/tingling, joint pain, dry joints, excess worrying and anxiety, insomnia, tremors, sciatica

PITTA

The word *pitta* is derived from the word *tapa*, which means "to heat." Thus pitta represents the energy, heat, or fire in the body. Pitta is the biological combination of heat (agni) and liquid (apas).

ELEMENTS fire and water

GUNAS hot, light, sharp, oily, spreading, liquid, fleshy/foul smell,

RASA (TASTE) salty, sour, pungent; balance with sweet and astringent taste.

SEASON summer

ASSOCIATION WITH BODY Nabhi (lower stomach, small intestine, solar plexus), skin, blood, liver, spleen, gallbladder, grey matter of brain, eyes, sebaceous secretions

ACTION IN THE BODY metabolism, body temperature, vision, luster of the body, appetite, thirst, taste, intelligence, reasoning

PHYSICAL ATTRIBUTES red cheeks; sharp, lustrous, penetrating eyes; pointed nose; heart-shaped face; tapering chin; lustrous skin

MENTAL ATTRIBUTES good intellect, keen apprehension/comprehension, great orators, charisma, confidence, perfection

ACTION, INTENTION, AND RHYTHM steady with intention and direction; clear goals, driven by direction; pittas like to know how, why, how long, etc.; results oriented

PACIFY moving with balance and harmony, positively challenging, staying cool in the fire, moving energy down and out (apana)

SIGNS OF IMBALANCE increase in body temperature, inflammation, irritation, perforation, bleeding disorders, thick bile, gallstones, sluggish gall bladder, heating headache, diarrhea, rash, hives, lactose intolerance, foul-smell in excreta, indigestion, heart burn

KAPHA

The word *kapha* is derived from the two letters *ka* (water) and *pha* (flourishes). Thus, kapha means that which flourishes in the presence of water. Kapha is derived from the physical elements of earth and water.

ELEMENTS earth and water

GUNAS static, slow, heavy, dull, cool, oily, dense, soft, cloudy

RASA (TASTE) sweet, sour, salty; pacified with bitter and astringent

SEASON late winter, spring

ASSOCIATION WITH BODY upper stomach, chest, plasma, white brain matter, throat, pancreas, bony joints, plasma, fat, nose, tongue

ACTION IN THE BODY lubrication, liquification, all secretions and fluids, cerebrospinal fluid, support, strength, stamina, structure, anabolic, repair and regeneration, fill space as liquid

PHYSICAL ATTRIBUTES large frame and bones, thick hair, large/round eyes, short/rounded/button nose, white/porcelain skin

MENTAL ATTRIBUTES slow movements and speech; attachment, devotional and spiritual; contentment, forgiveness, love, compassion

ACTION, INTENTION, AND RHYTHM slow, steady, easy going, attached, does not move easily or willingly

PACIFY energize, bright, uplifting, devotional, love, compassion

SIGNS OF IMBALANCE lethargy, weight gain, cold, congestion, stagnation in lymphatic system, slow metabolism, low agni, low thyroid, edema, excess salivation, excess sleep, increased cholesterol

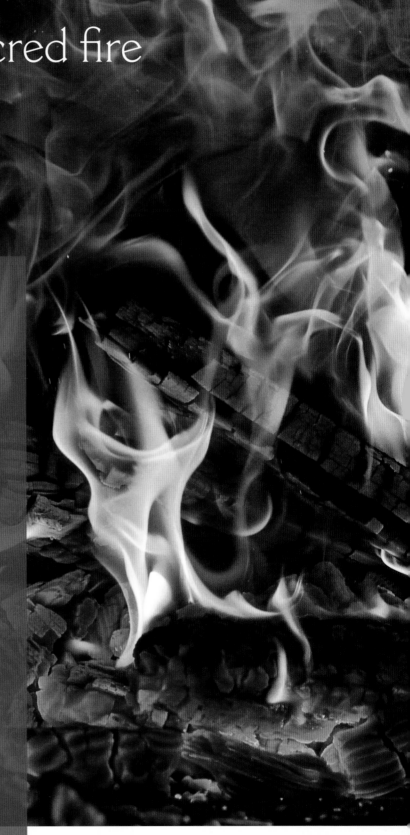

agni—the sacred fire

I offer into Agni—the Fire of Consciousness
Using the mind as sacrificial ladle, svaha.

I offer functions of the senses,
As oblation into the Fire which is Atman,
With the mind as ladle held by the handle
which is the path of Sushumna, svaha.

I offer all acts good and evil as
Oblation into the all-pervading Fire, fed by Time.
The two hands with which I hold the ladle are
Shiva and Sakti,
The ladle of the offering is Consciousness
(*unmani*), svaha.

I offer as oblation this universe of
thirty-six principles,
The first which is Shiva and the last earth.
Into the Fire of Consciousness which
through fullness
Is constantly burning within.

Svaha.

— KAULAVALINIRNAYA[6]

inner firekeeping ayurveda and the cultivation of tejas, ojas, and prana

In living vinyasa, the micro- and macrocycles of yoga and ayurveda both emerge from the fire altar. Agni—sacred fire—is revered as the divine consciousness and is understood to be both material and spiritual. In the body, agni performs much like the outer fire that burns wood. It is the metabolizing force of creation, and as such it requires physical fuel in the form of food, and spiritual fuel in the form of mantra and prayer. Agnideva, the personification of fire as a deity, has two faces: one creative, the other destructive. In its igniting capacity in the body, agni sparks cellular regeneration as well as the destruction of old cells to make room for the new.

Agni represents the fire at our core. Depending upon our constitution, lifestyle, and practices, it can be well balanced to support our evoution or lead to imbalances. When unbalanced, agni can burn us up and dry us out (known as excessive fire), manifest in low energy and lack of inspiration (weak fire), or oscillate in place, leaving us unable to move forward in life (wavering fire).

Ayurveda applies Vedic and tantric teachings on balancing the sun, moon, and fire within to maintain inner vitality.

Agni manifests as tejas—inner illumination—and governs all metabolic processes in the body. Because it involves heat, it is related to the sun's energy; it keeps body, mind, and emotions radiant. The moon of the Vedas and Tantras is soma or lunar nectar. It supports the cultivation of ojas within our physiology as a vital protective energy, a subtle substance providing luster and immunity to the system. Ojas nourishes the body in a way similar to the moon's effect on plant life. It soothes the emotions and the mind. The sun as vayu (wind) is prana, the life force, the flow of intelligence, creativity, and the circulation of vital energy. In cultivating your Heart Fire and creating a healthy life, you work to maintain balance between these qualities of tejas (fire), ojas (moon), and prana (sun) that is the core Vedic-tantric metaphor and practice of tending the fire in an altar or in one's spiritual or worldly life. The charts on pages 161–165 show ways in which tejas, ojas, and prana can go out of balance. They also offer life practices that can restore your radiance to a balanced state.

OJAS—CULTIVATING THE NECTAR

Soma represents the water element in the universe and ojas within the body. In firekeeping, a common substance we offer to fire is liquid ghee (clarified butter), a fuel that produces no smoke. It is considered to impart a healing, restorative luster reminiscent of ojas (think of a healthy baby's plump cheeks) and is an important part of ayurvedic cooking and medicine that is used to cultivate ojas. Ojas is the essence, like honey created by the essence of flowers, and is related to vitality and immunity. The accumulation of the flower essences is stored in the honeycomb, which in our body is like ojas, the pure essence of our dhatus, or bodily tissues. Ojas is considered to be generated from the original essence of para ojas in the heart, which then circulates via the heart and throughout the body for support.

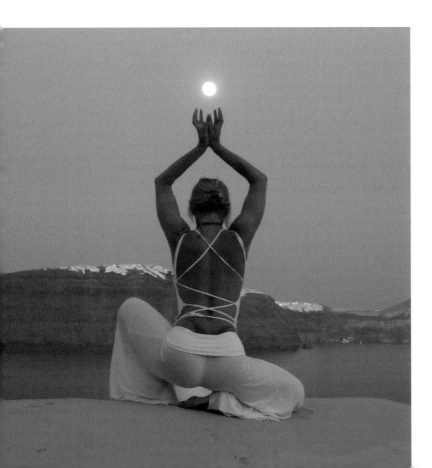

We are tremendously full of effort.
We try to get rid of anger, which is an effort,
we try to get rid of fear, which is an effort.
All efforts build stress and that
stress diminishes ojas.

— DR. VASANT LAD[7]

Ojas is the super-fine essence of *kapha dosha* associated with lunar cycles; it is therefore connected to regeneration. The qualities of ojas and kapha dosha are similar: liquid, sweet, and unctuous. Together they provide great support for the immune system and the reserves of life force.

There are two types of ojas found in the body. *Apara ojas* is the refined essence from digested food that circulates in the bloodstream, transforms the tissues of the body, and nourishes para ojas. Para ojas is a sacred essence found only in the heart. It consists of eight drops, or *asta bindu,* given by the mother during pregnancy. It is highly concentrated, with a powerful effect on the vitality of all the body's cells, tissues, and organs.

Meditation enhances and spreads para ojas throughout your being, circulating immunity, happiness, love, and compassion and emanating from your very self. Because of the vital nature of ojas's role in health, ayurveda encourages us to behave in ways that support it and to avoid actions that undermine it.

In that effortless state of awareness, you recognize
your true nature, which is peace and love, and that
state is supported in every cell by para ojas.
In other words, para ojas opens the door to God
consciousness, which is non-judgmental awareness.
Then para ojas becomes soma, which releases
molecules of bliss throughout the body.

— DR. VASANT LAD[8]

TENDING THE FIRE WITH OJAS

LIFE IMBALANCES THAT DECREASE OJAS IN THE BODY

> Stress that is from life circumstances or self-created

> Lack of heart-brain entrainment

> Dissonant thoughts and emotions; worry, anxiety, anger, jealousy, excessive pride

> Disconnection from the Heart Fire and the diminishing of love and compassion

> Shock and trauma, overexerting oneself, overdoing, exposure to extremes

> Late nights, insomnia, lack of proper rest

> Excessive travel, multitasking, draining technology rhythms

> Dieting, improper nutrition, malnutrition

> Excessive sexual release

> Eating unwholesome foods, incompatible foods, processed and junk foods

> Excessive smoking, alcohol, addictions, recreational drugs

Om Ojoyai Namah

I bow to the One who is overflowing with Ojas[9]

INCREASING OJAS

> Nourishing the Heart Fire with love *sukha* (intrinsic happiness), and santosha (contentment) in your life

> Cultivating aesthetics, beauty, the arts, peaceful rhythm, and enjoyment of the art of living

> Balancing solar-lunar rhythms in one's practice and life by doing solar activies at a non-depleting time (not at night or when you are tired) and bringing more relaxation into daily life

> Steadily following nourishing rhythms of dinacharya and rtucharya

> Nutrition with organic, cooked (for digestion), vegetarian food—not overly spiced

> Organic dairy or nut milks if vegan (almond, cashew), ghee, fresh butter, small amounts of cream

> Fresh nuts, honey, dates, whole grains and rice, vegetables, and fresh, sweet fruits

> Balancing sexual energy in accordance with the seasons and one's constitution

> Ayurvedic herbs and *rasayanas*—tonic drinks and jams like Chayvan prash

> Making rasayanas with the guidance of an ayurvedic counselor of herbs, including Ashwagandha, Bala, Brahmi, Kumari, Shankapushpi, Shatarvari, Shilajit, Yashti madhu

CULTIVATING TEJAS

The agni of the fire altar corresponds to tejas, the illuminating light that emanates from fire. In the human body, tejas creates our ability to see and is found in the light that we see in each other's eyes; the light of insight, knowledge, and imagination; and the clarifying light of awareness that brings consciousness into the flow of life. Tejas is our natural cellular intelligence and is connected to *pitta dosha,* including biological processes such as digestion, assimilation, metabolism, sensory processing, and regulation of body temperature. Cultivating tejas harnesses radiant energy and replenishes the fire. A person with good tejas is radiant, has lustrous eyes, and possesses clarity, insight, courage, compassion, and fearlessness. Tejas is the regulation of optimal energy flow (prana) and the reserve fuel of that energy flow (ojas). If the inner fire or tejas is dim, there is less creation of raw ojas—our natural luster, immunity, and joy. When the tejas is too high, it will dry and burn ojas—the ayurvedic understanding of "burning out," leading to the condition of excess fire or *tikshna agni.* Hence, ojas is dependent on the balancing of our inner fire or tejas.

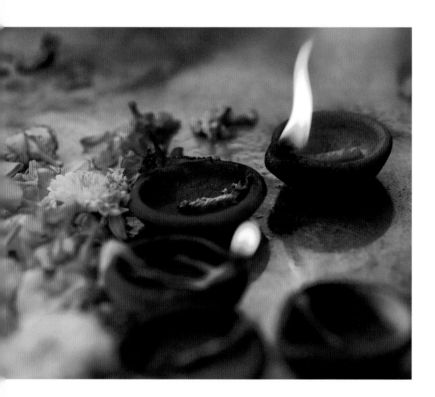

The principle of tejas embraces both light and heat. The illumination of the sun is tejas. Tejas is the primary energy involved in the digestion and transformation of everything we take in and experience. This includes food, liquids, thoughts, actions, emotions, and all else that comprises our human life.

—DR. VASANT LAD[10]

TENDING THE FIRE OF TEJAS

LIFE IMBALANCES THAT DECREASE TEJAS IN THE BODY

> A condition of tikshna agni—which burns all the nutrients that feed our body and tissues

> Pitta-aggravating lifestyle and diet: overly spicy, fried, or processed foods; too much doing from excess ambition and will

> Misuse of senses through the media— not being selective about what and when you watch, read, or listen

> Habits, conditioning, or life-circumstance which diminishes inspiration, joy, enthusiasm, and motivation for life

> Lack of intellectual stimulation

> Choosing activities and asanas that are always heating and stimulating

> Dissonant thoughts and emotions—excess anger, impatience, irritation, fast pace

Tejas is the burning flame of pure intelligence. Keep that flame alive and bright. That light is your true nature. That light is tejas.
—DR. VASANT LAD[11]

INCREASING TEJAS

> Listen to the body's intelligence

> Synchronize your rhythm with sunrise/sunset and absorb the morning sunlight

> Engage in activities that illuminate the mind (reading uplifting material, writing, study)

> Protect your senses from extrasensory stimulation, excess technology

> Follow the seasonal rhythms and the path of the sun to stay in rhythm with cosmic tejas

> Balanced Vira Rasa or solar yoga practice, surya namaskar, Agni Kriyas, core-strengthening that is heating and invigorating (fire-based practices)

> Gazing upon the fire, solar meditations, trataka, agni hotra practices

> Stimulating pranayama—bhastrika, *agni sara*, kapalabhati

> Eat a nourishing diet to support digestive fire, including warm foods with (tejas) spices like ginger, black pepper, cumin for digestion

> Herbs like Brahmi, ginkgo, sandalwood for the mind and elevated consciousness

TENDING THE FIRE WITH PRANA

Prana is movement, the flow of intelligence as the life force and as respiration. Prana is the great governor over ojas and tejas. It is connected with the vital energy of breath, the wind element, and vata dosha. A person with good prana has vitality, breath, circulation, movement, and awareness. Prana helps transform food into cellular consciousness and is the bridge between mind, body, and consciousness. If prana is low, ojas and tejas will also be low. Vata and prana both govern all life functions as the vehicles of intelligence, awareness, and energy. Both are responsible for activity, alertness, breath, and neurological impulses and processes.

The disturbance of prana is rife in the modern world; noise and air pollution are among the things that deplete it. This depleted state is described as "vata aggravation" or being "vata deranged," and can manifest as stress brought on by too much movement—too many thoughts, emails, texts, too much driving, multitasking. Actions that disrupt prana lead to *vishama agni,* or wavering fire.

Prana is a bridge between Purusha (soul)
and Prakriti (manifest matter),
male and female, solar and lunar energy.

— DR. VASANT LAD[12]

TENDING THE FIRE OF PRANA

LIFE IMBALANCES THAT DISRUPT PRANA IN THE BODY

> Multitasking, including excessive overdoing, overworking; excess technology rhythms that fragment life-energy

> Dissonant heart-brain thoughts or emotions, particularly excessive fear, anxiety, or worry

> Vata-aggravating diet and lifestyle: irregular rhythm, cold foods, raw, dry, or light foods in the wrong season

> Overdoing to the point of fatigue and exhaustion

> Multitasking and dispersing energy to various activities

> Losing focus and not completing tasks or projects

> Holding the breath, suppression of natural urges and rhythm

> Stimulating yourself when you are tired (drinking caffeine)

> Neglecting creative expression or avoiding communication

INCREASING PRANA

> Vata-pacifying diet and lifestyle: warm foods, regular dinacharya and rtucharya

> Moderating movement and cultivating a grounded, steady life rhythm

> Keeping steady focus and doing one thing at a time

> Cultivating expression in creativity and communication

> Slowing down and cultivating Shanti and Sringara Rasa in practice and daily life

> Maintaining balance between the solar and lunar currents (ida and pingala nadi) through solar and lunar yoga practices, meditation

> Pranayama (*anuloma viloma*, bhastrika, ujjayi)

> Grounding and fluid cardiovascular activities: walking, swimming, cycling

> Expansive herbs: Ashwagandha (to nourish), Calamus, Jatamamsi, and Shitopaladi

Om Pranaya Namah

I bow to the essence of Prana[13]

balancing the fires—*samagni* and dim, excessive, and wavering fires

The ayurvedic concept of *samagni*, or balanced fire, can be said to be the goal of our ayurvedic fire-keeping practice. While the focus is usually on the digestive fire, ayurveda also outlines the effects of imbalances in our lives more generally. Cultivating samagni gives us a healthy appetite for life, which we reflect through enthusiasm, inspiration, higher energy levels, creativity, sexuality, expressiveness, prosperity, love, and spirit.

When burned in the fire too quickly, agni leads to imbalances on the excessive fire side, called *tikshna agni,* and is connected to the quality of pitta. When we offer it too little, the fire goes out or we have dim fire, called *manda agni,* connected to kapha. When it is difficult to stabilize the fire, wavering fire (*vishama agni*) develops, which is connected to vata. Our goal is samagni, the balanced fire that supports our life force. In order to sustain a healthy fire, we must seek a balance between purification and rejuvenation, solar and lunar qualities.

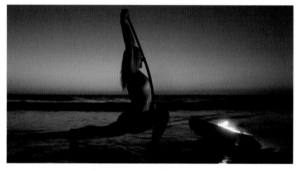

BALANCED FIRE—SAMAGNI
balanced metabolism, energetic, content, joyful, fearless, clear-minded, balanced, peaceful, blissful, enlightened, sustained by well-rounded practice

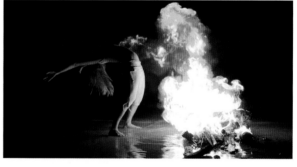

EXCESSIVE FIRE—TIKSHNA AGNI
extreme hunger, excessive body heat, aggressive, impulsive, angry, jealous, critical, self-righteous, fanatical, intolerant, balanced by Shanti, Sringara, and Lunar practice, cultivating Ojas, and balancing Tejas

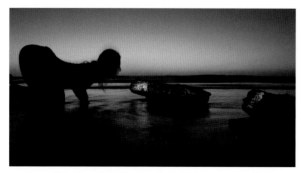

DIM FIRE—MANDA AGNI
poor appetite, low energy, depression, lethargy, dullness, lack of inspiration, spiritual darkness, balanced by Sringara, Vira, and Solar practice, cultivating Ojas while stoking the fire

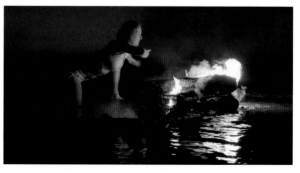

WAVERING FIRE—VISHAMA AGNI
irregular appetite and body heat, erratic breathing and energy patterns, moodiness, instability, indecision, inconsistent faith, balanced by Solar-Lunar practice, cultivating Prana, and Vata-pacifying lifestyle

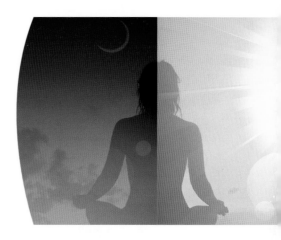

living
vinyasa

Cycles of Rhythm and Flow

SUNRISE SANDHYA

Rise near sunrise

Sacred time for your yoga/meditation practices

Dinacharya practices to harmonize with the day

> There are rhythms within rhythms within
> rhythms. And these drumbeats echo all around
> us and within us. We are not outsiders to
> the process; we are part of it,
> throbbing to the pulse of the universe.
>
> — DEEPAK CHOPRA[1]

NOON SANDHYA

Peak of the day

Largest meal with the strongest agni

Take a short walk to aid digestion

SUNSET SANDHYA

Sacred time: yoga/meditation with the sunset

Light evening meal around sunset

Ratricharya practices to harmonize with the moon

VINYASA IN ESSENCE IS EVERY CYCLE OF LIFE,

from the micro-pulse of the quantum and cellular pulse that emerges and dissolves in seconds, to the vinyasa of our inhale of receiving new life and our exhale of letting go, to the awakening of every morning to when we retire, and all of the mini-cycles that pervade the vinyasa of the day, week, and lunar/solar cycles. Ultimately our life from our conception to when our body dissolves is one vinyasa. Paying attention to the beginning of a cycle, the way it is sustained and builds, and the completion of a vinyasa is the open secret to living flow. Flow is equal to vinyasa just as an incomplete cycle is the absence of flow. Tending our fire is the intelligent awareness of and connection to all of the cycles of our life—inner as well as cosmic rhythms and flow. This chapter begins with the core to ayurvedic firekeeping of tending one's vital energy through the practices that guide the flow of the day (*dina*) and night (*ratri*) and ends with the ancestral connection to the solar and lunar rhythms that have affected life on earth for at least five billion years.

NIGHT SLEEP

Simple ratricharya rituals before bedtime

Giving thanks and generating love before sleep

Ideal rest time: before 10 p.m.

ayurvedic dinacharya and ratricharya practices for harmonizing the sun and the moon

How will you tend the rhythm of your life? Dinacharya and *ratricharya* practices offer ways to support your well-being and cultivate the rhythms of your daily life. Together they can be translated as "daily conduct" or "daily movement."

BEGIN THE DAY—DINACHARYA

Within the Tantras and ayurveda, the first waking breath of the day is a very sacred sandhya, a practice in itself for waking from the dream state in life. It is also a reflection of where your consciousness resides. You can engage in a series of practices, described below, to help align you and your Heart Fire with the fresh energy of morning and carry those rhythms into the rest of your day.

> The light has shone in the sky.
>
> Waking up in the morning,
>
> I see before my very eyes compassion
>
> flooding down
>
> — BAUL SONG[2]

Sahaja Yoga in Bed

Allow your body to enjoy a spontaneous, fluid, catlike motion that connects you to your instinctual body. Move in any way that feels natural to you—in ways your body yearns to move—at the very beginning of your day. Curl your spine, stretch, and invite the energy of your heart and emotions to express themselves through your body.

Generate Love

While you are still in that soft, dreamlike state upon first opening your eyes, invite feelings of love, kindness, and openness into your heart. It may be easier to do this if you select a "target" for your love. Embrace and generate love for whoever is there with you—your beloved, your baby, your dog or cat. Invite love into your state while the day is fresh and new.

Awakening with the Light

Learn when the sun rises in your location, whether you are at home or traveling. When you are not under stress or needing extra rest, try to rise before sunrise and complete the morning cleansing process so you can begin your meditation with the sunrise. If that is not possible, try to honor the sunrise by repeating a simple mantra and gazing at the sun as it rises, or toward the lightening sky in the east if the day is cloudy. Enjoy the stillness of this moment.

First Step of the Day

You have set the tone for your day in those first powerful moments when you emerge from sleep. Now it is time to set your day in motion. Step out of your bed and touch your feet to the earth, giving thanks for another day to walk upon it.

Morning Cleansing and Purification Practices

Now you can begin your daily cleansing and purification practices, preparing your body for the activity of the day. Bring the energy of love and kindness that you generated while you were still in bed into these practices.

Hydration

First, replenish yourself by drinking fresh, purified water (in ayurveda this is put into a copper cup the night before in order to receive the benefits of this trace metal). You can infuse your water with lemon for a hydrating and cleansing effect if you wish.

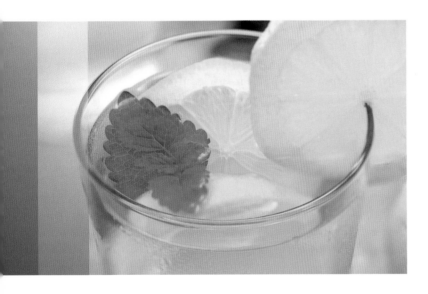

Caring for Your Sense Organs—Nourishing the Eyes, Ears, Nose, Mouth, and Tongue

Though all of these practices are nourishing and balancing, they are best undertaken with the guidance of a teacher or health practitioner. Avoid oiling, medicinal drinks or herbs, and the like if you are menstruating, pregnant, feel toxic, have undergone recent or have upcoming surgeries, or suffer from a chronic condition.

Prevent earwax and nourish the ears through *karana purana*, oiling the ears; it helps to put a few drops of sesame oil in each ear.

Nasya, or nasal drops, requires putting three to five drops of oil into each nostril as your head is tilted back, to clean the sinuses, improve the voice, strengthen vision, and increase mental clarity. (For vata, use sesame oil or ghee, or *vacha* (calamus root) oil. For pitta, use Brahmi, ghee, or sunflower or coconut oil. For kapha, vacha oil is preferred.)

Gargling with sesame or coconut oil twice per day is a practice that strengthens the teeth, gums, and jaw. To do this, hold the oil in your mouth, swishing vigorously. After spitting the oil out, massage the gums gently with a finger.

For the tongue, gently scrape its surface with a spoon or stainless-steel tongue scraper from the back to the front for seven to fourteen strokes. Tongue scraping removes dead bacteria from the tongue, aids in digestion, and stimulates the internal organs.

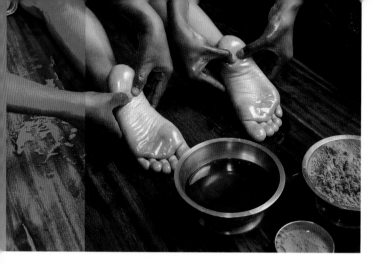

Abhyanga—Oiling with Love

Massaging warm, herb-infused oil into the body is one of the most nourishing, life-enhancing gifts of health you can give yourself for the rest of your life. Regular *abhyanga* is particularly welcome during the dry and cold months of the year and for people who travel often or exercise a lot.

For yoga practitioners—or really anyone interested in the vitality of his or her body— abhyanga is an essential method for both solar (purification) and lunar (regeneration) purposes. Daily oil massage, a lunar sadhana, is a great tonic against the drying and stiffening effects of stress and aging. Circular movement over the heart region and joints has a warming, soothing quality that releases stress and grounds the nervous system. The power of touch can help heal negative body attitudes by generating connection, loving touch, and awareness. Abhyanga also has the solar quality of circulating and purifying. When combined with dry-brushing, it wakes up the body and establishes healthy rhythms for the day.

When you share this practice with someone you love, abhyanga is a method of bonding and caring for each other's well-being. An oil massage on the limbs, spine, and tummy of a young child stimulates neurological and tissue functioning while creating a comforting cellular memory of the important bond between parent and child. For couples, giving and receiving abhyanga can be a beautiful ritual of care and love and a great way to tend the fire of your relationship bond. It's also a highly practical way to receive daily attention in sore areas of the body, to tonify, and to strengthen areas of weakness.

Enjoy Essential Oils

Applying a small amount of natural essential oils gives beautiful energetic support for your day. Vata benefits from the grounding scent of amber. Pitta benefits from sandalwood for men or jasmine for women. And for kapha, amber is a great warming scent, or you can use a stimulating scent such as eucalyptus or peppermint if it's not too cooling for the season.

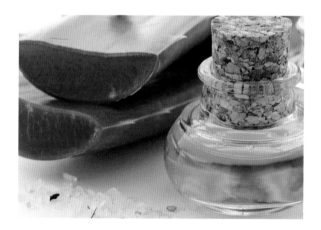

AGNI HOTRA PRAYER

At the point of sunrise, begin by chanting *Om suryaya swaha*, meaning "I realize the Sun." While you say *swaha* —the great fire-offering mantra—offer one part of the rice grains to the fire. Then chant *Suryaya idam, na mama,* meaning "This substance belongs to the sun, not to me," as a humble phrase honoring the life-giving power of the sun in all. Then chant *prajapataye swaha,* meaning "This offering is given to Prajapati, the Source of all Created," while offering the rest of the rice. Then finish the mantra: *prajapataye idam, na mama* ("This belongs to the Source, not me")

Finally, meditate on your inner Heart Fire and its connection to the energy of the rising sun. Meditate and generate energy within your heart and, if possible, until the flame goes out on its own. If you need to leave or continue your yoga practice in other forms, leave the fire burning and try not to blow the fire out. For tapas, or vigil with firekeeping, you can keep the fire burning all day and night in a safe place and reactivate it for noon and sunset meditations.

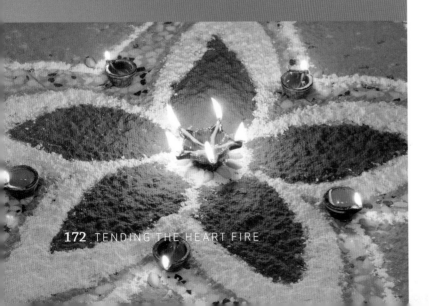

Solar Sandhya Practices

Honoring the sacred juncture when the day begins anew at sunrise is a ritual that is part of many spiritual cultures, particularly in yoga where the core meditative practice is synched exactly to the sunrise and sunset. Enjoyment of your yoga practice with these sandhyas, be they meditation, flowing yoga, walking, or prayer, will be heightened by practicing within forty-five minutes before or after sunrise.

Fire Offering: Agni Hotra

Agni hotra, or fire (*agni*) offering (*hotra*), can be a simple firekeeping practice stemming from the Vedic-tantric traditions and a universal way to align and elevate the energy of the day.

Simple Agni Hotra Sadhana

Ten minutes or more before your meditation, set up your supplies, which will include:

> Meditation seat, altar, or power place to see the sunrise or sunset
> Fire altar in the form of a small candle or copper *kund* (womb place of the fire) placed on a ceramic plate, rock, or heat-resistant support
> Fuel in the form of a soy or beeswax candle; oil such as coconut oil or ghee
> Fire twigs or dried cow dung (easier to get than you think)
> Ghee (plus a wooden spoon for offering) or rice, either plain or mixed with turmeric to be the color gold (use your hand)

For your morning *agni hotra sadhana* practice, find a place where you can face east and gaze at the sunrise. Create a fire kund with a small copper pot. Smear a few drops of ghee over two pinches of clean, unbroken rice grains and place them in your left palm or in a small dish. Divide the rice into two parts.

As sunrise approaches, chant *Om* and the mantra at left three times, or offer your own prayer.

RATRICHARYA—EVENING LUNAR SADHANA

Honor the Sunset

The time of day when the sun begins to drop in extraordinary glory upon the horizon is also a heightened sandhya for yoga practice and meditation. You can again come into any form of yoga practice or any of the heart or energetic vinyasa practices and feel the magical energy that is particularly transformative during meditative practice. If at all possible, try not to schedule mundane activities within one and a half hours of the actual sunset time, or at least in the twenty minutes around the sunset sandhya period. If you find yourself in line at the bank as the sun is going down, go into spontaneous meditation. If in traffic, chant and get in touch with your inner Heart Fire in whatever way you can. Be a keeper of your inner fire by inhaling the natural magic of the day and not missing a single opportunity to feel the extraordinary power of the sunrise and sunset—the times of great awe, epic scale, and potent realization freely emanating from nature.

Enjoy Loved Ones, Family, and Creative Time

In the last part of your evening, take time to be with your loved ones or enjoy reading, reflecting, or being creative. Be sure to keep your environment relaxed, and be mindful of connecting too much or at all to technology so that you do not become overstimulated before bedtime.

Lunar Energetic Vinyasa: Slowing Down for Regenerative Energy or Making Love

You can light your lamp and offer chandra namaskar —Moon Salutations—*shanti rasa vinyasa*, or meditation in candlelit darkness. You can also massage the soles of your feet with oil or knead them by rolling them on a tennis ball. If it's wintertime, wear socks over the oil. Enjoy a relaxing cup of tea, hot milk, or almond milk infused with cardamom, black pepper, ginger, or rasayana herbs recommended by an herbalist or special supplier. These include Brahmi, Ash-

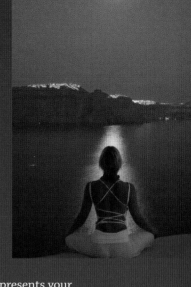

wagandha, or Shatarvari mixed with a natural sweetener. If you make love, you might want to drink your evening rasayana after love, adding a sprinkle of raw cashews and organic sweetener to nourish ojas. Rituals such as these are not some fairytale lifestyle. They are natural pleasures that can be woven into your life in anywhere from ten minutes to two hours a day.

Closing Meditation, Practice, Prayer of the Day

If you read in bed, consider that this represents your last vibrations of the day to take into the dreamtime. Offer a prayer of gratitude before going to sleep. Enjoy some sahaja yoga in your bed and settle into blissful sleep. Hug and generate love with your partner or kids. Be aware of your dreams, and sleep deeply in peace (even under the moonlight during the summer months). You have embodied the cosmic cycle with a day and are linking your body to the natural source.

EVENING AGNI HOTRA

For your evening agni hotra practice, follow the sunrise agni hotra offering but with the following prayer. (The offering practice on swaha is still the same whether morning or evening. The only difference is the invocation of Agni, which sustains the light of the sun in the evening by the fire.) The mantra goes as follows:

> *Om Agnaye Swaha*
>> I honor the fire
> *Agnaye Idam Na Mama*
>> This offering which belongs to the fire and not me
> *Prajapataye Swaha*
>> I honor the Source being
> *Prajapataye Idam, Na Mama*
>> This Source, not the individual ego me[5]

Meditate or leave the fire safely going until it goes out naturally, or keep it burning all night in vigil.

ida and pingala rhythms: honoring the dance of shiva and shakti

When the yogin or yogini gives herself
over to Shiva/Shakti the sun and moon
come up in the central channel.

— YOGA SPANDAKARIKA[6]

The microcosm of the sun and the moon are experienced in the body through the alternating rhythms of ida (the lunar current) and pingala (solar current) and the sushumna nadi (the central channel around which they wind), representing the integration of the two. These have multiple correspondences in the bio-pulses of the body through the nadis. Nadis are the subtle channels (there are more than seventy-two thousand of these) of energy flow through the subtle body. The ida current relates to inner experience, the parasympathetic nervous system, and the right hemisphere of the brain, while the pingala current is the activating, outward-moving energy of the sympathetic nervous system and the left hemisphere of the brain. The yoga system that tunes you to these rhythms, known as *swara yoga,* focuses on synchronizing your inner and outer rhythms.

Our energetic focus alternates brain hemispheres every hour and a half—a shift we can experience by acknowledging the natural ebb and flow of our energy throughout the day. Whenever you feel yourself naturally moving inward—to relax, reflect, or meditate—you are naturally moving into *ida nadi.* When you feel raring to go and are drawn to stimulating activities, you are experiencing *pingala nadi.*

DISRUPTING THE NATURAL FLOW

In the modern world, we constantly override these fundamental natural rhythms. When we wake up tired, we get some caffeine. When we feel wired, we use something external to calm us down. The key to living vinyasa is to instead synchronize our natural internal rhythms as we move through the day. We need to honor both ida and pingala if we are to be in balance and functioning in our highest state. This is the union of the sun and the moon in the fire of the heart, the rhythmic balance of inhalation and exhalation, of the oscillating universe that pulses through our body.

IDA NADI

> Associated with parasympathetic nervous system

> The left channel of the nadi system

> Associated with the moon and nurturing force in all beings

> Correlated functions: moving inward, restoration, relaxation, conserving energy, increasing serenity, calming the mind, nourishing

> Connected to the flow of creativity, artistic expression, and intuition

> Alpha-wave state, nine to fourteen waves per second: a heightened state of well-being; non-focused body awareness; a creative state; body self-healing

PINGALA NADI

> Associated with the sympathetic nervous system

> The right channel of the nadi system

> Associated with the sun and activating force in all beings

> Correlated functions: the energy for physical movement and activities, vitality and power, mental quickness, constructive actions

> Stimulates vital energy, rational, analytical, and logical thinking

> Beta-wave state, fifteen to forty waves per second: high mental activity; strong concentration

CHECKING OUT YOUR IDA-PINGALA FLOW

You can tell which nadi is dominant at any given moment by which of your nostrils is dominant. Close one nostril at a time to see which one carries a stronger flow of breath, or hold your hand underneath your nostrils to feel the breath flow. Now that you know which nadi you are experiencing, as much as possible, match your activity to that nadi. This could mean engaging when you're feeling sluggish or doing a calming practice if you are feeling agitated. Respect your authentic energy.

You can bring natural flow to your day by learning to honor your oscillations instead of going against them—or, if circumstances do not allow this, by at least being compassionate with yourself when you have to go against the grain. This is a very important part of living vinyasa.

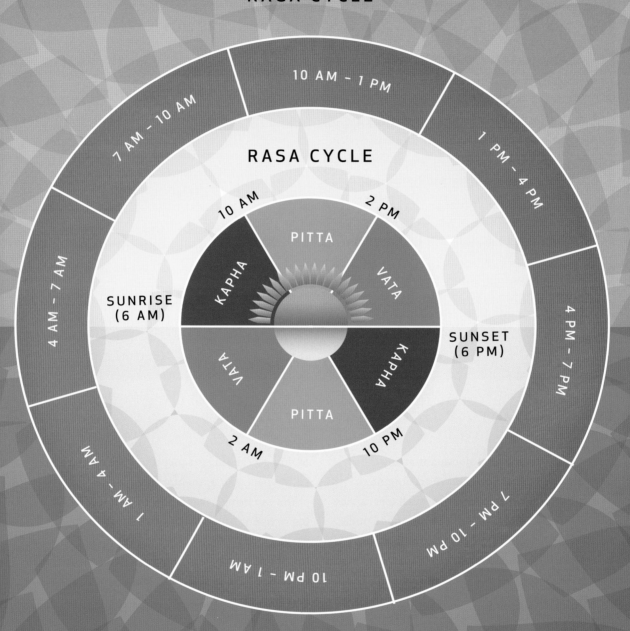

RAGA CYCLE

10 AM – 1 PM

7 AM – 10 AM

1 PM – 4 PM

RASA CYCLE

10 AM

2 PM

4 AM – 7 AM

PITTA

KAPHA

VATA

SUNRISE
(6 AM)

SUNSET
(6 PM)

4 PM – 7 PM

VATA

KAPHA

PITTA

2 AM

10 PM

1 AM – 4 AM

10 PM – 1 AM

7 PM – 10 PM

rhythmic cycles of the day

THE DAILY CYCLE OF RAGA-RASA RHYTHM

There is a beautiful understanding of the rhythm of the day from the Natyasastra: that there is a *raga*, or melodic sound, that is matched with a rasa, or general energetic quality, and that these occur together at certain times of the day. In this understanding, the day is broken into eight three-hour periods (*prahars*), with specific ragas for each. The first-cycle raga, for example, corresponds to the sacred twilight hours before dawn, or *bhramamuhurta*.

If you study the way musical notes unfold, you realize that they synchronize with the nature of our bodies, beginning with the low bass tones that resonate in the pelvic region and rising into the higher-frequency tones of the upper chambers of the brain. The different combinations of notes and the patterns in which they are played have very distinct effects on our emotions.

AYURVEDIC CYCLES OF THE DAY

In the ayurvedic system, every four hours there is an oscillation of the doshas: kapha, pitta, and vata. The transition times between the doshas occur at sunrise and sunset, and at midday and midnight.

> **Vata** encompasses the hours between two and six o'clock
> **Kapha** usually runs between six and ten o'clock
> **Pitta** is strongest between ten and two o'clock

This ayurvedic time clock reflects the natural energetic cycles that our bodies absorb from and reflect back into the natural environment. Vata is the principle of movement and air and is strongest during the transitions between day and night, light and dark, warm and cool. Pitta, the fire principle, is strongest at the warmest time of day, again at the peak of external coolness, and within the body when hormones and enzymes are repairing and rebuilding the body. Corresponding to the earth element, kapha is present during the building, rising transitions of midday and midnight. Thus, within the cycle of a single day, the three energetic doshic forces of vata, pitta, and kapha dance to the rhythm of nature, affecting our bodies and minds in various ways. Ayurveda offers lifestyle recommendations to enhance and work with these natural rhythms and forces.

> The secret to living flow is to see and feel your life as waves of vinyasas—rhythmic cycles— that connect throughout the flow of the day.
> — SHIVA REA

weekly rhythm
planetary days of the week

Feel into the rhythm of the week and experience the alternating flow between activation and rest. Build energy in balance and find your natural optimal flow as each week slightly or dramatically changes.

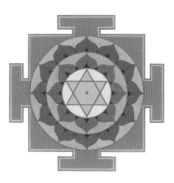

SUN
SUNDAY

Color: Orange/Red/Gold

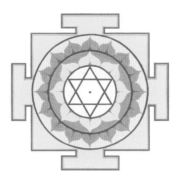

MOON
MONDAY

Color: White

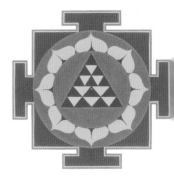

MARS
TUESDAY

Color: Red

The flow of the week is a natural rhythm that links us to the cosmos, honored through time and across cultures: in ancient Greece and Rome, Norse and Celtic cultures, and the Hindu-Yogic culture of India, among many others. The seven days of the week are named for the seven planets of classical astronomy, and thus we have *Sun*day and *Moon*day.

Generally, Sunday and Tuesday are the main solar days, associated with the sun, with the fiery planet Mars, and with fiery colors. Monday and Friday are natural lunar days, associated with the moon and the planet Venus, and linked across cultures to the flow of love and beauty. Monday, for example, has a beautiful, restorative, lunar energy, and this is perhaps why so many people do not feel in a "solar mode" on Mondays.

In India this natural cycle of planetary energy is used as a guide for sadhana. Devotees dedicate

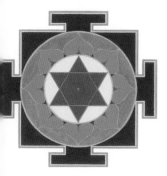

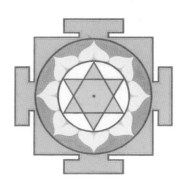

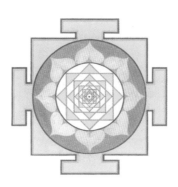

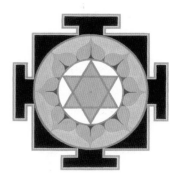

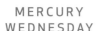

**MERCURY
WEDNESDAY**

Color: Green

**JUPITER
THURSDAY**

Color: Yellow

**VENUS
FRIDAY**

Color: White/Pastels

**SATURN
SATURDAY**

Color: Blue or Black

and deepen certain practices, such as retreat, mantra japa, or fasting, on Monday, dedicated to Shiva; or on Friday, dedicated to Shakti. Observe the natural flow of your own energy as you move through the week.

Another practice is to observe the effects of the colors we wear in conjunction with the days of the week and incorporate the mantra of each planet into our daily awareness: a simple sadhana that

ayurvedic teachers like Dr. Vasant Lad recommend to help people attune to the macrocosmic effects of the planets (reflected in these colors in the seven yantras of the planets). You can also explore the energetic effects of solar-lunar dynamics by wearing cooling blues, purples, or white to bring a lunar calm energy to your day, or by using bright, warm colors such as orange, red, and green for a warming, activating effect.

lunar rhythms—the creative power of the thirteen moons

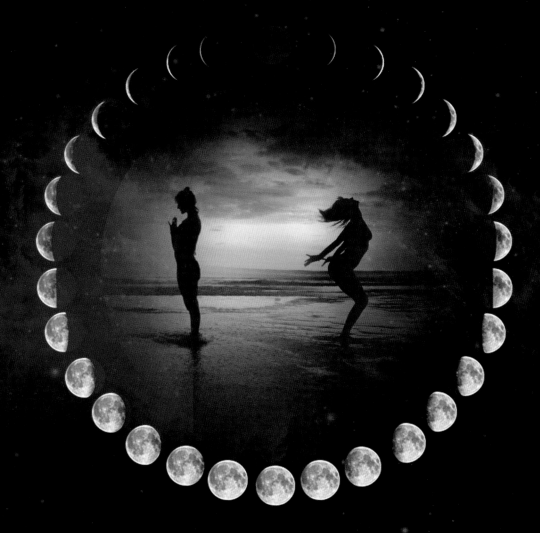

Moonlight floods the whole sky from horizon to horizon.

How much it can fill your room depends on its windows.

Grant a great dignity, my friend, to the cup of your life.

Love has designated it to hold His eternal wine.

—RUMI[7]

In the West, most people living in urban settings are unaware of the phases of the moon, but for our ancestors, the waxing and waning of the moon offered important guidance. Planting crops, tending the fields, harvesting, organizing communal life, and cultivating healthy energy were all done in accordance with the phases of the moon.

Known as a tithi in the Vedic calendar, each phase of the moon is associated with certain favorable activities. There are two main phases of lunar light. The first half of the lunar month is the fifteen-day period of waxing moon, beginning with *amavasya*, the new moon (the last day of the dark half of the lunar month). It ends at *purnima*, the full moon. These are the tithis of *shukla-paksha* (the word *shukla* means "white"), which mirror the solar period of increasing light. All auspicious activities such as initiations and beginning new projects are best done here. This is the "inhale" phase of the lunar month.

The second main phase is the waning phase, beginning on purnima and flowing back to amavasya. The tithis of this half of the lunar month are *krishna-paksha* (the word *krishna* means "dark"). This is the "exhale" of the cycle, a good time for "housecleaning," completing projects, and settling any unfinished business. A naturally inward-moving time of increasing darkness, it is also a time to conserve energy.

The following lunar mandala shows the essence of the general effects of the lunar tithis in eight phases that mirror the solar cycles, which we will delve into a little further on: initiation, fruition, death, and renewal. Included are suggestions for working with each phase for optimal flow.

THE CREATIVE CYCLE OF THE MOON

New Moon—amavasya—fertile darkness (day one). For sadhana, the day of the new moon is a powerful time to ignite or renew any aspect of your inner or outer life: spiritual study, relationship bonds, creative projects. This is a good time to clear the space to plant seeds for the next creative cycle.

First Quarter Moon—(days one to three)

Crescent Moon—light emerging—the germinating seed (days three to seven)

Half Moon—waxing energy—building the organic structure for what was planted to emerge (days seven to fourteen)

Full Moon—peak creativity and fulfillment (day fourteen)

Waning Moon—krishna—harvesting the fruits (days fifteen to nineteen). Moon rises in mid-evening and sets in midmorning.

Third Quarter Moon—light and dark in balance, with darkness increasing (days nineteen to twenty-three). The moon rises at midnight and sets at noon. As the last waning cycle begins, it is a good time to focus on completing creative projects.

Balsamic Moon—completion, and processing the shadow (from day twenty-three until the new moon). This is a time to release, compost, and integrate any shadow work that is arising before the next lunar-month cycle begins. This is the most powerful phase for personal retreat time to digest and understand the wisdom gained through the last cycle, to cleanse and to envision, and to set intentions for how you will enter the coming moon phase. The symbolic seed contained in the fruit of the full moon now returns to be reborn again with the new moon.

THE WOMAN'S MOON CYCLE AND THE CREATIVE JOURNEY

All of these energies associated with each phase of the moon are reflected in women's lunar cycles.

The new moon and the few days that follow are often when a woman "receives her moon" or begins menstruating. As the waxing moon moves from new moon toward crescent moon (days three to seven), a woman will feel her energy rebuilding and her creative energy begin to take focus. This is a time of "light emerging" as the womb prepares for the possibility of new life. As the waxing cycle of the moon continues into half moon (days seven to fourteen), light is balanced with darkness. A woman's energy begins to shift with the coming ovulation, and she feels more sensual and has a greater sense of beauty and luster than she did in the new-moon phase. More energy is now available for outward creative expression and for building the structures to support it.

The full moon (day fourteen) can align with a woman's ovulation. Now she is at her sexual peak, and she can feel her own radiant splendor and channel it into creative powers. The fullness of the moon is mirrored by the flowering or ripening of her creative fruit.

The waning-moon phase (days fifteen to nineteen) is a time for inner cleansing and to gather energy. The tended plant flowers and then passes its peak, and this is mirrored in the womb. The unfertilized egg creates a hormonal shift that can generate a subtle sense of "grieving" for the life that did not arise, especially at midevening when the moon rises and when it sets at midmorning. This is the most potent time for moving inward.

The third quarter moon (days nineteen to twenty-three) is a turning point when most women begin to feel a tugging inward to process the "dark" or shadow aspects of their inner landscape, their home life, and the world around them. The dark increases and gives way to a "composting" of whatever needs to be released or returned to the earth, the Great Mother. As the moon continues to wane during the balsamic moon (from day twenty-three until the new moon), the creative cycle for women continues inward with a sense of "moving into the temple," or the womb.

Sometimes a woman is opposite the cycles, having her moon cycle linked with ovulating on the new moon and menstruating on the full moon. Here the opposite can work in polar balance—relaxing on the full moon and revving up with the new moon. Moonbathing is one of the recommendations for women with a wavering moon cycle, along with herbs, nutrition, and lifestyle changes as ways for a women's body to re-synchronize with the lunar light.

The rhythms and energies of the doshas are also found in a woman's lunar cycle, providing a beautiful way to go with the flow and, along with food and herbs, heal any premenstrual stress and imbalances.

DAYS OF BLOOD FLOW—VATA PHASE

Follow a vata-balancing lifestyle during this time that is grounding. Stay at home, rest, and save "solar activating" practices for after your blood flow ends.

END OF FLOW TO OVULATION— KAPHA PHASE

This is the best time in the month to follow an ojas-cultivating mode of practice, and the period in which a woman feels her solar power.

FROM OVULATION TO BEGINNING OF FLOW—PITTA PHASE

This is the best time of the month to balance pitta through calming, grounding, and excessive-fire-balancing practices.

BEING A MOON QUEEN

In many parts of the world, a woman on her moon cycle does not do any housework or cooking or any active, pingala nadi types of activities. In places such as Kerala, India, which has a strong reverence for the goddess and ayurvedic practices, a woman is honored during her moon cycle and is allowed to rest completely. Ideally, premenstrually and on your moon cycle, it is good to reduce your solar activity as much as possible and to even completely go within, particularly avoiding activities that aggravate vata and pitta, like computers and phone calls, travel, overstimulation, imbalanced food choices, or anything you find stressful. Follow the lunar cycle and gradually begin to pull inward as you become closer to your cycle, taking time to enjoy a lunar retreat for as long as you can, particularly on the first day of your cycle. Take up to three days of retreat and meditation practices to restore your natural essence.

MEN'S MOON CYCLE

I have come to observe through life, love, and anecdotal conversations that men have their own equivalent to a woman's "moon cycle" that is related to the release of their seed.

Within the theory of ayurveda, men's *shukra*, or seminal fluid, is the energetic equivalent to women's *pushpa*—the blood of their womb as well as female sexual fluid (also shukra). These fluids are distilled through many days of work from foods and liquids to become precious life-creating substances.

Although semen is created daily (eighty-five million sperm per day per testicle), it takes seventy-two to ninety days to develop mature sperm.[8]

Leaving aside the many theories and practices about men withholding and releasing their seed—which is really very individual, seasonal, constitutional, and unique to every man—there is a wonderful period of absolute lunar, yin, receptive, relaxed, content, open, loving space that men enter into after lovemaking that is wonderful for women to relax into and honor in men. For those precious few hours to a few days, men can be adored as "Moon Kings" too, just as the "Moon Queens" are to be respected and nurtured.

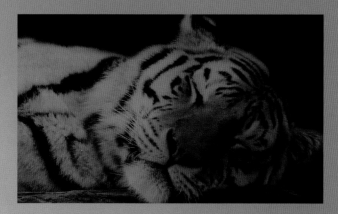

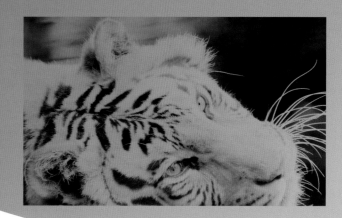

rhythms of love—
the balancing of ida and pingala
nadis for men and women

The union of moon and lotus
is by the act of Divine Love alone.
Where there is real passion
There is Divine Love.

— SONG OF BHAVA[9]

For men and women who are in a relationship, harmonizing your changing rhythms is an important aspect of the relationship, creating greater flow, more balance, and closer bonding. Amid the fluctuating rhythms and constant demands of householder life, particularly when you have children, the Heart Fire of your partnerships can easily waver. By becoming aware of the solar and lunar dynamics at work within the relationship, including when each partner goes into ida nadi (the inward-moving current) and pingala nadi (the outward-moving current), you can learn to respect each other's natural way. When men and women honor ida nadi within each other and within their union, a harmonization of solar and lunar rhythms takes place that can significantly reduce tension and stress among all family members. The entire household benefits by honoring the moon cycles, including children and teenagers, who naturally savor their "down time" to play and relax.

Communicate with your partner when you feel yourself shifting into ida nadi—whenever you're naturally recovering your life force, whether it's at the end of a long work day or in the quiet, inward times of the lunar cycle. Find your own way to communicate this to your partner. When you acknowledge your true energetic state, it allows your partner to support you, as he or she hopes to be supported when in ida nadi. Equally important is to honor the solar expression of pingala nadi: passion, adventure, and the desire to take action and manifest that arises naturally, as well as the joy of sharing and collaborating together in partnership.

TIGER TIME TOGETHER

Wherever you experience satisfaction, the very essence of bliss will be revealed to you if you remain in the place without mental wavering.

— VIJNANA BHAIRAVA TANTRA[10]

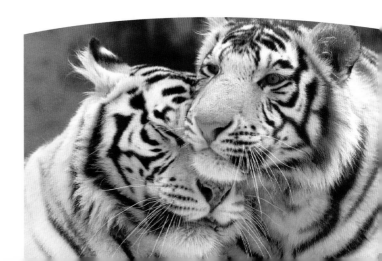

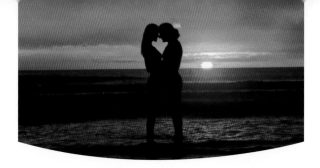

When you and your partner are both in ida nadi, this is the perfect time to bond, offer and receive affection, and enjoy the nonverbal space of hanging out together. Honor a love sadhana in the mornings and evenings when you can relax in each other's arms or massage each other for your daily abhyanga. Enjoy the nourishing power of touch. This "tiger time" of deeply surrendering your bodies to the earth and to each other is one of the great joys of life. Many busy adults pass this opportunity by, but you can reclaim it.

> It is easy to make love
> First put aside individuality
> Then you and I will fall in love
> This very lifetime.
> — SONG OF BHAVA[11]

MAKING LOVE IN ALL FORMS

Making love takes place in many forms, as our senses are vehicles for appreciating and embodying our connection to life. In a loving relationship, lovemaking takes place all day long in the form of subtle communication, tender affection, and rituals of love or sexual union. A tremendous charge is generated through lovemaking that is not just the electrical release of orgasm but literally the synchronization of rhythms together. Lovemaking, like other forms of firekeeping, generates heat and passion that melts the tension and agitation that can suddenly erupt between partners.

> At the start of union, be in the fire of
> energy released by intimate sensual pleasure.
> Let thought reside in the quivering of your
> senses like wind in the leaves and reach the
> celestial bliss of ecstatic love.
> — VIJNANA BHAIRAVA TANTRA[12]

Male and female orgasm naturally produce a cascade of oxytocin and a regenerating rhythmic entrainment between our brainwaves and our heart rhythm, creating the feeling of a downward stream of bliss that is so healing for every level of our being.

The relaxation that follows after reaching this peak is a sacred time for men to experience the healing power of ida nadi—the "lunar current" of our parasympathetic nervous system—by resting in whole-body surrender. Women's sexual release creates the same melting-into-being but is often energizing, as it is not anywhere near as "depleting of essence" as for men. Hence the rhythmic differences that can emerge post-union.

Men and women can authentically recognize the beauty of ida nadi within the *shukra-pushpa* (seed-ovum) release cycle and give that support and love to each other by creating a natural rhythm of serving the Moon King-Queen. This can be done in the smallest of ways, such as feeding your lover in bed or making him or her a special ojas tonic. (Ayurveda recommends warm almond milk with honey and cashews sprinkled on top.)

Creating space for the rhythms of love is an important art in householder life. While the tantric view of lovemaking has been exaggerated from the original tantric teachings, tantrics have always recognized the love union at the heart of creation: a union symbolized in the stories of the mother and father of the universe: Shiva and Shakti. One can be celibate and still cultivate the ability to sense their mythic dance in the divine current and rock in the natural sway and flow of love.

rtucharya—tending the fire of the seasons

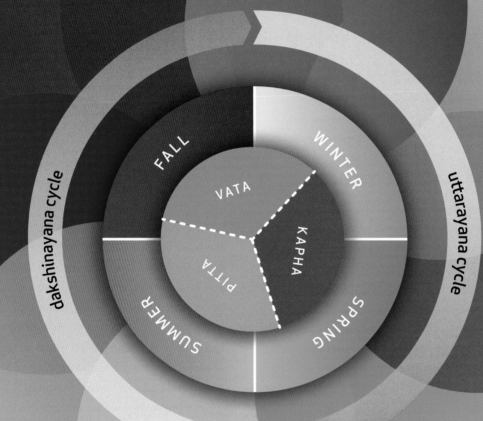

dakshinayana cycle

uttarayana cycle

FALL

WINTER

SUMMER

SPRING

VATA

KAPHA

PITTA

In ayurveda, the term *rtucharya* describes the cycle of the seasons through the year. The word is based upon the root *rtu* from the Vedic *rtam,* meaning "cosmic rhythm." In remembering the Vedas through the use of this word, we return once again to the ancient fire altars that first linked our inner rhythms with the outer cosmos. Within the great mandala of the yearly cycle, the earth completes its orbit around the sun, bringing cold and heat, dark and light to our environment, including all creatures and our own bodies. And just as the three doshas are associated with lunar cycles, we find them in the annual cycles as well.[13]

The *uttarayana,* the six-month period that begins with winter solstice, is a time for the great exuberance of life. The plant world grows from seed to fullness with the waxing light of the sun, which strengthens and intensifies until summer solstice. During the six-month *dakshinayana* cycle, after the summer peak, the sun's energy wanes and the moon's energy increases, releasing water and cooling energy back to the earth. This is vital nourishment that can also cause dampness of spirit or health that's common toward the end of the dakshinayana period of late fall, when many people are vulnerable to depression and getting sick.

WINTER

Winter can generally be divided between the vata and kapha energies. The early part of winter, marked by wind and dryness, shifts to the colder, damper aspects of winter. In this cycle it becomes important to stay in alignment with the forces of nature as we move from the lightness of fall to the heaviness of later winter, then yield to spring.

SPRING

This is a time of renewal and rebirth for all cycles, offering awakening, warmth, and growth. Kapha predominates during this time, as the forces of earth and water are strongest and exert their influence upon the earth and our bodies. Pitta emerges in later spring as the sun begins to peak.

SUMMER

This season initiates the pitta time of year, bringing heat and dryness to the wetness and heaviness of spring. The pitta principle of fire is strongest during this time of year when the sun's rays are strongest and hottest. And just as Earth is absorbing maximum solar energy at this time, so are our bodies.

FALL

The vata season of fall is marked by entropy, dryness, and decay as the harvest of the year begins. The heating energy the earth and we have absorbed slowly begins to cool. The last harvests of the year offer abundant and bright colors—red apples and trees, orange pumpkins—while inside we cultivate warmth for the coolness that is to follow. This shifting and changing creates motion, increasing the wind principle in our bodies.

SAMHAIN
NOV 1

Celebrated after the harvest

Growth Cycle: letting go—
the seed releases and
returns to the earth

WINTER SOLSTICE
(YULE) DEC 21

The rebirth of the sun and the
shortest day of the year

Growth Cycle: rebirth of the
spark of life in the seed

AUTUMN EQUINOX
(MABON) SEPT 21

Day and night are exactly
the same length

Growth Cycle: the end
of the harvest

And still, after all this time, the Sun

has never said to the Earth, *You owe me.*

Look what happens with love like that.

It lights up the sky.

— HAFIZ[16]

LAMMAS
AUG 1

The time for ripening

Growth Cycle: fruits ripen

SUMMER SOLSTICE
(LITHA) JUNE 21

The longest day of the year

Growth Cycle: the flower
opens and is fertilized

the solar cycle

**CANDLEMAS
FEB 1**

The melting and quickening

Growth Cycle: first sign of
new life as the bud emerges
from the winter branches

**SPRING EQUINOX
(OSTARA) MARCH 21**

Day and night are exactly
the same length

Growth Cycle: seedflowers/seed
comes back to life
(resurrection)

**BELTANE
MAY 1**

Flourishing and new birth

Growth Cycle: plant grows
in harmony with environment

Every day offers a new sunrise, a new start. Nature is forgiving that way. We get many opportunities through the year to renew our inner fire. As we are now a diverse and global community, both in terms of our cultural practices and our spiritual backgrounds, we have a unique opportunity at these junctures to connect with the collective ritual wisdom of the holy days of the solar vinyasa—a cycle that mirrors the moon, from the birth of new light at the beginning of the winter solstice, to the peaking of light in the summer solstice like the full moon.

OUR EXTRAORDINARY SUN

Our solar system was formed about five billion years ago from the "stellar nursery" of enormous clouds of dust and gas that were compressed by gravitational forces to give birth to our solar star.

One of three hundred billion stars of the Milky Way galaxy, the sun transforms five million tons of itself into light every second, and it emits energy that we receive some ninety-three million miles $(1.5 \times 10^8$ km) away—a continuous process of creation and dissolution.[14]

It would take one hundred trillion tons of detonated dynamite every second to match the energy produced by the sun.[15]

Through the magnificence of solar power and the process of photosynthesis, we are given the air to breathe, food to eat, and water to drink. Sunlight is indeed the divine source of prana. We are literally made of the sun, our great star.

The sun's radiant energy produces six thousand times the amount of energy used by all human beings worldwide, and it would take only .001 percent of its energy to power all of the world's current energy needs for a day.

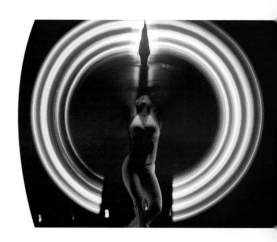

time
out of time

Sacred Retreats for
Energy Regeneration

the ritual art
of retreat

Our explorations of the many rhythms found in our bodies, our planet, and the cosmos bring us to the art of retreat—the power of the inward pull, the time in between. **Life is a ritual from sunrise to sunset every day throughout the day, time outside of time, within the pure presence of one cycle of breath.** We can experience the essence of ritual this way, following the nature of our own bodies. Human culture has developed around these timeless cycles, and the festival and retreats we have created back through time have always reflected these rhythms of nature. It is natural to honor these rhythms by pausing occasionally to regenerate, and all of nature does this: the tiger at rest on the savannah conserves her energy instinctually.

Just as we waste more energy than we actually use in the United States, we often "waste" the most precious times for experiencing heightened energy. This chapter describes the retrieval of the power of retreat—no matter who you are or what your life circumstance is. In Part Four, we will journey around an entire yearly cycle to follow the seasonal rhythms and the ritual holidays that are synched with the solstices, equinoxes, and new- and full-moon cycles. These sandhyas have been retreat periods as far back as human history and beyond.

FIVE RHYTHMS OF RETREAT

In my life and as I have led global retreats over the past twenty years, I focus on five aspects of retreat, whether I am creating a group offering or one for my own daily life. These retreat elements are sacred time, sacred space, natural ritual, spirit of sadhana, and sacred activism—the power of something positive being generated through that retreat time. Just the act of "unplugging," taking time off the technological grid every day, has positive repercussions for our energy future.

Five Flows of Retreat:

> **Sacred time**—setting an intention and setting time aside within the flow of life

> **Sacred space**—awakening to the space around you, tending your inner and outer altar

> **Natural ritual**—ways of connecting to the natural process of change

> **Spirit of sadhana**—ways of integrating practice into your retreat

> **Sacred activism**—energy Sabbaths—unplugging as a way of energy activism

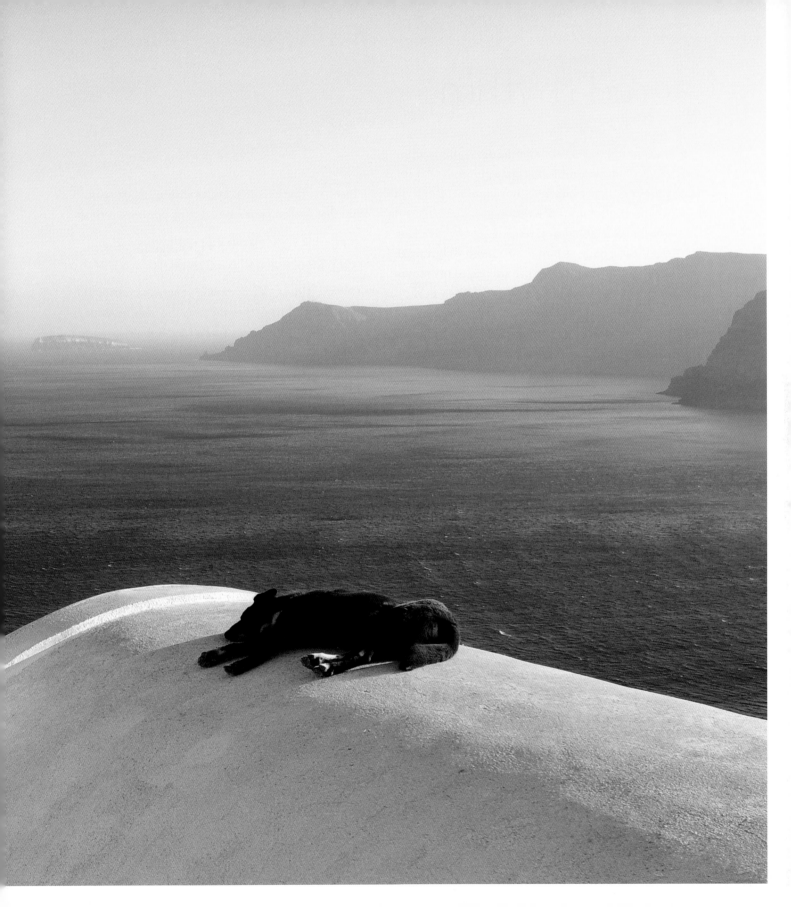

sacred rhythm

The natural waxing and waning of life offers all kinds of opportunities to create personal retreat time and allow yourself to move into harmony with whatever may be arising within you. You can create a sacred retreat at any given moment by honoring the breath, daily at sunrise or sunset, or during the cross-cultural holy days that are tied to the movements of the sun and moon through the wheel of the year. You can answer the call for retreat whenever you see auspicious signs that the time is right, or when you sense a warning that you need some regenerative time. This listening creates your intention, or your dedication, for your cycle.

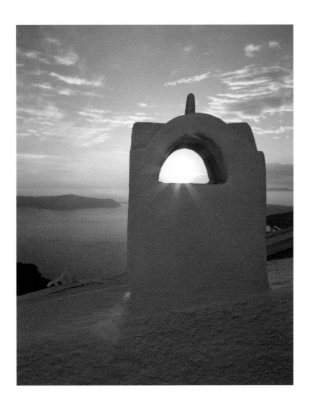

There are three natural cycles within the pulse of life that we can emphasize during our retreat times:

CYCLES OF INITIATING— RHYTHMS FOR BEGINNING ANEW

Optimal times: On an inhale; at sunrise; during the new moon; during the wheel-of-the-year festivals of winter solstice, New Year's Day, Imbolc, or spring equinox; any time you are initiating a new phase in your life, such as a project or a relationship.

CYCLES OF SUSTAINING THE PEAK—HONORING AND CELEBRATING FULLNESS

Optimal times: On an inhale retention; at noon and sunset; during the full moon; at summer solstice; during waxing solar sandhyas (spring equinox or Beltane); any time you are sustaining a challenging project in your life.

CYCLES OF LETTING GO— HONORING COMPLETION, DEATH, AND SHADOW WORK

Optimal times: On an exhale; at sunset and night-time; during the waning period three days before the new moon; at Samhain (the last six weeks of the year); any time you are completing a process or working with shadow healing, death, or letting go.

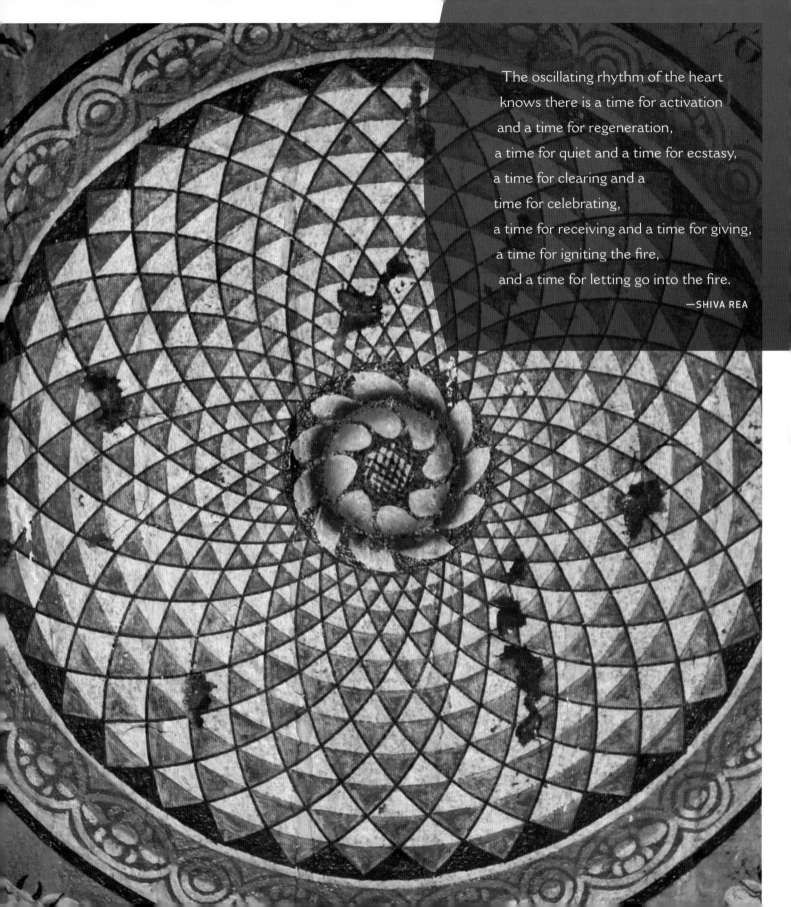

The oscillating rhythm of the heart
knows there is a time for activation
and a time for regeneration,
a time for quiet and a time for ecstasy,
a time for clearing and a
time for celebrating,
a time for receiving and a time for giving,
a time for igniting the fire,
and a time for letting go into the fire.

—SHIVA REA

sacred space—
tending your home altar

Tending your inner fire is an important aspect of cultivating the sacred space of your retreat, and this process is reflected in your home altar. Your personal altar is a great nexus—a navel that connects your inner and outer worlds—a conduit for your prayers, and a reflection of your inner space and what is stirring within your heart.

Every altar has a central focus—a primary symbol—which can take any form: an image, a sculpture, a natural object such as a stone or feather, or anything else that you find meaningful.

Throughout our lifetimes, various symbols come to us; sometimes they are given to us, sometimes we find them, and sometimes we must search for them. Often they come our way before we are fully ready to understand their meaning. So remain open to the possibilities.

Beneath this central symbol we may place an altar cloth made of any natural material of any color. We can have several of these and change them with the seasons, with the lunar cycles, or whenever it feels appropriate.

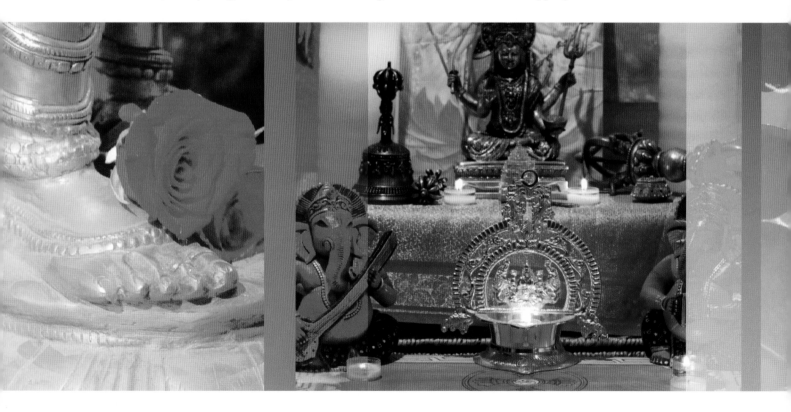

Also on the altar we often include symbols of the elements. Earth can be represented by fruit, a rice bowl, living plants, or flowers. Water can be placed in a separate bowl and changed daily, or it can serve the purpose of keeping flowers fresh in a vase. Incense is the most universal way we invoke the element of air, or feathers can be used. Space can be represented as a container or a vessel in which intentions or symbolic objects can be placed. Fire can take the form of candles or lamps—you can let your spiritual tradition be your guide.

PURIFY YOUR SACRED SPACE

Honor the sacred space of your altar by regularly cleaning and refreshing it. Before your dedicated retreat time, clear away any objects that may have served their purpose. Remove dust, wilted flowers, or ashes or wax left from burning. You may bathe sacred objects in water or dust them with a special cloth that you only use for your altar. You can do this daily or weekly; each time invoke the new beginning that is connected to this symbolic ritual of revival.

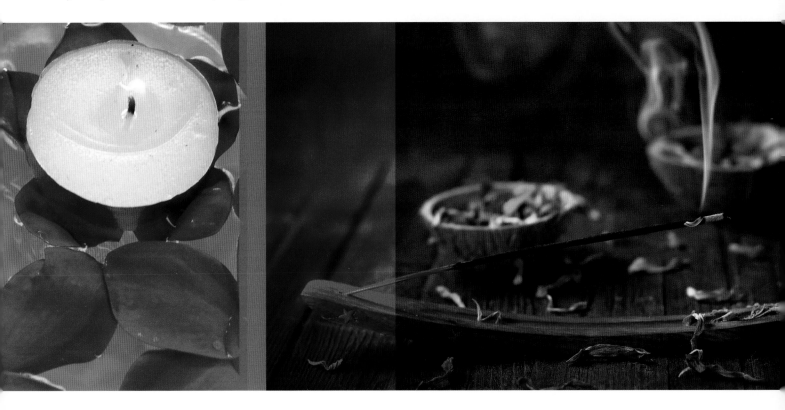

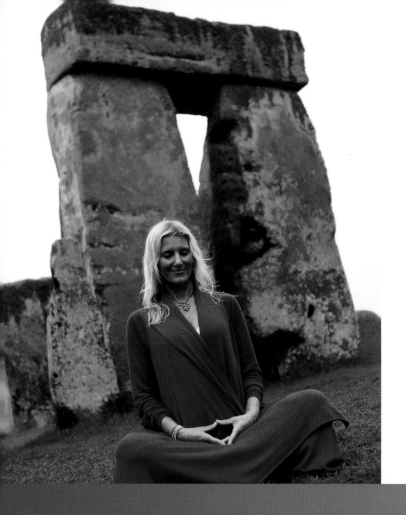

INVOKE THE MANDALA OF THE ELEMENTS AND DIRECTIONS

Invoking the elements and directions is a way to create a mandala or sacred circle for your retreat time—a universal sense of creating a sacred container that can be integrated at the beginning of your daily meditations. This ritual is found cross-culturally and in different spiritual systems, and you can do this according to your own spiritual tradition.

Various traditions associate colors with the elements and directions, and you can incorporate these into your altar. In our yearlong living yoga sadhana program, we go into depth on the changing art of one's sacred space. Here is an invocation of the sacred directions and elements that you can adapt as you wish for your own unique ritual.

THE ELEMENTS AND DIRECTIONS IN VARIOUS TRADITIONS

	NORTH	NORTHEAST	EAST	SOUTHEAST	SOUTH	SOUTHWEST	WEST	NORTHWEST
HINDU/VASTU	Green	Shades of Yellow / White	White	Silver / White	Pink/Coral Red	All Shades of Green	Blue	White
		Water		Fire		Earth		Air
CELTIC	Brown / Green		Yellow		Red		Blue	
	Earth		Air		Fire		Water	
NATIVE AMERICAN	White		Yellow		Red		Black	
	Air		Fire		Water		Earth	
VAJRAYANA BUDDHIST	Green		Blue		Gold/Yellow		Red	
	Air		Water		Earth		Fire	
TAOIST — FENG SHUI	Blue / Black	Beige / Light Yellow	Brown / Green	Brown / Green	Red / Orange / Purple	Beige / Light Yellow	White / Gray	White / Gray
	Water	Earth	Wood	Wood	Fire	Earth	Metal	Metal

INVOKING THE MANDALA OF ELEMENT AND DIRECTIONS

> To begin, upon the threshold of your invocation, face toward the east, and affirm your intention to call upon the elements and directions.

> Stand or sit and connect to your heart center. Now, turning your body to face each direction, gaze as far as you can toward each point, embracing all and emanating from your heart. You can honor the four cardinal directions, all eight directions, or all of these, including the directions of above and below as well.

> For a simple invocation, you could sprinkle water or light sacred herbs such as sage, copal, or incense and silently turn and honor each direction. You can also offer the mantra *Om, Om Shanti* (peace), or *Hum Phat* from the Yoga tradition to

each direction. In the Celtic tradition, you might repeat a prayer while facing each direction: "May there be peace in the east," "May there be peace in the south." Make your invocation for each direction and the element connected to that direction, using any words, prayers, sounds, or thoughts you like to welcome that direction and element into your mandala. Continue to the south, west, north, and finally above and below. As you turn in each direction, allow your gaze to extend as far as you can envision, encompassing all of creation, people, and nature.

> Now, with the directions and elements encircling and permeating your space, engage in any practice of your choosing, feeling the power of ritual space.

> At the end of your practice dissolve the mandala by bringing everything back to your heart.

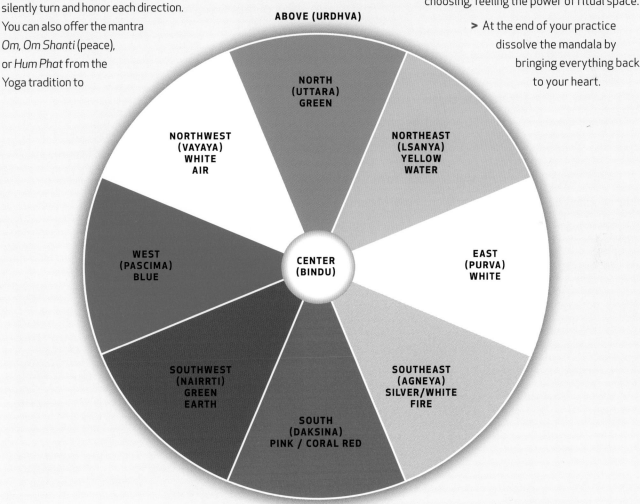

ABOVE (URDHVA)

NORTH
(UTTARA)
GREEN

NORTHWEST
(VAYAYA)
WHITE
AIR

NORTHEAST
(LSANYA)
YELLOW
WATER

WEST
(PASCIMA)
BLUE

CENTER
(BINDU)

EAST
(PURVA)
WHITE

SOUTHWEST
(NAIRRTI)
GREEN
EARTH

SOUTHEAST
(AGNEYA)
SILVER/WHITE
FIRE

SOUTH
(DAKSINA)
PINK / CORAL RED

BELOW (ADHO)

MY FIRST GOURD ALTAR

One evening I was driving home from teaching yoga, singing along with some lively kirtan that I had playing on the stereo. I entered an intersection where the light had just turned green and—BAM!—something smashed into the driver's side of my little Honda. The next thing I knew, blood was pouring down my face and my legs were pinned to the center console by the crumpled door. I hadn't seen the other car coming, so I had no fear hormones swirling in my body; it was simply that one moment I was singing and the next I was covered in blood. Time unwound as people came to help me. Everyone around me seemed like bodhisattvas or angels—I especially remember the fireman who helped me get loose and onto a stretcher.

After three days in the hospital unable to move, I was sent home to heal my broken pelvis. Myself. By being still. There is no way, it turns out, to put a pelvis in a cast. If your pelvis is broken, you may not walk for a week, and your return to full movement will take months.

At the time this happened, I was twenty-seven and a third-series Ashtanga practitioner doing intensive asana practice two hours a day, six days a week. Now, suddenly, I could move only my toes and my upper body.

This is how I learned the power of mudra vinyasa. I found that despite my immobility, I could support the reknitting of my bones through positive and benevolent coaxing, using my breath and the immense circulatory energy of the Heart Fire. Drawing on the power of the subtle, loving movement of breath and pulse, day after day—and with the help of my husband's herbs—I made the transition from feeling great pain and weakness with even the tiniest of movements to enjoying a full range of motion and a stable base.

This intuitive awakening of prana yoga gave birth to the movement art form I now teach, as I literally embodied the rebirth that follows a death or an initiation. In this case, it was my muladhara chakra that was being reborn.

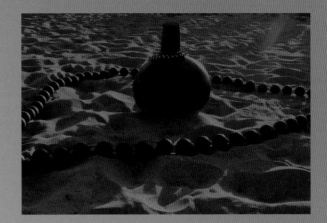

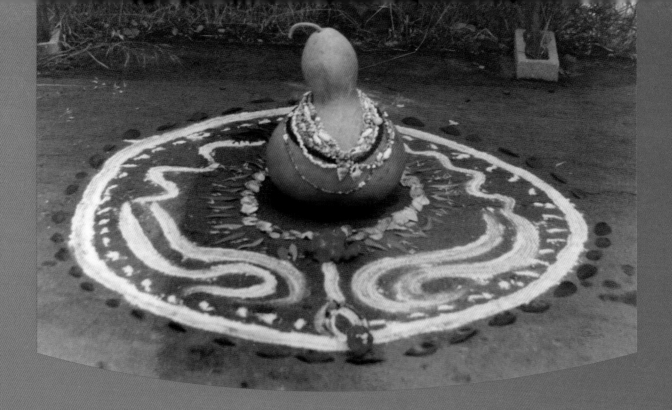

While I recovered, I was drawn to placing on my altar beautiful gourds that people brought to me from the farmer's market. These were primordial, voluptuous Great Mother shapes, wombs holding the space for my rebirth. With so much time spent in stillness—I moved very little for a month—I went deep into the fertility of soul healing, creating not only a new body but a new life. I felt a vastly more subtle connection to my own living energy and found the emergence of new forms within the limitless creativity of yoga. And I experienced a transformation from pain and immobility to the flowering of a new body.

Gourds—with their feminine shapes and in their array of bold and subtle colors—became the anchors of my altar, symbols of an organic connection to my reemerging life force and a new life.

the spirit of offering: puja—natural rituals to integrate into your retreat

A puja is a heartfelt offering. There are probably an infinite number of ways to make a puja, and even if you always follow the same steps, it will have a different quality or feeling each time. The following twelve-step puja is a method of altar care that can be practiced in the flow of yoga based upon the guidance of Sreedevi Bringi, and includes many beautiful elements. You can choose to complete all twelve steps or do a shorter form that stops after step five, at which point you can begin meditation or another practice.

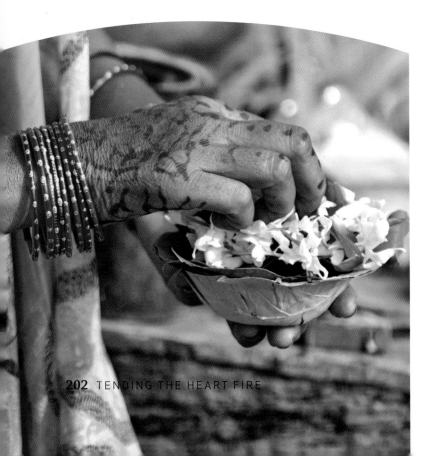

STAGES OF A PUJA OFFERING

Krama One—renew yourself and sacred space—*atma shuddhi*—purification of the soul

Before you begin your puja, take a bath or splash water on your face and change into fresh clothes. Clean and refresh your altar space so that everything is vital and alive. Chant *Om* for three rounds and offer a prostration to become connected to your heart. Then offer this mantra, sipping water from your right palm after each repetition:

> *Chant* Om *three rounds and then* Om *achutaya namah, Om anantaya namah, Om govindaya namah*
>
> *I honor the Divine, the Infinite Divine, and the Source of the Senses*

Krama Two—balance and purify your energy field through your breath—*nadi shodhana pranayama*

> *Do three or seven rounds of alternate-nostril breathing (nadi shodhana pranayama).*

Krama Three—invoke your puja

You can invoke your puja and connect to your outer and inner altars using any of the meditation practices from Part Two, such as the invocation of *Om* with mudra or the use of a mantra or the mandala invocation. Across yoga traditions, the auspicious current embodied in the energy of Ganesha is often the focus of the invocation step; he is revered as the remover of all vibrational dissonance and obstacles on the path.

Recite Om gam ganapataye namah
to invoke the auspicious current.

Krama Four—offer your intention, or *samkalpa*

Every time you enter into ritual space is an opportunity to declare and affirm your intention for this sacred time. This can be a simple connection to the living sacred or a specific dedication or samkalpa for a ritual period.

Bring your hands together with your left palm placed on top of the right for samkalpa mudra.

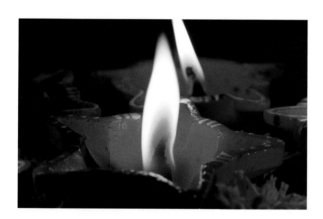

Krama Five—ignite your altar

Offer a prayer as you light your candle (use a non-polluting kind such as soy or beeswax) or oil lamp (containing pure oils or ghee), with reverence for the fire element and the fiery flow of consciousness. You can:

Offer the mantra Om dipayai namah *or offer your own prayer as you light the flame.*

You can end your puja ritual here if you like and move directly to mantra japa or meditation, or to your closing prayer. If you choose to continue, the following stages of the puja will allow a deepening connection to the Heart Fire.[3]

Krama Six—honor the Divine Self within—*atmapuja*

Embody the art of nyasa (touch with awareness and mantra). You can use your touch by itself or with healing herbal powders such as sandalwood, sacred ash from a ritual fire (*vibhuti*), red turmeric powder (*kumkum*), or essential oils. You can touch your heart, throat, third eye, and then crown of the head, accompanied by your own prayer or with the mantras that follow. Pause and connect to each part of the body with the mantra, meaning, and intention of deep communion. For the last nyasa, you can also offer a flower with reverence for the Supreme Self within you:

Om Atmane Namah
 Touch heart: I honor/bow to/realize the Divine Self (atma)

Om Antaratmane Namah
 Touch throat: I honor/bow to/realize the Divine Self (atma) existing within all (antar)

Om Jnanatmane Namah
 Touch third eye: I honor/bow to/realize the Wisdom (jnana) Self (atma) within

Om Paramatmane Namah
 Touch top of head: I honor/bow to/realize the Self (atma) beyond all conceptions (para)

Om Atmapuja Samarpayami
 Place a flower on top of your head: I worship and love with devotion the Divine Self within

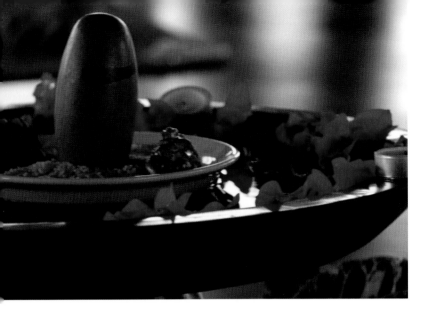

THE SPIRIT OF OFFERING IN PUJA

Krama Seven—offer water (*achamaniyam*)

In this practice, you offer a spoonful of water to your central altar image or just to the heavens, and then while sipping the water recite the mantra and visualize yourself being nourished by the sublime flow of love.

Offer the mantra Om namaha achamaniyam samarpayami *while sipping water.*

Krama Eight—offer flowers (*pushpanjali*)

The offering of flowers or leaves or any living substance is an intrinsic conduit of the heart. You can change the flowers you offer with the season. I often use fresh wildflowers from the nearby hillside. It is the heart exchange that matters, which can also be just within one's mind, with the most extraordinary flowers referred to as the highest offering from one's heartmind (*manaspuja*).

Offer flowers or flower petals from your heart with a prayer or a mantra of your chosen ishta devata.

Krama Nine—offer food (*naivedyam*)

Sprinkle water upon your food offering (*prasad*) of fruit, rice grains, or a prepared dish, and chant the following mantras, honoring the movement of life (*prana*) that is manifested from food. This is a wonderful mantra to say before a meal as well, while visualizing the movement of prana through your body.

Chant the movements of life as you offer fruit or food.
Om pranaye swaha: *I honor the in-drawing, rising energy within all creation*
Om apanaye swaha: *I honor the downward, rooting flow within all creation*
Om samanaye swaha: *I honor the energy that contracts to the core within all creation*
Om vyanaye swaha: *I honor the energy that expands omnidirectionally from the core within all creation*
Om udanaye swaha: *I honor the energy that rises and moves outward within all creation*

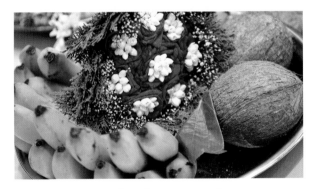

Krama Ten—awaken heart consciousness (*hridaya nyasa*)

Place your right hand in *tattwa mudra* (touching the thumb to the base of the ring finger) and place it over your heart. Gaze into your heart and combine mantra and touch as a form of hridaya nyasa.

Offer the mantra Om aim hridayaya namah: *I bow to the sacred Self in the heart chakra.*

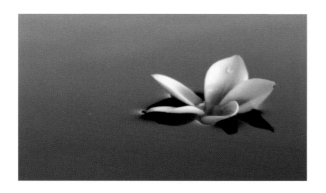

Krama Eleven—make offerings through meditation, or mantra japa

Now, here within the sacred ritual rhythm and space of the puja, you can enter meditation, including mantra connected to your seasonal sadhana and what is arising from within your heart or dedicated practices. You may also offer something from your altar to your heart—a flower or some rice—with each repetition of the mantra; if you have an image on your altar that symbolizes a deity, a teacher, or an ancestor whom you wish to honor, you may offer flowers or rice to this symbol instead. Remember that offerings can come in all forms, from the pure vibrational substance of feelings and intentions, to the universal altar materials of flowers, rice, incense, fruit, and nectars (holy water, milk, or honey). Also remember that all outer offerings are also inner offerings.

You can release difficulties as offerings as well. Offer challenging states of being, thoughts, emotions, objects symbolizing life challenges, sour-hot fruits such as lemons or chili peppers, or written prayers for letting go. These are equally beautiful offerings because they represent the full spectrum of life.

Rest in meditation or offer the mantra of your choosing for nine, eighteen, twenty-seven, fifty-four, or 108 rounds in full connection to your heart.

Krama Twelve—offer light, or arati, with mantra, kirtan, or prayers

There are many ways to end your puja. One firekeeping way within yoga and many spiritual traditions is to wave your candle or lamp above and around your altar in an offering of light—a ritual called arati. Chant a mantra, sing or make joyful music (kirtan), or pray. All of these are ways to celebrate the time you have dedicated to communion with your Heart Fire as you draw your puja to a close.

Offer the light, or arati, with Om *or a mantra, kirtan, or prayer such as* lokha samastaha sukihinoh bhavantu *or* Om shanti, shanti, shanti—Om *peace, peace, peace.*

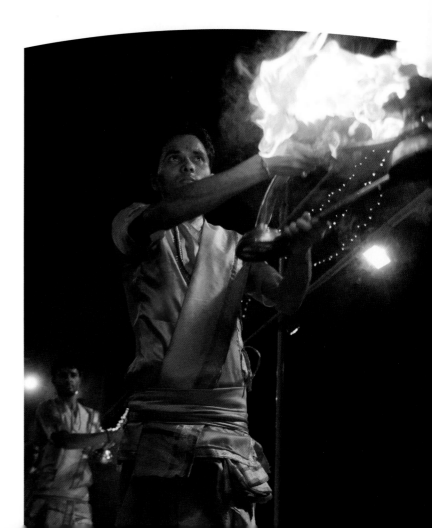

practice offering a yoga mala: 108 surya namaskar or sun salutations

THE POWER OF 108

The number 108 has long been considered sacred in yoga and many other spiritual traditions around the world. Roger Boese explains: "Renowned mathematicians of Vedic culture viewed 108 as a number representing the wholeness of existence. This number also connects the sun, the moon, and the earth: the **average distance of the sun and the moon from the earth is 108 times the sun's and moon's respective diameters.** Such phenomena have given rise to many examples of ritual significance."[4]

There are 108 chapters of the Rig Veda, 108 Upanishads, and 108 primary Tantras; 108 *marma* points, or sacred places of the body; 108 classic dance postures. There are even 108 steps leading to the Devi Chamundi Hill in Mysore, India.

In 2007, the Global Mala Project was started as a way to bring people around the world together to work with the collective heart field by synchronizing breath, intention, and global awareness in yoga practice connected to 108 (from surya namaskar, to mantra japa), to raise consciousness and funds for good causes. It has since traveled around the world through more than fifty countries and continues every year on the United Nations' International Day of Peace, which takes place around the fall equinox, and at any time ritual activation is needed.

The Source of Love shines in the heart of all.
Seeing one in all creatures
the wise forget themselves in the service of all.
The world is their joy, the One is their refuge;
such as they are lovers of the One.

— MUNDAKA UPANISHADS[5]

Offering a collective yoga mala practice is a powerful experience of heart entrainment as people move together for eighteen to 108 rounds of collective movement around the breath pulse we all share. Empower yourself in your own practice first, on ritual holidays, before leading a group.

Krama One—create a sacred space for your practice

If possible, bring everyone into a mandala circle to practice around a community altar. The circle empowers the community and is symbolic of a mala, but not all spaces lend themselves to a circle. If yours does not, don't let this deter you.

Krama Two—create mala counters

Create two bowls to count from. In Bowl One, place twenty-seven seeds, and leave Bowl Two empty. Every time you go into a forward bend, put one seed into the empty bowl. If you choose to do the full 108 rounds, then reverse, taking seeds from Bowl Two and placing them into Bowl One. After four cycles you will have reached 108.

Krama Three—introduce the yoga mala

Unify the group by chanting an invocation of *Om* or by chanting a mantra. Some communities may want to include a talking circle in which everyone has the opportunity to offer a dedication before you begin. Allow the first three rounds of the mala to be about getting everyone in synch around the power of their breath.

Krama Four—offer dedications and rounds of the mala

This step is done during the first position of the namaskar when the hands are placed in front of the heart in anjali mudra. Open your inner ears and listen to your heart teacher—an offering of a dedication will emerge spontaneously as a revelation. Meditate on this dedication as you move with your breath in heart-brain synchronization. Circulate this dedication through the whole round of the namaskar until your hands return back to your heart for the next round.

You can offer the complete mala of 108 namaskars in four rounds of twenty-seven, or six rounds of eighteen. Over the past twenty years, I have adapted a four-round process that moves from the microcosm within outward to the Source.

> **Round One**—Dedications for personal transformation and realization. This round is for you: prayers for your own personal activation, healing, and fertilization, and for the manifestation of the potency of your life.

> **Round Two**—Dedications for family, friends, and "precious jewels" (anyone you have an unresolved conflict with).

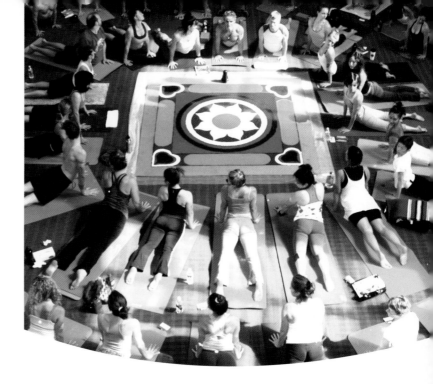

> **Round Three**—Dedications for the world. This is the bodhisattva round in which we pray for what we care about in the world and actively participate in transforming the world, whether we want to end war or global warming, to focus on healing of a disease, or to serve our own community's local needs. This is a very powerful round.

> **Round Four**—Dedications to the Source. This is a moving prayer that can be filled with nonverbal praise, gratitude, and joy for your feeling-connection to the Source.

When all four rounds are complete, move into shavasana (relaxation) and meditation. Read sacred texts or poetry aloud if you wish. Complete your yoga mala with a closing heart mandala dedication and the mantra *Om shanti, shanti, shanti,* and bathe in the radiance and empowerment of this practice.

energy sabbaths—
unplugging as sacred activism

Sacred Activism is a term, teaching, and approach coined by Andrew Harvey and refers to how we can align our actions with our heart, particularly in addressing any issues of the times. Global warming is one issue that has no borders, as everyone is "downwind" from someone else and toxic energy affects the soil, water, air, and ozone layer of all beings on planet Earth. Becoming conscious of your energy use so you can transform any toxic or unconscious energy usage in your home, workplace, and beyond is one of the simplest and most positive actions that everybody on the planet can take.

ENERGY SABBATH—DOING NOTHING TO DO SOMETHING

It is possible that our ancestors understood that "doing nothing can be doing something"—the universal teaching that being is a form of acting, that repose and reflection are often the best course of action. Our last section offers the "Mandala of the Year." The twenty-six new and full moons, eight solar festivals, and sunrise-sunset daily and weekly rhythms are potent times to unplug, tend your energy, and listen deeply to your heart.

These sandhyas are the rhythmic legacy of our ancestors that often involve returning to natural light outdoors, creating bonfires, special lighting of candles, and letting go of work life and interruptions from the outside world. This rhythm of

retreat—referred to as the Sabbath in Western spiritual culture—offers a new form of sacred activism, a kind of energy activism that can be offered to the transformation of our energy future that must happen within our lifetime. It must happen now because today we are wasting more energy than we create, and the toxic forms of that energy are destroying our environment and hurling us into the throes of climate change.

Even though our ancestors used carbon-releasing fuel to tend a living fire, it is nothing compared to the waste of energy we have today.

We are actually wasting 54 percent of the energy we create—throwing away more than we use.[6] This is perhaps the price of the ease of electricity: we are no longer gathering wood and valuing our resources. We must stop wasting our outer energy just as we must learn to cultivate and honor our own life-energy. This loss is a disconnection from the rhythms of nature and a split between our brain and heart, our being and nature, that we can all feel and observe within ourselves and in the world.

THE POWER OF UNPLUGGING

Central to an energy Sabbath or energy activism is unplugging—turning off electronics for a set period to create a ritual container free of distractions. This is an offering not only to saving and being more conscious of our energy intake—in the way that fasting attunes us to being more conscious of our food choices—but also toward restoring our own inner energy, which is continually pulled in many ojas-depleting directions.

One can commit to taking an energy Sabbath for three to twenty-four hours (sundown to sunrise, sunrise to sunrise, or sundown to sundown), or longer periods any day, or in synch with the special retreat days already aligned with the solar/lunar rhythms that Part Four of this book honors. In addition, one can take care of one's waste and be conscious of water use, not as an austerity but as a waking up and a reclaiming of our home as the foundation for our firekeeping—the essence of living our energetic heart by caring for the energy we circulate.

SOME ENCOURAGEMENTS:

> Turn off and unplug all electronics and appliances (except the refrigerator)

> Take a technology fast—let your family and friends know in advance

> Take time for yourself or gather with your loved ones, family, and friends in creative and rejuvenating ways

> Use ghee lamps, soy or beeswax candles, or solar-charged lamps for necessary light—create light from natural sources

> Create meals that use less processing and fuel to cook

> Go for zero or as little waste as possible

> Reduce packaging—cook with whole, organic foods

> Park your car—ride your bike or walk

> Reduce water consumption: flush one less time and/or cut two to six minutes off your shower

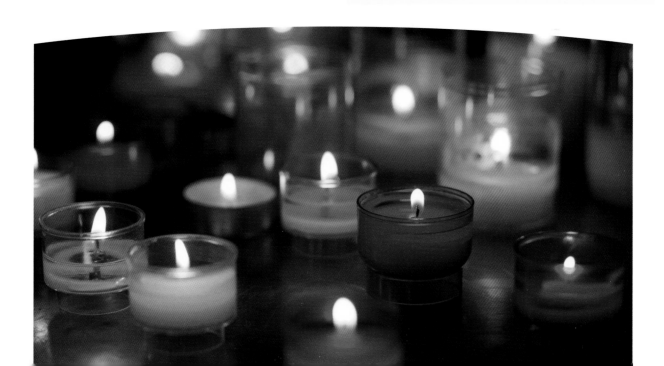

living vinyasa

The Solar-Lunar Mandala of the Year

WINTER SOLSTICE

Life is the Shrine,
the Journey and the Way.
—BAUL SONG[1]

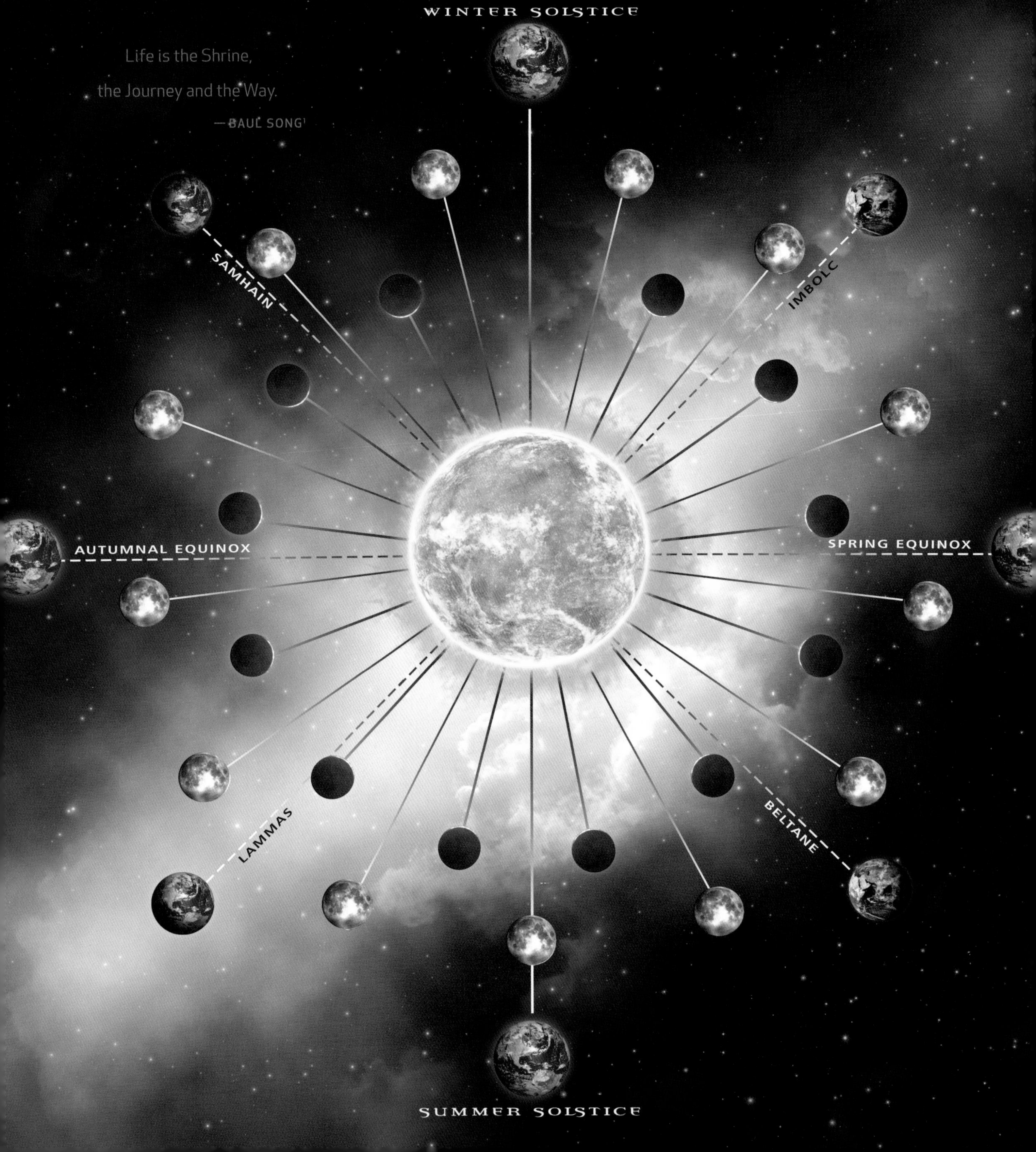

SAMHAIN

IMBOLC

AUTUMNAL EQUINOX

SPRING EQUINOX

LAMMAS

BELTANE

SUMMER SOLSTICE

The center of the mandala is the bindu, or human heart, that connects with the heart center of our solar system, galaxy, and all the universe. Contemplate the mind-blowing journey that is before us all: your circumambulation around the great fire of the sun. From where you are now in time and space, know that after 7,884,000 breaths, 365 sunrises and sunsets, 26 new and full moons, and the many changes the shifting seasons of the year will bring, you will return to the turning point of the year as a different person.

Part Four is an invitation to take this journey with full awareness of each sacred juncture of the year so that you may live vinyasa in harmony with the solar and lunar rhythms. This new calendar, the Solar-Lunar Mandala of the Year, is designed to help you envision your journey around the sun in tandem with the cycles of the moon and to synchronize your own rhythms with the many holy days that are celebrated worldwide at new and full moons and at potent solar junctures of the year.

Your journey will begin at the nadir of the year, in the fertile darkness of the winter solstice. From there it will flow around the sun and the moon through the eight cross-quarter festivals, equinoxes, and solstices (represented by the earth in eight stations around the sun). Whenever you look at this mandala or sacred wheel of the year, try to visualize this journey you are taking. What phase are you in in the flow of this journey?

All the hemispheres in existence

Lie beside an equator

In your heart….

the Great Circle inside of You

— HAFIZ[2]

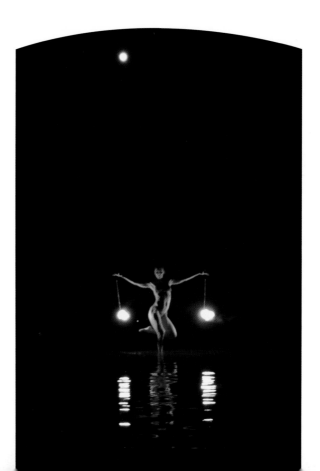

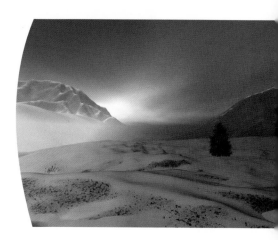

winter solstice

Rebirth of Light

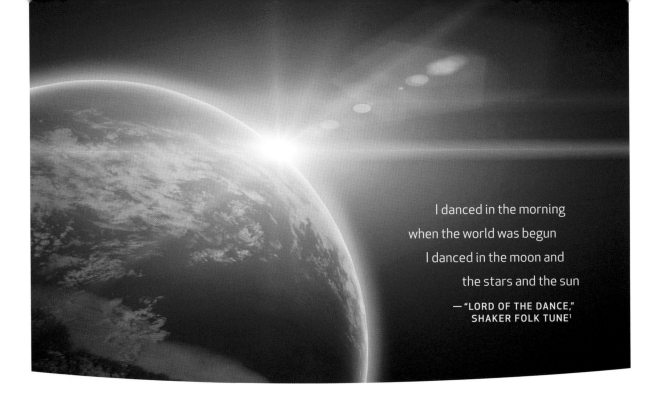

I danced in the morning
when the world was begun
I danced in the moon and
the stars and the sun

—"LORD OF THE DANCE,"
SHAKER FOLK TUNE[1]

At winter solstice, the darkest point of the year, light begins its journey of reemergence. This great cosmological rhythm sets our internal clocks, our biorhythms, to the subtle flow of slowly increasing light. In our spiritual and creative process, we begin our own gradual awakening and reemergence from the dark, fertile soil of winter.

This biological and spiritual *attunement to light* is what has made the many cosmological temples, with their ritual periods of connection to the sun, so powerful through the ages.

Can you imagine the impact of the winter solstice less than a hundred years ago when we lived life primarily in natural light? At the nadir of the year, we were sustained by the living fire of candlelight and by bonfires when, in some places in the world such as Scandinavia, a day might consist of as much as twenty-three hours of darkness. And we were sustained by celebration—the twelve-day festival of yule and other rituals of its kind—in which we came together and made merry and honored the promise of the lengthening days ahead.

We have marked the all-important sadhya of winter solstice, the rebirth of the sun, with the literal birth of a son. Myths about the return of the sun king at this time of year have been recorded as far back as ancient Sumeria and Egypt. The birth of Christ and of the Lord of the Dance of the seasons reflect an extraordinary diversity of winter solstice holidays that celebrate the rebirth of the light through the mirror of human birth. In fact, there are more cross-cultural celebrations at this point in the wheel of the year than at any other time—from Scotland to China, from Tibet to Antarctica—as we turn to one another for comfort, solace, and the shared joy that comes from bonding together to celebrate the return of the light.

at the point of greatest darkness, the sun-son is reborn

The winter solstice ceremony of the druid tradition is Alban Arthan: "the light of Arthur." In this ritual, the sun god dies and is reborn as the Celtic "son of Light."[2] Ancient ritual sites such as Stonehenge and Newgrange align with the sunrise on this shortest day of the year. Contemporary ceremonies under the open sky or around symbolic altars echo these ancient ceremonies, aligning our bodies with the cosmic rhythm.

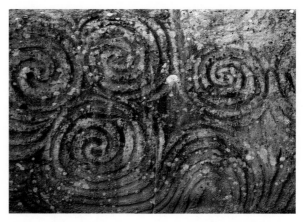

In Newgrange, Ireland, the spiral at the end of the central chamber lights up with a shaft of the winter solstice sunrise.

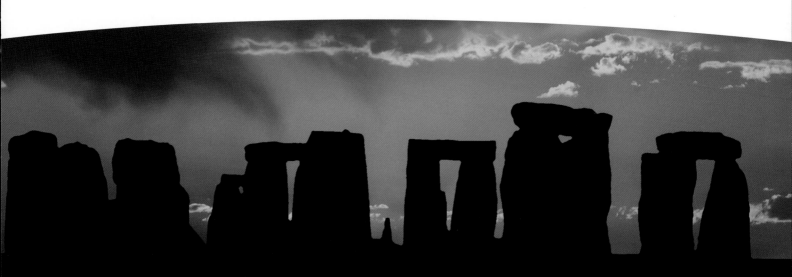

The Winter Solstice ceremony begins in darkness, mirroring the fertile darkness covering the earth. At Stonehenge, the departing winter sun sets through the southwest stone trilithon structure and is reborn through the southeast trilithon.

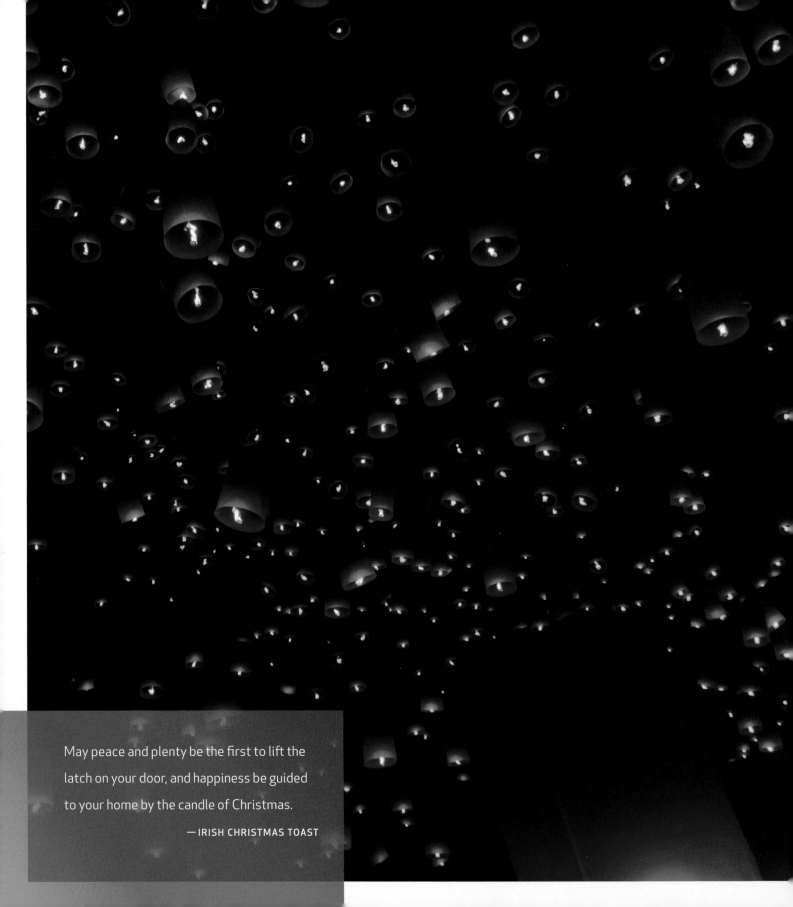

May peace and plenty be the first to lift the latch on your door, and happiness be guided to your home by the candle of Christmas.

— IRISH CHRISTMAS TOAST

YULETIDE

Yuletide is memorably described in the song "The Twelve Days of Christmas." The word *yule* means "wheel," and these twelve days are a ritual period set aside to celebrate the birth of the Son as Christ at a key turning point on the wheel of the year, a wheel symbolized by the sun in the center of our Solar-Lunar Mandala.

There is an unbroken stream of ritual and celebration connected with Christmas that dates back thousands of years, yet many of us are unaware that these traditions are so old. From the time of the Roman emperors through Martin Luther and Puritan culture, the merrymaking of the season and the bonds with the evergreen trees and all the old ways were nearly extinguished. Where they survived, they had often been reduced to shorter festivals. But we can view all of the holidays from December 21 through January 1—winter solstice, Christmas, and the New Year—as a continuum marking this period of turning of the solar yule.

Good health, every day, whether I see you or not!
May your cup overflow with health and happiness.
May all your days be happy ones. We dance a jig
for a Merry Christmas and a Happy New Year!

— GAELIC CHRISTMAS BLESSING[4]

Nollaig Faoi Shean Is Faoi Mhaise Dhuit

Knoll-ig f'wee haan iss f'wee shun-ah g-with

"A Christmas of Happiness and Joy to you"

— OLD IRISH SAYING[5]

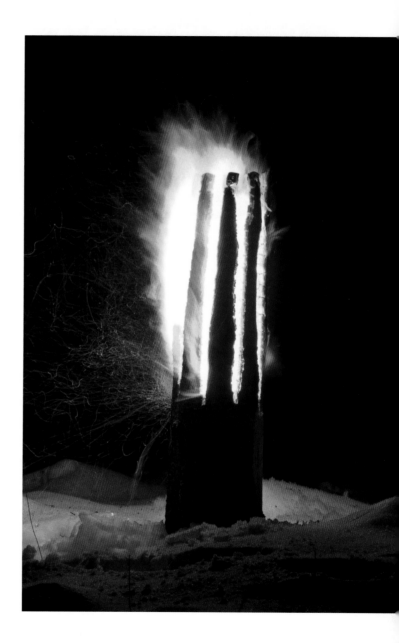

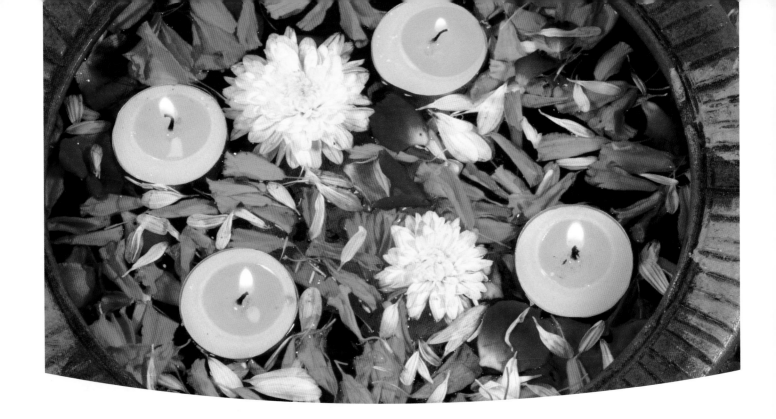

MAKAR SANKRANTI—REBIRTH OF THE UTTARAYANA CYCLE

The Hindu tantric calendar begins on January 14 with *makar sankranti,* a time of honoring the emerging light. This day marks the shift into waxing light—the six-month journey of increasing solar energy—considered auspicious for creativity, growth, and all kinds of sacred manifestations. The Sanskrit *sankranti* refers to the transit of the sun from one sign of the Indian zodiac (one *rashi*) to another, such as the movement of the sun from *dhanu rashi* (Sagittarius) to *makara rashi* (Capricorn). All over India on makar sankranti, the sun is celebrated with fire rituals, festivities, and feasts as an invocation of the kindling of enlightenment, prosperity, and happiness during the six months

of growing light. Makar Sankranti has lots of variations to celebrate this growing season, from honoring and ritually decorating cows for Pongal, to bathing in the Ganga in Bengal. The enormous bathing ritual of Kumbha Mela always begins on Makar Sankranti, as it is now the time to initiate auspicious practices for the next six-month cycle.

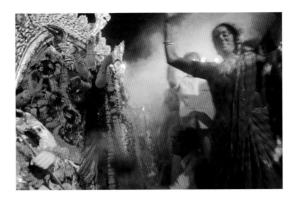

PERSONAL STORY: WINTER SOLSTICE, SPIRALS, LABYRINTHS, AND COWRY SHELLS

On the morning of my winter solstice retreat in 2011 in Nosara, Costa Rica, I woke up with unusually clear direction: "Collect 108 cowry shells." This seemed an impossible task, as before, in all my many travels, I had collected only a small number of cowry shells—less than a handful. I had found a precious few in Bali, Brazil, Kerala, and in Nosara, where I have made a pilgrimage for the past few years, and I had found another few during New Year's visits to Costa Rica in a magical place that is a sanctuary for turtle eggs.

I began my morning with a long ritual walk on the beach, a time for reflection. I walked for three hours. In between the ebb and flow of the tides, every few steps I found cowry shells. It was as if they had been strewn along a magic trail. Each shell was empty of its former inhabitant and each seemed to me like a tiny yoni, a symbol of woman's creative power. After the walk I had more than 108 cowry shells. I put them all in a case I had bought in Bali as a place to gather offerings.

On the long walk back, I came upon a local artist creating a large labyrinth on the beach, an ancient pattern. She began it by drawing three lines at the center; these then expanded outward and returned to connect back to the center. This is a symbol of the spiral journey of our adult life, where we are unsure whether we are going forward or backward but always make our way to the center, with faith.

That evening my partner and I built our own labyrinth using the cowry shells as an offering. At the moment the sun dipped below the horizon, its final beams shone directly upon the center point of our labyrinth before disappearing on the horizon. We gazed at one another in reverence for the magic-making on the Solstice—the return of the light.

When we begin our day of retreat prepared to open ourselves to whatever presents itself, we can never be sure what magic will unfold.

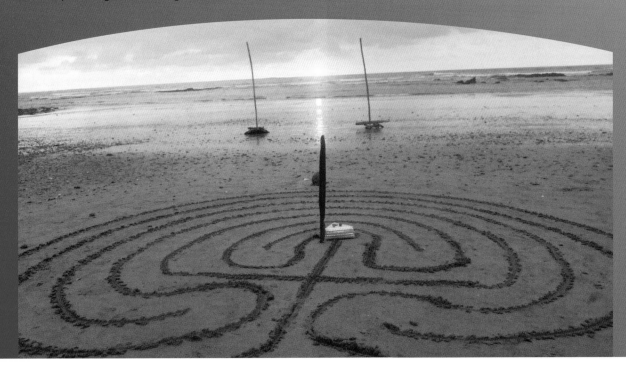

the sacred rhythm: reflection for the new cycle

As we reach the end of a cycle, we feel the teachings of completion—what is dying to be reborn, an awareness of the shadow side of ourselves to be "composted" and transformed. The solstice/New Year offers a mirror of every new cycle that will arise—new moons and changes in seasons. Much as people often make New Year's resolutions, we can reflect upon our seven fires (see the next pages) as a way to complete the old and ignite seeds for the new cycle—not just for New Year but for all the junctures ahead.

These new cycles are part of collective time synched with the greater alignment of the waxing-waning sun and moon to clear out the old and invoke the energy of the new. This is a time to refine our *samkalpas*—our will and our motivations—by holding and burning them in the fire of the heart.

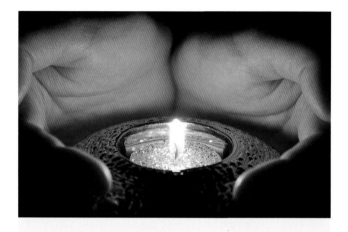

FIREKEEPING PRACTICE— IGNITING A NEW YEAR AND NEW CYCLE

During any new cycle, but particularly at the winter solstice–Christmas–New Year cycle, you can ignite a special candle that can last through the whole year (or a shorter cycle if you wish). This candle is lit only during special holidays and represents the concentration of your life-energy fuel, intentions, and dedicated tending of the fire through that period. You can offer this as a gift to others or yourself. You can make the candle by hand or simply enjoy the color, size, and symbolism of one you have purchased, as a powerful offering to your altar and ritual life. It will bring continuity, passion, peace, and clarity through the fire of consciousness that you ignite on the solstice, Christmas Eve, or New Year's Eve day. Create your own ritual way to ignite the new.

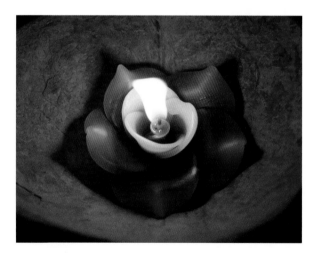

renewal of heart fire reflection— tending the seven fires

The seven fires of the seven chakras provide a map for our reflection, for the New Year or for the beginning of any new cycle. The chakras represent the movement from the foundation of our presence here upon the earth to our capacity for creative manifestation and the fires of love, including our enlightened vision: a capacity to see through the veils and understand on increasingly intimate levels what the alchemical journey of the year holds for us.

Renewing our fires takes place at both cellular and symbolic levels. The New Year is our opportunity to be born again. We must listen deeply during this time of the emerging light and become quiet as the earth, engaging in a coiling, inward process of revitalization and renewal. The following reflection can be done at the turn of the year or at the beginning of any new cycle.

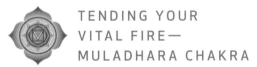

TENDING YOUR VITAL FIRE— MULADHARA CHAKRA

Feel into the state of your physical fire now, including your health and vitality. Reflect upon any imbalances you may find. What's going on with your health? What do you want to stoke with your physical fire? What imbalances do you want to address? What do you want to transform and nourish within your physical fire? Establish your "seed goals" for your vitality and what you want to cultivate, and write down one to three seed intentions for your physical fire in the new cycle to come.

TENDING YOUR CREATIVE-SENSUAL FIRE— SWADHISTHANA CHAKRA

Meditate upon the state of your creative process, upon what is being born and manifested through you. What aspects of your creative-sensual fire, inner or outer, need to be ignited? What is calling to be nourished? What inhibitions or states of neglect are blocking your flow?

Write down one to three seed intentions for your creative-sensual firekeeping in the new cycle.

TENDING THE FIRE OF AWARENESS— MANIPURA CHAKRA

What do you feel is calling to be manifested? What needs to be cleared or supported in connecting your inner world to the outer world? What limiting self-concepts block your sense of self? What ways is your ego disconnected from your core fire? What needs to be sustained and completed through sacred will—the sustaining power of manipura chakra? Write down one to three seed intentions for your manipura energy center and its heart connection in this new cycle.

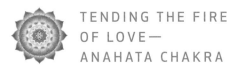 TENDING THE FIRE OF LOVE— ANAHATA CHAKRA

In anahata chakra we move into our full emotional fire and the core cultivation of love within our being. What are you radiating from your heart in your relationships, home, and community? Now write one to three seed intentions for your heart center this cycle.

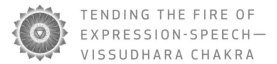 TENDING THE FIRE OF EXPRESSION-SPEECH— VISSUDHARA CHAKRA

Streams of butter flow from the ocean

of the heart . . . our words flow together

like rivers, made clear by understanding

deep within the heart.

— VEDAS[6]

Listen within for what needs to be healed from any miscommunications or misunderstandings, as well as which truths need to be spoken. How can you use your voice for healing and moving forward? Who do we need to reach out to? Who or where in the world are we called to support? What do you need to reach out to? Write down one to three seed intentions for the fire of your expression.

TENDING THE VISIONARY FIRE AND SPIRITUAL FIRE—AJNA AND SAHASRARA CHAKRAS

Reflect upon your highest vision for the next cycle. What limited views need to be released? In what ways do you feel disconnected from the Source? Reflect upon your *svadharma*, or unique purpose. Call forth a vision of the next cycle that is connected to your dharma and what you need to attend to in the next cycle. Write down one to three seed intentions for manifesting your vision.

SOLAR-LUNAR MANDALA OF THE YEAR

Take a moment now and look back at what you have written. These are the seed intentions of your new life, guidance for your evolution in all of your aspects: the container of your body, your sensuality and creativity, your will, your loving heart, your expression in the world, and your connection to Source. These seeds are your samkalpas, your navigating vision and intention, synching your life's rhythms with the deep knowing in the heart. Draw a circle-mandala with the sun in the center and visualize the flow of the year. You can plant any "seed qualities" to gestate in the center of the mandala, and any specific projects as radiating around the mandala to represent the natural progression of how the year may unfold. At every sacred juncture, you can reflect back to this to refine, change, and evolve.

vital rhythms—ayurvedic rtucharya: nutrition and lifestyle for winter

The inward-turning season of winter is ideal for nourishing our inner fire. The early part of winter follows the path of autumn, in which vata and kapha doshas are predominant, so the cold and dry qualities of vata are present in the body and the environment. The latter part of winter initiates the cold and damp qualities of kapha. Winter therefore becomes a delicate balance between these two doshas, requiring that we pay close attention to our environments—inner and outer—to keep our inner fire from growing dim or wavering.

The gunas, or qualities, of winter that we seek to balance are:

> Cold with warmth
> Heaviness with lightness of spirit
> Static energy with circulation
> Dullness with inspiration
> Excess dampness with dryness

When these qualities are balanced, the winter season can be nourishing and fortifying. When out of balance, kapha qualities accumulate within body and mind, creating heaviness of spirit, weight gain, poor digestion, depression, lethargy, and weakness in the immune system that leads to colds and flus. These can all be exacerbated by diminished digestive fire.

Winter is the time to build and restore. Just as nature draws inward to rest and renew, so too should we. Our bodies respond physiologically to cold weather by drawing our inner fire, agni, deep inside to protect the vital organs. We absorb nourishing lunar energy, and agni is the "cook" that rebuilds and replenishes the body from the inside out. Use this quiet, dark, reflective time to nourish your fire.

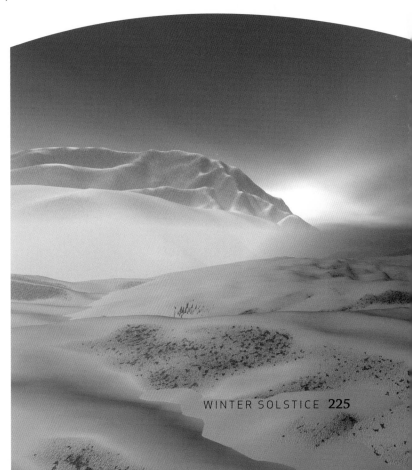

THE ESSENTIAL WINTER RTUCHARYA RHYTHM

1. Your digestive fire is strongest and most powerful during this time of year, and this is the season to build ojas, so eat nourishing and fortifying foods.

2. Avoid complete inactivity. This is the time of year to build strength and stamina without depleting your ojas.

3. Enjoy quiet time for introspection and meditation. Make use of the heavy qualities of winter to sit and read, write, and contemplate. Cultivate plans for the year ahead and plant "seeds" that will sprout in the coming spring.

4. Nourish ojas, the moist lunar energy, so it will be available to you for the expansion to come in the spring and summer. Good ways to do this are through daily abhyanga; warm, regenerative tonic teas or rasayanas; and warm, ojas-building foods.

5. Stay warm and dry to protect the body from the excess kapha qualities of the outdoors.

> To build ojas and strength, favor: ghee; warm, wholesome organic milk or almond milk; nourishing grains; and rich, warm, cooked foods. This is not the season to detox or lose weight but rather to rebuild and strengthen. Your body will actually want to gain or maintain your current weight at this time.

> Favor sweet, salty, and sour foods.

> Spices to favor: ginger, black pepper, pippali, cardamom, cinnamon, ajwan, cloves, licorice.

> Honey is the best winter sweetener because it is heating and pacifies kapha.

> For a kapha tea, add fresh-grated ginger and honey to your favorite tea. Tulsi-ginger tea is another good hot drink that strengthens the pulmonary system. Ginger plus cinnamon is another favorite combination.

> Because the sun sets earlier now, it is best to eat your last meal of the day earlier. Avoid eating later than an hour after sunset.

> Some favorite winter foods are yams, winter squash, cabbage, pumpkin, beets, brussels sprouts, chilies, garlic, and tomatoes. For fruits, cooked apples, bananas, dates, and figs are great. Eat tangerines for sour and sweet tastes. Good winter grains are amaranth, oats, rice, and wheat.

> The best herbs for controlling kapha in the winter season are Punarnava, Kutki, and Triphala Guggulu.

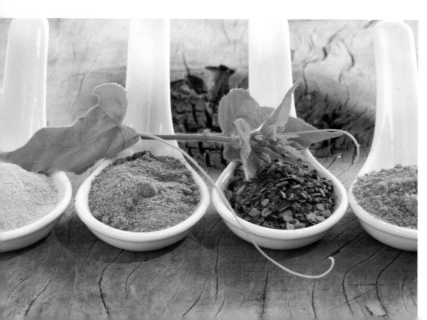

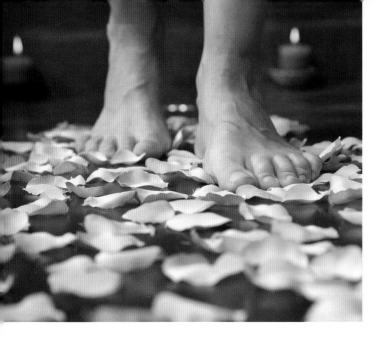

The winter season is the best time for these ayurvedic practices:

> *Sneha*—oiling the body, nose, and ears in the evening is nourishing and fortifying for the muscles and connective tissues. As our bodies are exposed to cold and wind, our pores and fascia tighten and roughen in response. Oiling the orifices of the head helps the sensory pathways stay balanced. Favor kapha massage oil, Ashwagandha-Bala oil, or sesame oil.

> Do dry-brushing a few times a week to invigorate the tissues and move stagnant lymph and blood.

> *Shiroabhyanga*—friction-rub the scalp to release dull, stagnant, heavy qualities of kapha in the head. Great to do in the morning.

> *Padabhyanga*—oiling of the feet. Do this at night, using sesame or Bhrami oil.

> Good winter scents are rosemary, cinnamon, ginger, grapefruit, pine, bergamot, lemongrass, and rose geranium.

Kala—From the winter solstice onward, the winter season is the best time to synch with the sunrise (unless you are depleted and need to rest) and to honor going to bed after sunset.

Desa—Cultivate a warm place for practicing the flame of your inner and outer altar, carrying the warm colors of fire—red, orange, and ochre earth colors—in your home and dress (hats, scarves, and footwear) to keep the inner fire alive.

Bhava—Follow the sun and begin to gradually increase your outward energy and activity so as to store energy (ojas) and at the same time keep your fire (tejas) and life-energy (prana) circulating; be calm, joyous, positive, and inspired.

Dosha—The winter season is the most vulnerable time for those with dim fire or manda agni, kapha dosha, or those experiencing a stagnant lifestyle, depression, or lethargy due to less solar energy.

Yoga Practice—Cultivate Vira and Sringara Rasa practices, solar and lunar practices to balance the firekeeping within your body. Solar practices with the New Year; waxing energy and lunar practices with the evening and waning energy.

Enjoy solar and lunar namaskars. Build stamina in heating but grounding ways such as long standing-asana sequences, inversions (headstand, shoulderstand, handstand), and longer periods in backbends to keep the lungs and chest stimulated and heated (to prevent excess kapha or phlegm). Honor lunar energy in earthy forward bends and hip openers to store energy for spring. Meanwhile, heating pranayama such as bhastrika can help lungs and sinuses stay strong and clear during cold and flu season, and these practices help release any excess kapha mucous from this area.

imbolc: the six-week fire festival beginning february 1

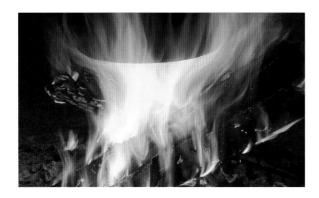

Ancient White that covers All—
Stars of Light that melt in sky—
Winds that howl, Oreads Sing—
Keep your Candles lit and high—
Imbolc-tide but once a year, Make light
the dell, enchant good cheer.

— ALEAF BACHAROUS[7]

Imbolc marks the six-week mark of each new year, a halfway point between winter solstice and the spring equinox. Seeds within the earth begin to stir, and buds emerge upon the seemingly dead branches of winter. The solar fire deep within the seeds slowly begins to emerge in the miracle of life.

In Celtic culture, Imbolc is the first of the sacred fire festivals of the year, dedicated to the Mother Goddess under her many names but primarily to Brighid, the lady of the hearth. A ritual that follows honors the Mother by bringing together fire, symbolizing the emergence of life, and a container of water, representing the womb of the sacred feminine. The holy days of February include several festivals that celebrate love and union and that call us to invoke the power of devotion that will keep the fires burning through the remaining months of winter—a time for the gestation that is required of all creative processes and generative acts.

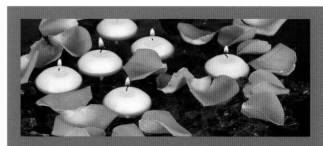

A FIREKEEPING RITUAL— FIRE AND WATER

Make a special offering on your altar with a bowl of water. Add eight floating candles, or place in the bowl candles that are sturdy and tall enough to be above the water. These represent the eight junctures of the solar cycle of the year. Each person in your household can participate in lighting the candles while offering a prayer as a way of eliciting the alchemy of fire and water and the fertile blessings of this first fire festival, just as the buds of coming spring begin to emerge.

FEBRUARY HOLIDAYS OF LOVE

SARASWATI PUJA—CHINESE-TIBETAN NEW YEAR—YEMANJA DAY
VALENTINE'S DAY—SHIVRATRI—MARDI GRAS—HOLI

A sequence—vinyasa—of interrelated holidays flows from late January to early March. Among them is one honoring Kamadeva, the tantric form of Cupid, visualized as the deity of human love or desire and represented as a young, handsome, winged man who wields a bow made of sugarcane. His bow is often depicted as a string of honeybees with arrows that are decorated with fragrant flowers. Trees dedicated to Kamadeva are often planted near temples as symbols of love, particularly in connection with Krishna and Radha, or with Shiva.

The story is told that one of Kamadeva's flower arrows pierced the Mahayogin Shiva as Shakti in the form of his soon-to-be consort Parvati. As the arrow hit Shiva's side, his eyes of bliss opened directly into the eyes of Parvati, who had been in deep meditation upon Shiva with burning devotion for millions of years. As Kamadeva was inciner-ated by Shiva's third eye, the heat of Shiva's lingam ignited in union with the great yoni of Parvati, an event that continued with such energy that the centrifugal force of their union needed to find outward expression, as the cos-mic coiling between the two was bound to release. With Kamadeva restored from the ball of ash that was his body,

Shiva and Parvati emerged as the eternal cosmic couple. The creative union of their heartbeat is part of the rhythm of Sringara Rasa, which seems so appropriate to the quickening as spring begins to stir and be expressed in the various relationships to devotion, love, and eros.

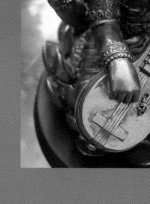

A related holiday is Saraswati Puja, the day for honoring Saraswati Devi. On this day, people place their musical instruments on the altar for a blessing, wear yellow, chant, dance, and play music to honor "She who flows." Saraswati Puja is when lovers called into their new love enter a sadhana of Kamadeva mantra japa. This period is also when Valentine's Day emerges—a wonderful kindling of the passion of lovers embodied in Kamadeva, who is honored for stoking the fires of eros, from the cosmic level to here on earth.

Kamadeva finds echoes in Cupid from Roman mythology and Eros from Greek mythology. Cupid's sweet arrows pierce the heart, and he is the central figure associated with Valentine's Day. Throughout the world there are many holy days dedicated to love.

ASH WEDNESDAY/LENT— THE FORTY-DAY PERIOD OF PURIFICATION BEFORE EASTER

Lent is a period of purification and fasting with roots in the New Testament. Jesus is said to have fasted in the desert for forty days and nights before beginning his ministry, and at this time of year we take the same number of days to purify ourselves and to cleanse ourselves of actions and habits that impede our growth and that could inhibit our spir-it's resurrection. Prayer and sacrifice are hallmarks of this period. The root word for Lent is the Old English *lencten*, meaning "spring," and this period of preparation is designed to move us into the full-ness of that season in a more purified state.

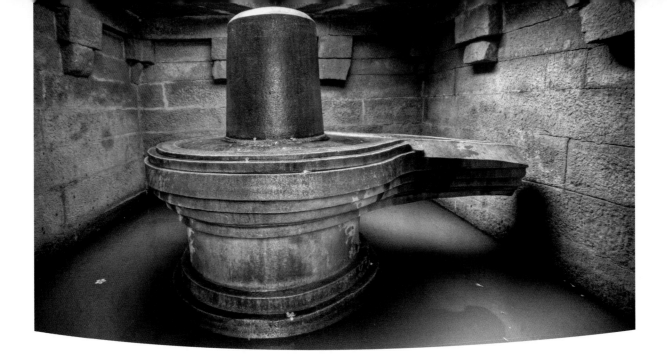

FIREKEEPING RITUAL—
ALL-NIGHT VIGIL FOR SHIVRATRI

This retreat can be adapted to any new or full moon or to any time of personal transformation. An all-night candle vigil is part of the spirit of *tapas*.

The word *tapas* can be translated as "burning, unwavering devotion," and "transformation through dedication." In tending the Heart Fire, a tapas practice is anything you dedicate yourself to for a cycle of transformation. Maha Shivratri is a tapas-oriented, nightlong festival that has been celebrated for thousands of years by hundreds of millions of devotees of Shiva around the world.

Held on the night before the new moon in the month of February–March, Maha Shivratri honors the night (*ratri* means "night") that Shiva performed the *tandava nritya*—the dance of primordial creation, preservation, and destruction—and the night of the marriage of Shiva and Shakti. Householders stay up through the night chanting mantras, bathing

lingam forms, offering puja, and in meditation for the Mahadev, King of the Yogis, Lord of the Dance, bathed in the light of lamps burning ghee. Devotees fast on water, milk, fruits, *kitchari*, or special fasting foods from sunrise until dawn the next day.

Maha Shivatri is considered an auspicious time for women. Married women pray for a long, prosperous marriage and the well-being of their husbands and sons. Unmarried women pray for a husband who is like Lord Shiva—spouse of Kali, Durga, and Parvati—considered the ideal husband for his devotion; virility; and loving, enlightened, wild, and fun ways of being—and for his ability to transform poison into nectar.

This festival is an outer and inner pilgrimage, the tending of the lamp fire and the fire of consciousness through the night. All yoga practices are said to have emanated from Shiva, particularly those having to do with internal transformation, and Maha Shivratri is a vigil of awakening consciousness.

SHIVRATRI: THE NIGHT I MARRIED SHIVA

The days before *shivratri*, the darkest days before the new moon, can be intensely transformative. My first shivratri in India was in 1990 when I spent a year as an exchange student at the University of Delhi. I was also studying Odissi, an Indian temple dance form that blends the strong dynamic footwork of Shiva's *tandava* and the flowing form of curves and bends of Shakti's *lasya*. When I came home from dance practice, my roommates greeted me at the door looking desperate and pale. One of my dear friends had just returned from a Vipassana retreat and was in the midst of a nervous breakdown—I was shocked to learn that she was trying to gouge her eyes out. Together we held her through this terrible, dark passage as further help came to her aid.

The next day as I was walking to the bus stop, I passed by a man lying dead on the street with his guts spilling out. My own body was on the edge, dealing with intestinal amoebas. I felt the death cycle everywhere around me, and the dark days before the new moon shook the ground beneath me. The world seemed surreal, hurtling toward dissolution. My father had named me Shiva. It seemed I was fulfilling the name now in the aspect of Shiva's meditation in the cremation grounds.

I felt fortunate to have Ramachandra Gandhi, grandson of the great Mahatma Gandhi, as one of my teachers. I continued on my journey and met him for tea, telling him all that had transpired and that I felt my world was embodying a dark aspect of Shiva right now. "Your name is Shivaaaa," he said, "pronounced with a long *a*. You are the wife of Shiva."

I left our tea with this reverberating in my heart and walked to the dance academy. A little shop caught my eye, and in the window I found the most beautiful *murti*, or divine image, of Shiva. He was meditating on a tiger skin with the most beatific expression. I felt the awakening in my heart of a primordial love at the center of the center of my being: a sudden flash of recognition.

This became my first altarpiece, and along with a garland of flowers I brought it to my dance lesson. My teacher saw my murti and, more importantly, a shift within me. He beckoned me to place the murti on the altar and drape the garland over it. Then he said, "Ahhh. Now you will be married to Shiva, as tomorrow is shivratri, the great night for realizing Shiva."

On that night, I stayed with my murti and I felt an effortless surge, my first intimate experience of chanting truly pouring from my heart in a flood of devotion. *Namah Shivaya Namah Shivaya Namah Shivaya Jai Shiva Shankara Nataraja!*

The dark nights before shivratri often involve death or dissolution in some form, making way for the fire of rebirth and a deeper union to emerge out of the darkness. The all-night firekeeping of this special holy day is a threshold to transformation, to the reigniting of the fires of realization.

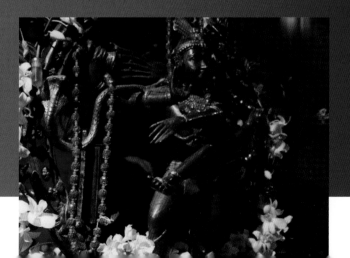

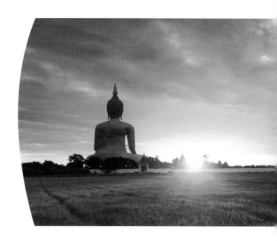

spring equinox

Reemergence of Life

signs of life— spring bursts forth

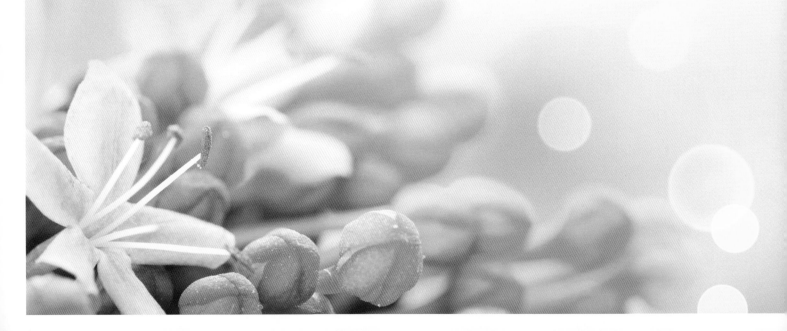

The first signs of spring are the breaking open as death gives way to life: buds bursting from the trees, shoots leaping from the earth, a great rising amid the debris of winter. For nature, renewing herself through dying is the only way she can be reborn. And this rebirth is what links Easter, Passover, Purim, and the Goddess festival *vasant navaratri* to the spring equinox. There are both gradual and sudden metamorphoses of new light and life. Now is the time to give full power to the seed dreams you incubated in your Heart Fire during the darkness of winter. The spring equinox is a powerful time to care for the earth and shed any limiting or toxic behaviors. During this time of tremendous growth, let us all take care to protect the precious seedlings that have emerged from the depths of winter. Let us honor the fiery energy of new life.

To say "yes" means to allow a thought
or circumstance to flower, to let go and expand.
The trees say "yes" to every season.
When spring comes, they say "yes"
and they flower. Then summer comes,
they say "yes" and become dry and thirsty.
When fall comes, they say "yes,"
change color, and are ready to drop
their leaves. To say "yes" means to
surrender—to every thought, feeling and
emotion. It means let go, and letting go
is a journey toward the heart.

—DR. VASANT LAD[1]

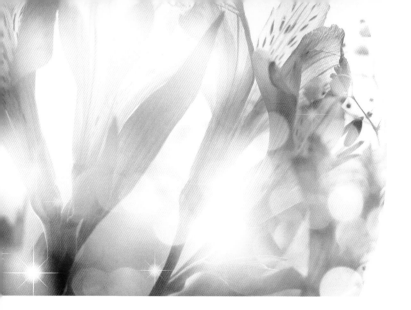

The sun is Love.

The Lover, a speck circling the sun.

A Spring wind moves to dance

any branch that isn't dead.

Something opens our wings.

Someone fills the cup in front of us.

We taste only sacredness.

— RUMI[2]

ALBAN EILIR—SPRING EQUINOX

Alban Eilir, "light of the earth," is the balance point between the winter and summer solstices and between Imbolc and Beltane. The spring equinox is one of two times during the year when the tilt of the earth's axis is parallel to the sun. On this day the forces of darkness and light are equally matched, but light is on the increase. It is a time of great fertility and hopefulness, containing the promise of abundant crops and burgeoning creativity. Spring equinox is aligned with those holidays connected to the reigniting of the candle flame, from the Jewish culture's Passover as a time of liberation to the Christians' Easter as a time of the resurrection of the light. Mayan temples, too, affirm the cyclical process of time: the serpent of light Kulkulkan descends and manifests at the spring equinox and then returns back in the cycle of death with the fall equinox. The connection to the triumph of light is also reflected in the Festival of Color of Holi and of the celebration of the strength of Hanuman.

PASSOVER

The springtime festival of Passover celebrates the liberation of the Israelites from Pharoah's rule. The festival lasts for eight days. The first two and last two days are full-fledged holidays. Celebrants light holiday candles, perform the kiddush blessing, and serve lavish holiday meals. In strict observance, during these four days of ritual work, observers refrain from working and engaging in many other everyday activities; all focus is on the many varied elements of ritual and on contemplation.

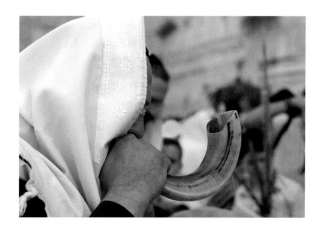

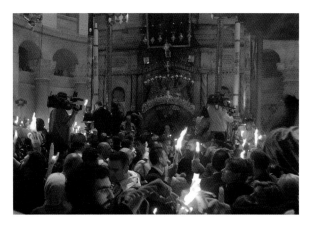

EASTER

Easter is a celebration of the triumph of light over darkness, and it marks the end of Lent, a fast broken by the feast celebrating Christ's resurrection. The name Easter hails from Eastre, the Teutonic goddess of spring and dawn. The full moon of the vernal equinox represents the "pregnant" phase of Eastre, the bearing of the fruit of summer that gives birth to the sun's offspring. The Easter egg symbolizes creation, the cycles of nature, and the union of masculine and feminine.

The Festival of Holy Fire takes place at the Church of the Holy Sepulchre in the walled Old City of Jerusalem. Each year on the day before Pascha (Easter), at noon on Holy Saturday, a miraculous light appears from the core of the Holy Sepulchre, from which the patriarch of Jerusalem lights thirty-three candles from the deep center of the tomb and then offers this light to reignite candles all over the world. The flame of the Church of the Holy Sepulchre is considered by many to be the longest attested annual miracle in the Christian world.

REEMERGENCE—CHICHEN ITZA

For the spring equinox of 2012, I made the pilgrimage to this extraordinary site, which aligns with the spring and fall equinoxes. Here, mostly local Mayans and Mexicans from throughout the region come to this ancient pyramid built nearly a thousand years ago to witness the descent of the "serpent of light," or Kulkulkan. All gather at the moment when the shadow play creates this effect. Thousands raise their arms in joyous celebration, a heightened experience of collective alignment that is not led or dictated by any leader. It is instead a spontaneous experience in the moment that hovers and lasts for that peak few moments and then dissolves into the general auspiciousness of the spring equinox—the entry point into the following season of greatest waxing light.

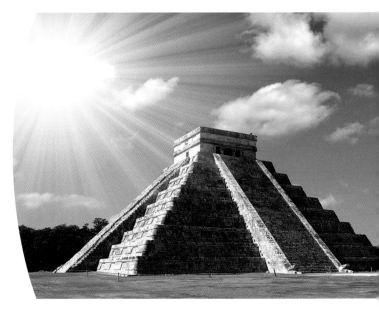

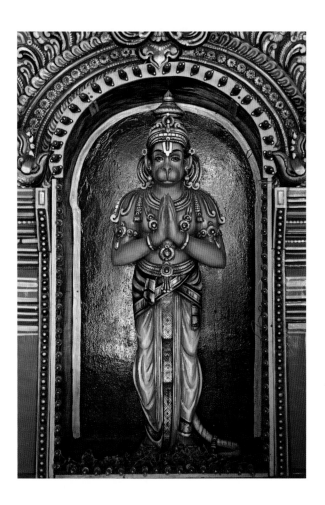

HANUMAN JAYANTI

Hanuman Jayanti is a celebration of the monkey god Hanuman of the Ramayana, who represents strength, energy, resourcefulness, and devotion. It, too, is celebrated around the spring equinox. On this holy day, devotees fast, read the Hanuman Chalisa, offer *seva* (service), and spend the whole day in the *japa* of Ram-Nam, Ram Ram Ram.

FIREKEEPING PRACTICE— COLLECTIVE IGNITING OF THE HEART FIRE

For the past twenty years in the collective meditations I have led in the evening, I have been part of many beautiful experiences of the "passing of the flame," mirroring the cross-cultural, ancestral practice of symbolically lighting each other's candle or *dipa* (small lamp) from one central source. I have witnessed this in the city of Thiruvanathapuram, Kerala, where more than a hundred thousand women light their central cooking fires one by one from the central fire of the Attukal Devi (Goddess Temple) during the spring festival period.

Whether it is a small family gathering or a larger meditation circle, you can ignite the central candle with one primary flame along with a silent or vocal prayer or chant. From there, either "pass the light" with smaller candles that then circulate or have everyone present come forward and light from the central flame.

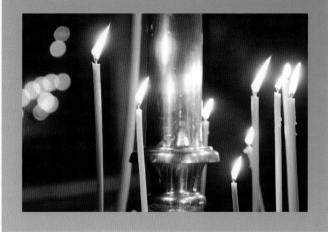

vital rhythms—ayurvedic rtucharya: nutrition and lifestyle for spring

Spring is the time to be reborn and to flourish. Following the rhythm of the nature burgeoning around us, we awaken into the light and warmth of the season and allow the nourishing rains to cleanse us of impurities. This juncture in time is considered one of the most optimal to clean and detoxify the mind and body. Ayurveda's famous Panchakarma system offers a wonderful way to move out toxins, balance the doshas, and release stagnation in the tissues and organ systems of the body.

According to ayurveda, springtime is marked as kapha time, which brings the gunas, or qualities, of heavy, dull, liquid, dense, slimy, and oily. These qualities have been prevalent since the winter season (another kapha time), and now whatever quality was increased in the winter and is not brought to balance during the spring will adversely affect your health. Most people are familiar with spring allergies, congestion, and sinusitis. This is nature's way of melting away the inner "snow" of the body. Just as mountain snows are now melting into the rivers and swelling their waters, our bodies respond in much the same way at this time of year.

The gunas, or qualities, of spring that we seek to balance are:

> Heavy and dull with stimulating
> Static with activity and movement
> Oily and liquid with astringent and bitter
> Smooth and dense with dry and rough

When these qualities are balanced, we can look forward to a time of renewal and invigoration during the spring season. Excess kapha in spring will bring allergies, asthma, sinus infections, colds, and chest infections, leading to a mucus-producing cough and excreta.

THE ESSENTIAL SPRING RTUCHARYA RHYTHM

1. Melt your inner snow with invigorating and heating practices and activities.

2. Change your eating habits toward a preliminary cleansing. To decrease excess kapha, favor lighter and drier foods that are bitter, astringent, or pungent. Clean up your diet and avoid sweets, refined sugar, dairy, and wheat, all of which increase the heavy, dull, and dense qualities in the body.

3. Spend time outdoors and soak up the radiant and increasingly abundant solar energy known as *atapa seva* (sun bathing) in ayurveda.

4. Exercise outdoors with plenty of cardiovascular activity. This is a great time of year to sweat and begin to move winter stagnation out of the body. The best way to move excess heaviness and mucus is to move the lymph and blood that circulate throughout the body. This is best done in the morning between 7 and 10 a.m.

5 Start to wake up one hour before sunrise and bring greater circulation to your daily dry-brushing with more invigorating ayurvedic self-massage (see Body Rhythm, below). Kapha time begins around 7 a.m.; to avoid increasing kapha qualities in the body, it is important to be up and moving before the sun rises in order to move toxins and stagnant lymph that have accumulated over the night. Notice that sunrise will continue to come earlier during this time, so stay present to this change.

Food Rhythm

> Warm water with honey is great first thing in the morning. For excess kapha, add apple cider vinegar.

> Agni becomes weaker now, and you can tend toward lethargy or feelings of heaviness after meals. It is important to properly spice food and to not overeat or indulge in rich foods. Eat light, dry, and heating foods.

> Favor bitter, astringent, and pungent foods. Avoid heavy foods like wheat, avocado, cucumber, dates, banana, melons, and potatoes.

> Favor vegetables like sprouts, dandelion greens, kale, mustard greens, Swiss chard, endive, collard greens, and spinach. Eat light and astringent fruits such as apples, pears, cranberries, pomegranates, and dried fruit. Avoid sour and juicy fruits like watermelon and oranges.

> A good spring tea is ginger, lemongrass, and honey. Other good teas are dandelion, cardamom, cinnamon, orange peel, and hibiscus. Cumin, coriander, and fennel tea is a natural diuretic for any excess water weight that might accrue in the spring.

> Use oil sparingly, and choose mustard, sunflower, and safflower oils as they are light.

> The best grains for spring are amaranth, barley, quinoa, and rye.

> Spices for flavor include black pepper, pippali, clove, ginger (fresh), nutmeg, sage, thyme, rosemary, cayenne, and turmeric. Trikatu (black pepper, pippali, ginger) is an ancient herbal mix that increases digestion and removes toxins from the body.

Body Rhythm

Spring body care is centered on moving lymphatic stagnation, invigorating the tissues and skin, and lightening the body. Choose stimulating and invigorating scents and avoid heavy and earthy scents, because kapha is predominantly earth and water.

Abhyanga is done very sparingly (if at all) during this season and generally with much less oil. The technique of "friction rubbing" is recommended, where the massage strokes are brisk and quick rather than long and smooth. Favor light oils—like sunflower oil or mustard oil—for the body.

Spring essential oils/scents include clearing and stimulating ones such as eucalyptus, tea tree, turmeric, peppermint, and rosewood.

> Enjoy dry-brushing the skin with silk gloves or a loofah to bring blood to the surface and to begin the detoxifying process.

> Use a *neti* pot to keep the sinuses free and clear. This is a great practice to emphasize in the spring to prevent allergies.

> Take saunas or steam baths as a favorite detox practice to decrease kapha and *ama* (excess toxins) in springtime.

ENERGETIC VINYASA FOR SPRING SEASON

Kala—Continue to synch with the sun (unless you are depleted and need to rest), gradually getting up earlier before the sunrise. This is the peak time of growth, so synch your movements with that waxing light.

Desa—Spend more time outdoors to absorb the fresh prana of spring; be aware of the oscillation between warm and cold days with the birthing of spring so keep carrying the warm colors of fire— red, orange, ochre earth colors—in your home and dress to keep the inner fire alive.

Bhava—Begin to increase your expression mirroring the emergence of the plant world towards the ecsatic celebratory energy of late spring; radiant, joyous.

Dosha—The spring season is the most vulnerable time for those who burned too much energy during the winter to become sick or run out of steam (vata-pitta imbalance) or for those whose fire grew dim to feel sluggish and lacking power for creative manifestation (kapha imbalance)

Yoga Practice—This is the best time of the year for wise solar or Vira Rasa to assist in preparation of spring cleaning and activating one's creative and manifesting power; when you are engaged in spring cleaning be sure to cultivate lunar or shanti rasa practices so as to support your body's detoxing practices by resting all other forms of output.

Enjoy the solar, dynamic, and alchemical balancing of lunar namaskars. Begin to slowly move from heavier practices to lighter practices (March to June). This is the best season to do arm balances; deeper backbends; and activating, heating inversions like handstand or headstand. Utilize the strength you cultivated in the winter to sustain more challenging asanas.

Enjoy stimulating pranayama practices at this time: kappalabhati, bhastrika, surya bedhana.

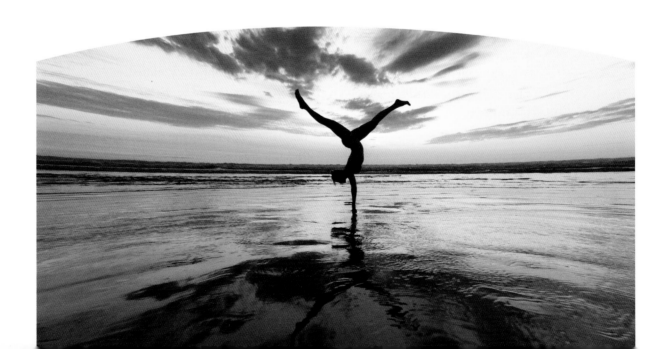

sacred rhythm and holidays—
beltane, buddha's birthday

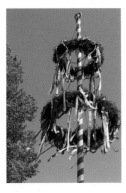

BELTANE: SIX-WEEK FIRE FESTIVAL BEGINNING MAY 1

Beltane is the third spring celebration in the druid tradition. By May 1, the season has truly emerged, and spring growth is in full flower on the earth and in our own bodies.

Fertility is a main theme of Beltane. May Day is the time for dancing around the maypole, a phallic symbol rooted in the earth, which is the female symbol of the yoni, our creative power. Beltane has been a time for ritual dances and races through mazes—rich symbolism reflected in spiral labyrinth carvings found in a number of prehistoric burial chambers.

The original meaning of Beltane is "the good fire," connected to the fire of the Celtic or proto-Celtic god known as Bel, or Beli. Bel was "the Bright One," the god of light and fire, and "Bel fires" were lit on hilltops to celebrate the fertility of the season and coming of new life with the spring. All over the countryside in the United Kingdom at this time, bonfires are lit, often from a central fire built for the Beltane ritual of jumping over the fire. Young people leap over this fire to bring themselves husbands or wives; travelers jump over it to ensure a safe journey; pregnant women jump over it to have an easy delivery; young women leap to ensure their fertility.

FIREKEEPING PRACTICE— JUMPING OVER THE FIRE

By May, the celebratory energy of the earth is in full bloom, and an outdoor celebration with a bonfire is a way to connect to the ecstatic energy of spring that is rising in our own bodies. We all, from young people to adults, can embody vigor and joy as we leap (check the height of the fire!) through the flames without fear. I have enjoyed this practice in collective retreats supported by the fun and boisterous support of the community—we leap into our fertile potentiality that Beltane ignites.

BELTANE FIRES

From South and North

in polar spheres twin fires reign,

one issued from male desire,

the other fueled by female flame.

Like attraction dancing, sparks fly,

passions edge closer together.

The two unite.

—KAAREN WHITNEY[3]

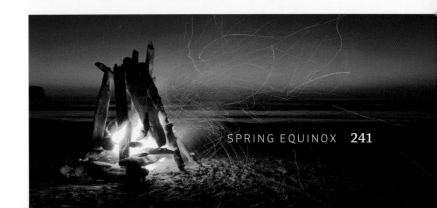

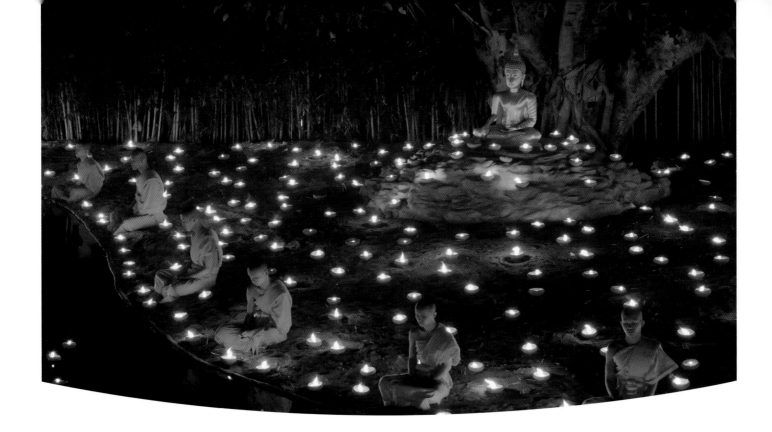

BUDDHA'S BIRTHDAY

Thousands of candles can be lit from a
single candle, and the life of the candle will
not be shortened. Happiness never
decreases by being shared.

—THE BUDDHA SIDDHARTHA GAUTAMA[4]

The birthday of the Buddha Siddhartha Gautama
is celebrated as the day of his enlightenment.
Offerings and meditations are undertaken around
the world, particularly in Bodh Gaya, in northern
India, where the "granddaughter" of the original
Bodhi Tree (where the Buddha awakened) is a site
for prostrations, meditation, and remembrance.

CHAPTER TWELVE

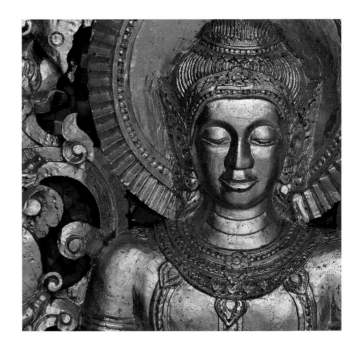

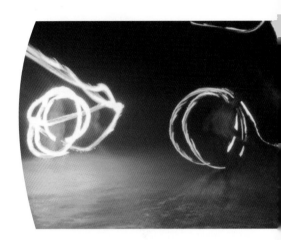

summer solstice

Peak of the Light

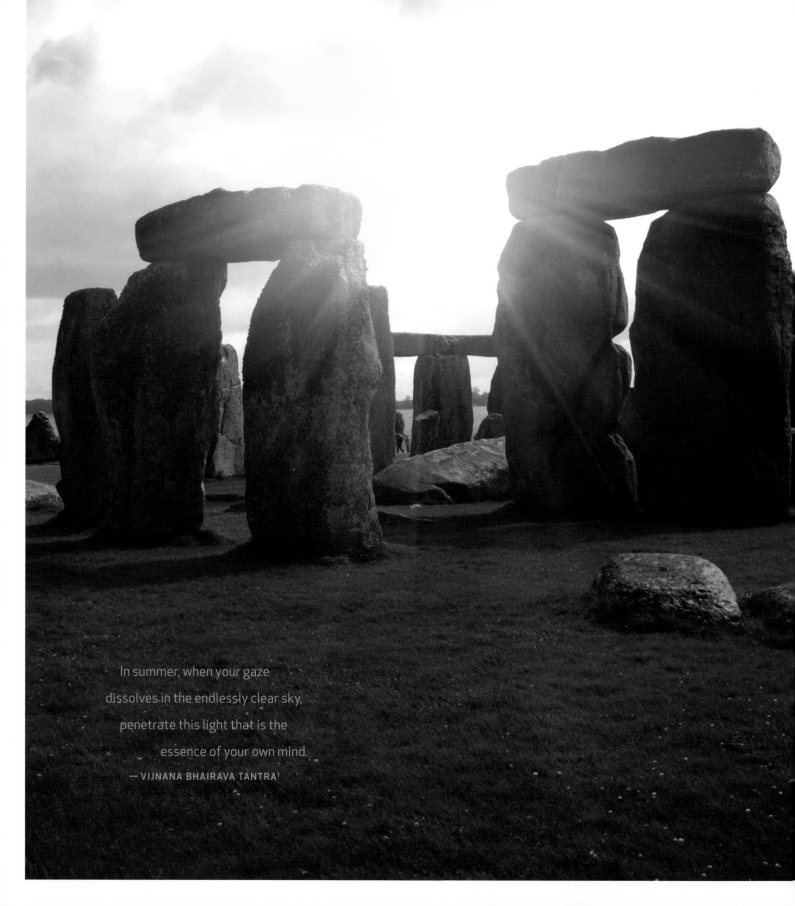

In summer, when your gaze
dissolves in the endlessly clear sky,
penetrate this light that is the
essence of your own mind.
— VIJNANA BHAIRAVA TANTRA[1]

cross-cultural summer solstice celebrations

Summer solstice celebrations have occurred worldwide for millennia. In Celtic tradition, the celebration of the apex of the light symbolized the crowning of the Oak King, God of the Waxing Year.[2] In ancient China, the earth, the feminine, and yin forces were celebrated. In ancient Gaul, the people celebrated fertility, sovereignty, and agriculture.

Ancient tribes in Europe (Germanic, Slavic, and Celtic) lit bonfires to "boost the sun's energy," hoping that it would remain potent throughout the rest of the summer and provide an abundant harvest. Within Christianity, the Feast of St. John the Baptist mirrors at summer solstice the celebration of Jesus around the winter solstice. In India, the summer solstice marks the beginning of the dakshinayana period, when for six months the earth moves in the southern, or *dakshina*, orbit of waning light.

During this period the sun is at its peak in the northern hemisphere, reflecting the abundance of fruits and the fertility of the earth. According to tradition, the full moon in June is the best time for harvesting honey; this is why it also known as the Honey Moon. The sacred union of the Goddess and God at Beltane during May made June a traditional time for weddings, a time to bring to fruition the powerful union of earth, moon, and sun.

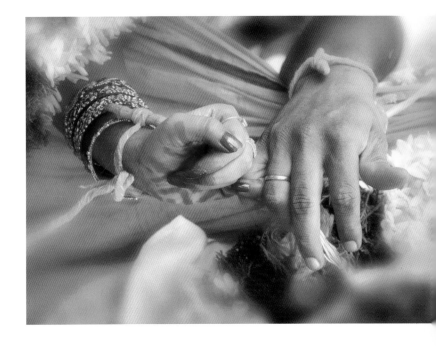

summer solstice sacred retreat

Prepare your home altar with the colors of the sun: choose brilliant golds, reds, and oranges for fabrics, fruit, and candles. Celebrate the wildflowers of your area by including them on your altar, making sure to water any plants from which you gather flowers. Choose a symbol to honor your ancestors, whether from your immediate family or cultural symbols of the past. Adorn your body with the sun's colors to bring brightness and radiance into your being.

In a journal or in meditation, reflect on your journey over the past six months. Remember the intentions you planted at winter solstice, the seeds fertilized at Imbolc that began to flower with the spring equinox, that rose up in fullness with the Beltane maypole, and that now peak with the summer solstice. What has transpired for you in this first half of the journey around the sun, the period in yoga known as the *uttarayana?*

Place a jar or bowl filled with water in the sun to be energized by the solstice sun. Drink it in the afternoon to receive the vital energy of the sun. Place any gold jewelry you may have near a window to be recharged and blessed by the solstice sun.

Bring the light into your heart and feel the power of completion and renewal. Continue to follow that energy all the way into the next new-moon cycle.

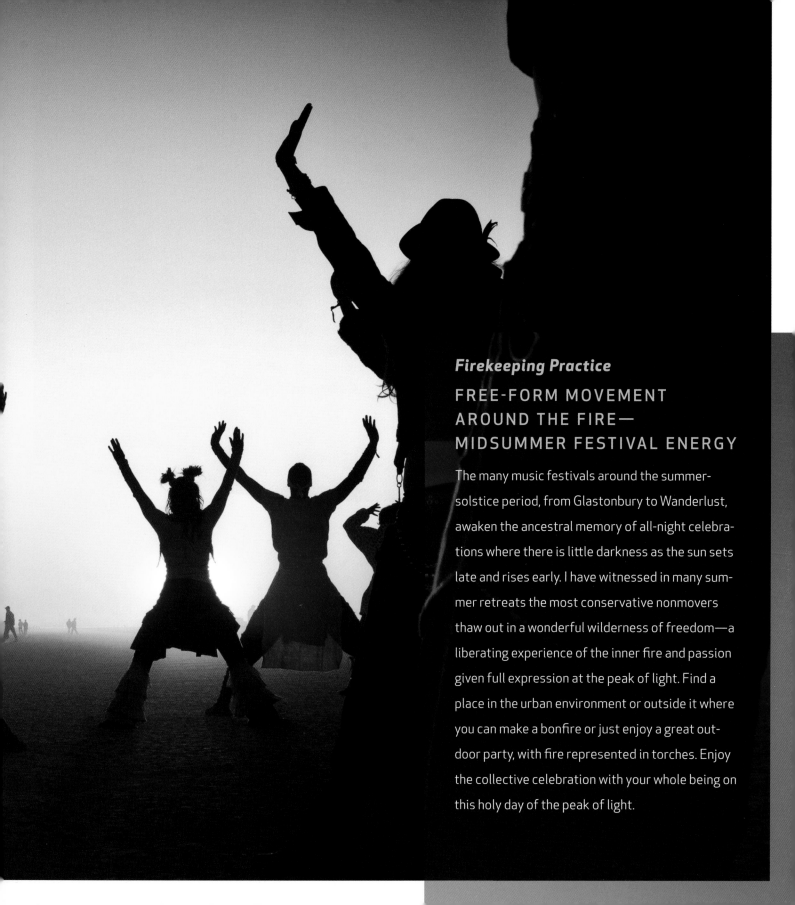

Firekeeping Practice

FREE-FORM MOVEMENT AROUND THE FIRE— MIDSUMMER FESTIVAL ENERGY

The many music festivals around the summer-solstice period, from Glastonbury to Wanderlust, awaken the ancestral memory of all-night celebrations where there is little darkness as the sun sets late and rises early. I have witnessed in many summer retreats the most conservative nonmovers thaw out in a wonderful wilderness of freedom—a liberating experience of the inner fire and passion given full expression at the peak of light. Find a place in the urban environment or outside it where you can make a bonfire or just enjoy a great outdoor party, with fire represented in torches. Enjoy the collective celebration with your whole being on this holy day of the peak of light.

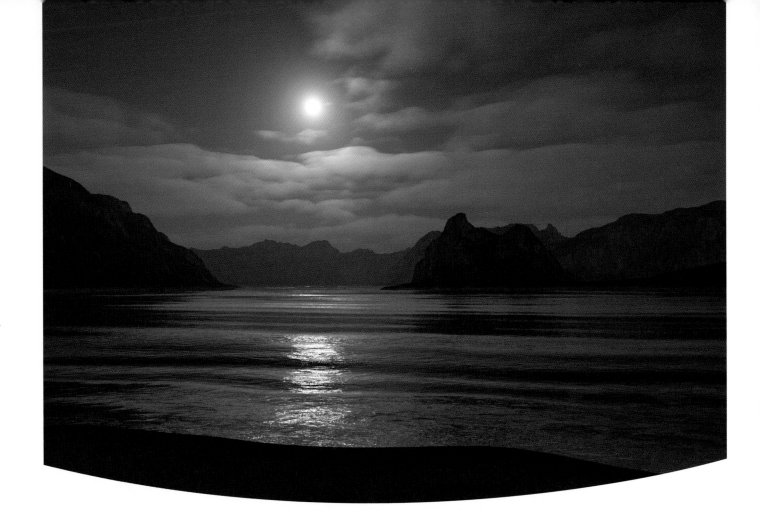

guru purnima

Guru Purnima (Full Moon of the Guru) is the day for disciples to offer worship and respect to their spiritual teacher, or *satguru*. The mother is considered to be a child's first guru, and mother and father together are responsible for the child's upbringing. Later in life, a satguru initiates deeper spiritual training. The guru embodies everything the spiritual seeker aspires to be, allowing the student to see his or her own infinite potential.

Guru Purnima is considered the beginning of a four-month initiatory cycle and is an auspicious time for spiritual advancement and for beginning new endeavors. You can create your own initiation at this time. Connect with all forms of the Guru that are in your life now. Look into your own heart for the Guru's perfection.

balancing the fire— summer ayurveda rtucharya

Summer is a time when the earth is most dry and arid, receiving maximum solar energy. All the radiant light is activating but depleting, and so we tend to be physically weaker during this time, and our digestive fire is also at its weakest.

Ayurveda considers summer a pitta season, with emphasis on the elements of fire and water. Pitta dosha is a radiant solar force, hot and sharp, and at this time of the year it is important to balance pitta because we can easily become dehydrated.

The gunas, or qualities, of summer that we seek to balance are:

> Hot and sharp with relaxation
> Oily and liquid with dry but nourishing

FIVE ANCHORS FOR THE SUMMER SEASON

1. Balance excess fire that overstimulates the pitta dosha by staying relaxed, calm, and cool and by tending the fiery emotions like impatience and irritation.

2. Shift your rhythm from manifestation to celebration. Take time to slow down. Enjoy life outdoors, but avoid activities that are overly exerting between 11 a.m. and 3 p.m. Stay cool and indoors.

3. Enjoy sleeping outside to breathe the fresh air and absorb moonlight. Try taking a moon bath: sit outside under the moonlight and absorb the watery, cooling nectar from the moon.

4. Summer body care is focused on cooling the skin with calming and soothing practices (see Body Rhythm, on page 250).

5. Eat and drink in ways that balance pitta dosha. Enjoy cooling fruits and vegetables in season (see Food Rhythm, below) and sip on warm water or herbal water to maintain and regulate body temperature.

FOOD RHYTHM

Due to the strong properties of the sun and the body's need to stay cool and release internal heat, our inner fire, agni, is pulled to the extremities to keep the body cool; therefore digestive agni is compromised, weakening our digestive capacity. That is why in the summer we are often less hungry and want to eat less. So it is good to eat lighter and smaller meals during this time of year.

> Drink a brew of cumin, coriander, fennel, and rose or mint tea to pacify the hot quality, improve digestion, and calm the mind.

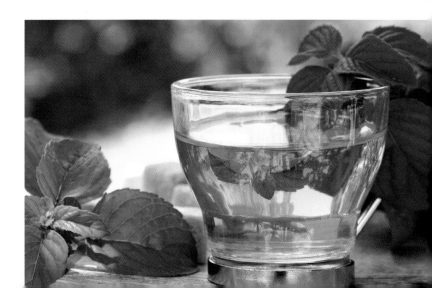

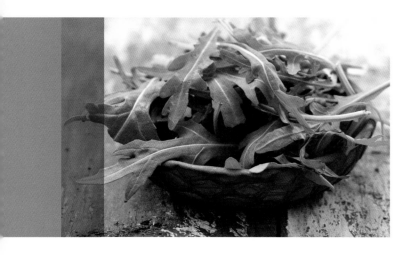

> Increase sweet, bitter, and astringent-tasting foods that are light in nature; eat plenty of bitter salad greens such as lettuce, arugula, radicchio, basil, and endive, all of which are particularly pitta balancing. Favor: coconut water, watermelon, cilantro, leafy greens, okra, zucchini, asparagus, olive oil, sunflower oil, coconut oil, ghee, cucumber, soaked/peeled almonds, kale, broccoli, pomegranate, apples, cranberry, mint, dill, fennel, cardamom, coriander, saffron.

> Avoid: tomatoes, eggplant, chili peppers, garlic, dry ginger, black pepper, fermented foods, spicy foods, sour fruits, heavy protein, mustard oil, molasses, coffee.

> Include cool drinks and raw foods in your diet, including cucumber, mango, and coconut water; natural fruit juices without added sugar; mint teas; and fresh berries.

> Reduce sour, salty, and pungent tastes.

BODY RHYTHM

> Give yourself a slow and loving full-body massage before taking a shower. Use pitta massage oil, coconut oil, or sunflower oil. Pitta season can create conditions for inflammation and overactivity of certain metabolic processes and secretions.

> A rose-water mist is a wonderful refresher for the face and body, as is a cooling milk-plus-mint bath, or milk-plus-rose petals. Make a sandalwood face mask with rose water. Have fresh aloe nearby for any pitta skin conditions that may arise, from sunburn to rash.

> Summer essential oils/scents include: sandalwood, rose, lavender, jasmine, lotus, gardenia, khus, and vertivert.

> Wear clothing of light texture and color. Excellent choices would be cotton, linen, and silk of white, blue, and green hues. Red and yellow shades tend to increase the fire that is already present.

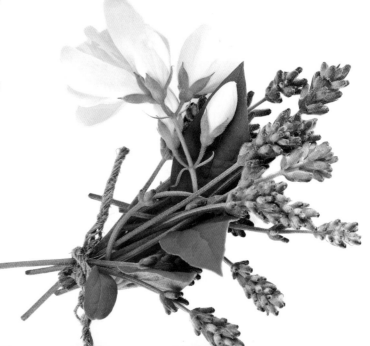

ENERGETIC VINYASA FOR THE SUMMER SEASON

Kala—Continue to synch with the sun, gradually getting up earlier before the sunrise; this is the peak time of growth, so synch your movements with that waxing light. Offer yoga outdoors in the shade so you can take in the fresh prana of the elements at this time.

Desa—Relate to the transition from spring to summer according to your ecology. In Southern California, we often have June gloom, and the peak of summer's heat doesn't get started till mid-August into September. If you are already experiencing the heat of summer, be aware of the effects of summer on excessive fire in your body. Begin to wear cooling colors and white to stay in the bhava of summer.

Bhava—Bask in the summer joy but be aware that the sun has reached its peak in the northern hemisphere and has begun its journey of waning for the next six months. The relaxing, easygoing quality of a more lunar, fluid nature can be integrated into the expansiveness of summer qualities—celebratory, sukha (intrinsic happiness), loving appreciation of the best of life—and the ease you feel in your body.

Dosha—The summer season is the most vulnerable time for those who did not cleanse fully in the spring to experience accumulated ama, or toxins, which can burn "impurely" during the excess heat imbalances of summer. The summer yoga practices and a proper clean-food sadhana can, with some mild cleanses, help you feel more balanced and clear in the prana flow of your body, which is the most open during the summer.

Yoga Practice—This is the best time of the year for Sringara Rasa, which nourishes the water element, balances excess heat, and helps us tend the fires of love and appreciation. Cultivate lunar or Shanti Rasa practices if you are feeling the blissful, lazy quality of a natural shift into ida nadi or the lunar current. This is the best season for flexibility and ease of range of motion, which you can enjoy by doing fluid backbends, namaskars to increase flow and agility, and Sringara Rasa circular movements for increasing the love flow.

> Enjoy stimulating but cooling practices at this time: *sitali* (hissing breath), slow and deep ujjayi pranayama, nadi shodhana. Reducing activity to light exercise will prevent pitta from building up in the body; avoid intense aerobic exercise at this time.

> Recommended exercises include those that are more cooling, such as restorative walking.

> Asanas that remove excess heat from the body, such as forward bends and mild backbends, are most suitable. Avoid asanas that build heat. Do cooling pranayama such as *sitali sheetkari, chandra bedhana,* and nadi shodhana.

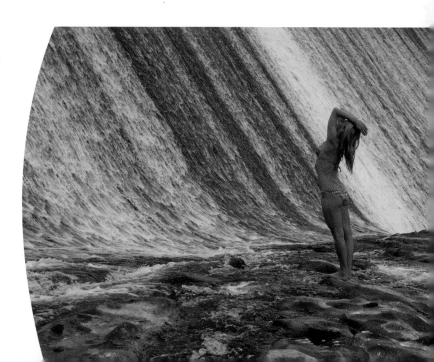

sacred rhythm—august 1 lughnasadh fire festival

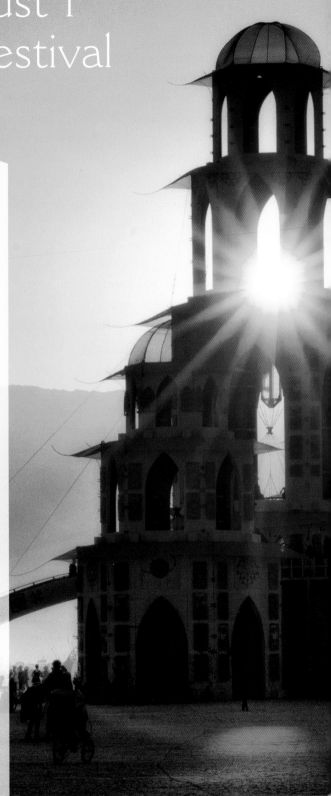

LUGHNASADH or Lammas is the third of the cross-quarter festivals, and it marks the halfway point between the summer solstice and fall equinox. Pronounced *loo-nus-ah,* Lughnasadh means "the commemoration of Lugh." As a god of fire and light, Lugh's name may well come from the same root as the Latin word *lux,* meaning "light," and summer is a time when we may feel the peak of light even more fully.

August 1 marks the apex of summer, the beginning of the harvest, and the age-old ritual of storing food for the waning months of autumn and winter ahead. As we begin to reap what we have sown, it is a time to reflect upon the "vinyasa of our actions" and upon what will bring completion to all the hard work and to the fruits that we have gathered. This includes celebration. August was a time when the great outdoor bonfires of the hillside were a central part of harvest festivals; the bonfire represented the sacrifice of the first sheaf of wheat, which was ceremonially reaped and then baked into a loaf. This harvest recalls the legend of the fire god Lugh, who undergoes death and rebirth, as do the foods grown so the people may eat and live.

Bonfires offer a final praise to the power of the sun that begins to wane at summer solstice—a celebration that is funereal for the "Sun King," as the sunlight now starts to fade.

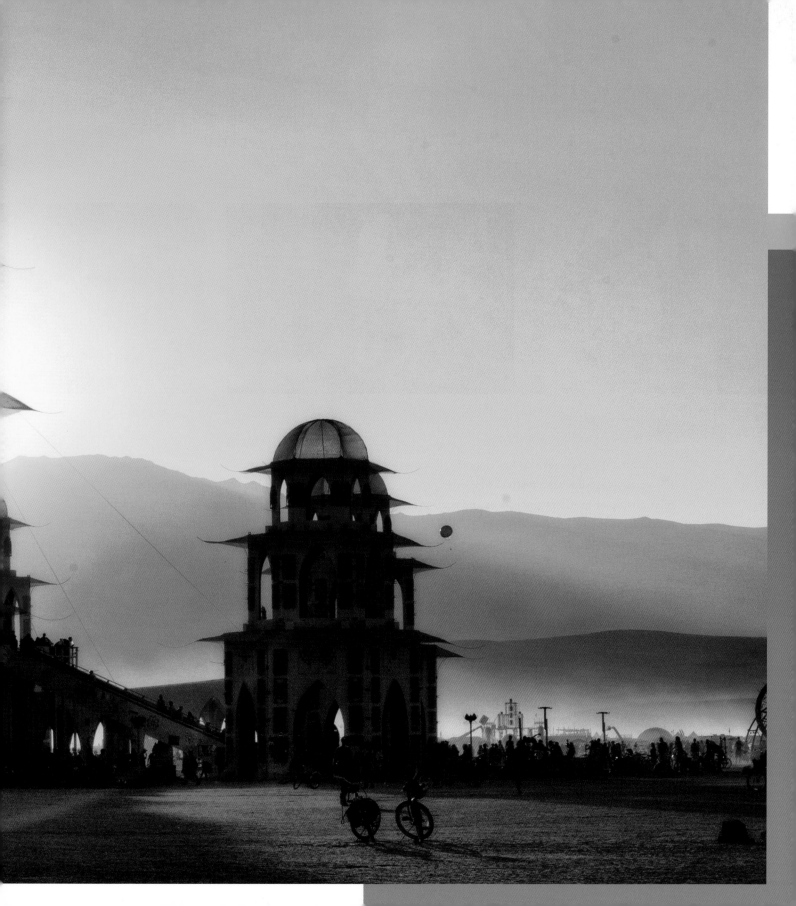

summertime hindu holidays

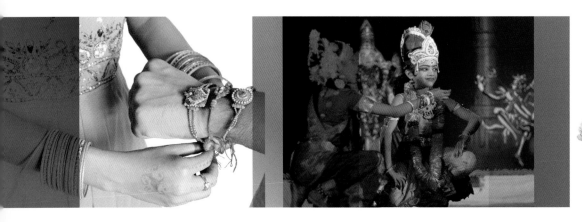

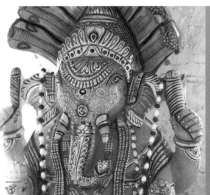

RAKSHA BANDHAN

The Raksha Bandhan festival has beautiful origins. It's usually described as a festival supporting the relationship of brothers and sisters and their protective bond with one another. It is symbolized in the giving of wrist ties between brothers and sisters.

KRISHNA JANMASHTAMI

Lord Krishna's birthday is celebrated in August with a daylong fast, often culminating at midnight when Krishna is said to have been born in prison on the eighth night of the waning moon. Usually depicted as the cow-herding, flute-playing, mischievous embodiment of love, Lord Krishna is also a spiritual warrior, slaying all that is against the flow of dharma.

Krishna dances in relationships: with his parents, his friends, his cows, and even the trees around him.

GANESH CHATURTHI

Ganesha is the son of Shiva and Parvati, lord of the muladhara chakra (root chakra at the base of the spine) and auspicious energy. He is depicted with the head of an elephant, denoting wisdom, and a human body representing the earthly existence of human beings. He removes obstacles, selfishness, and pride, and he opens the way for fruition. Ganesh Chaturthi is the day Shiva declared Ganesha to be superior to all the gods. It falls between mid-August and mid-September each year.

CHAPTER THIRTEEN

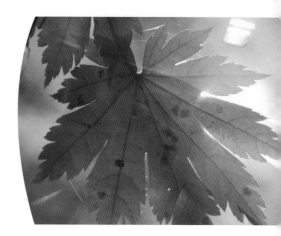

fall equinox

The Sacred Return

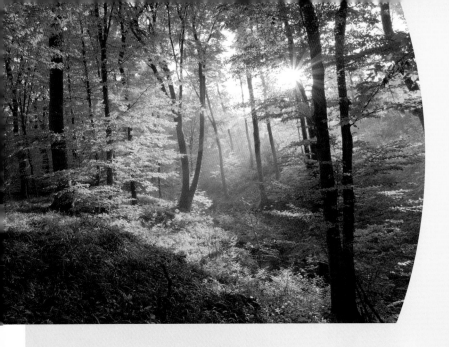

In the end

these things matter most:

How well did you love?

How fully did you live?

How deeply did you let go?

— THE BUDDHA SIDDHARTHA GAUTAMA[1]

As we begin the journey of the year at the fall equinox, or Alban Elfed in the Celtic tradition, we are given an opportunity to embody the meeting point of life and death; light and darkness; sun, earth, and moon that the cosmic body and earth are reflecting all around us. No matter if we're in a country or urban setting, the changes are occurring: the sun is rising and setting differently, the plant world is peaking and drying, the colors are changing, our activities are shifting, and the world at large is also at a turning point.

Fall is the season of the New Year in both Hindu and Jewish cultural traditions, which is why the New Year begins with the strong sadhana period of Navaratri-Diwali, Rosh Hashanah, and Yom Kippur. Both yearly cycles begin with a period of prayer, reflection, consumption of healing foods or fasting, and grounding into the mysteries of life (creation and dissolution). These are so embodied in the fall equinox moment of light balanced in equal darkness but moving toward the peak of greatest darkness mirrored in opposite in the spring. The spring movement toward greatest light and the fall movement toward fertile darkness is a theme that lives deep in our psyches—the mythic unconscious where our own shadow forces are churning to be held, understood, and released in the same cycle occurring within the earth.

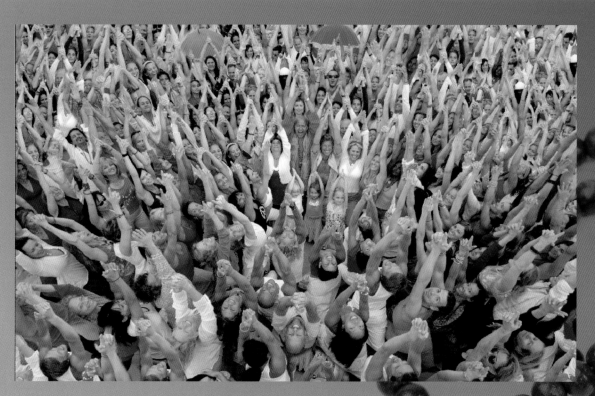

UNITED NATIONS INTERNATIONAL DAY OF PEACE AND THE GLOBAL MALA PROJECT

I wrote about the Global Mala Project in Chapter Nine—it was created to activate individual and collective awakening, empowerment, and unity. The Global Mala offers an opportunity to connect with the yoga community at large—across all borders, styles of yoga, and forms of yoga—each year on the fall equinox. This ritual goes beyond the norm, with practices of 108 sun salutations and 108 mantra japa. It combines yoga with action by offering the power of that energy and funds toward a greater purpose by supporting the organization of your choice. There is a profound vibrational ripple effect of students and teachers coming together as a mala—a circle of unity and peace—in yoga studios and centers across the globe on the International Day of Peace.

rosh hashanah

The festival of Rosh Hashanah—the name means "head of the year"—is observed for two days beginning on the new moon of the first day of the Jewish calendar. It is marked by the sounding of the *shofar*, the ram's horn, ushering in the first of the Ten Days of Repentance. The last day—Yom Kippur, the Day of Atonement—is considered to be the holiest day of the Jewish calendar.

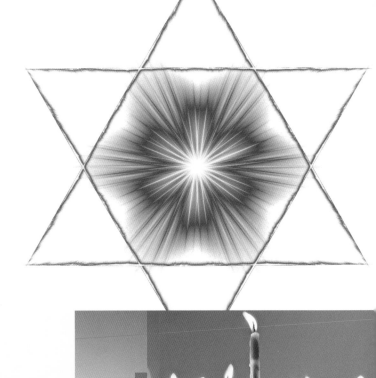

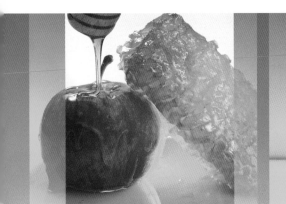
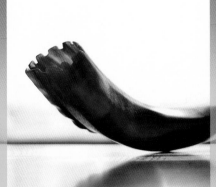
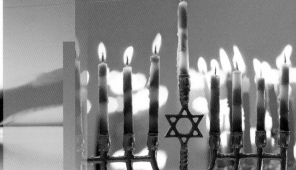

yom kippur

Everyone can symbolically participate in the Day of Atonement, whether you are Jewish or just want to connect to the inner process of atonement. There are two levels to this process: The first is your relationship with the creator—with God. Each of us has his or her way of returning to that original state or breath. The other level, which is very much customary, is to forgive and move forward, to speak to the people you may not have spoken to in a while—or to people who have wronged you. It's about unfinished business, and this is a good moment to clean up the situation, to make a phone call or send an email. There's a secret to the word atonement ("at-one-ment"): it's about being at one, looking beyond the situations that separate each of us, and finding what is common within each of us. Additional Yom Kippur practices include fasting and avoidance of bathing or washing. Wearing white clothing and going to temple or to a sacred place is traditional in order to symbolize one's purification on this holy day.

Whether you are Jewish, in relationship with a person of Jewish descent, or you just want to honor a beautiful firekeeping custom, the lighting of Shabbat candles eighteen minutes before sunset (or as close as possible) is a beautiful ritual with collective power, done every Friday night. As you light your Shabbat candles—the customary two white candles, a candle for each child in the family, or seven candles for each day of the week—visualize that light passing all around the world as millions of Jews observe a period of unplugging and restoration from sundown to sundown. You can light Shabbat candles while saying your own prayer, or use the traditional Hebrew prayer (below). Traditionally, after lighting the candles, the woman covers her eyes with her hands and recites her own prayer or this blessing:

Barukh atah Adonai Eloheinu, melekh ha'olam, asher kid'shanu b'mitz-votav v'tzivanu l'hadlik ner shel Shabbat

Blessed are You, Source of the universe, Who has made us holy through His commandments and commanded us to kindle the Sabbath light.

After the blessing is recited, the woman—the Shabbat queen of the family—uncovers her eyes and takes in the mitzvah, or special occasion of the weekly feast.

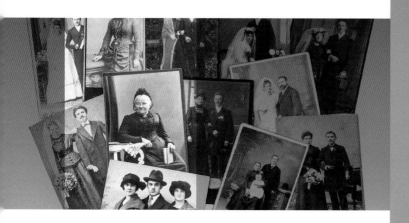

pitra tarpan

Pitra Tarpan is a time in India to honor your ancestors (pitra paksha). By offering ritual to them, we ask them to guide us in the maintenance of good health, peace, happiness, and enrichment. Create an ancestor altar: bring their spirits to your heart or altar. Offer light and a little nourishment (literally, food) on your altar, or give your memory from your heart as an offering. They will come alive in you. What they gave us with love—the light and the shadow—is a precious gift. Let us remember and offer back our life, our actions, and our tenderness and love.

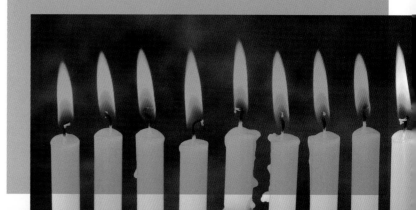

navaratri—
nine nights for the mother

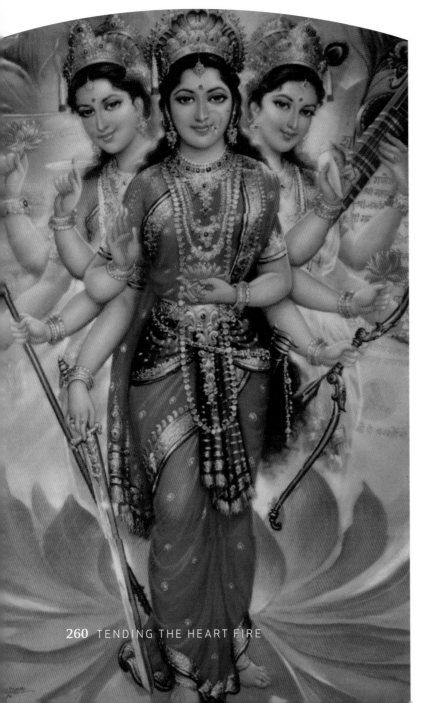

Navaratri is a nine-night (*nava* meaning "nine," *ratri* meaning "night") period dedicated to the triple form of the Shakti. It helps us to transform the shadow world during the changing of the fall season (Ma Durga), to celebrate the sublime creative flow (Ma Saraswati), to realize abundance of love, beauty, and generosity (Sri Lakshmi), and to celebrate the victory of consciousness as the culminating point of the sadhana period (Vijaya Dashami). While this celebration is additionally honored in the spring season, the autumn festivities often come with more grandeur.

The first three nights are dedicated to Ma Durga. She is often on a tiger or a lion; she is resplendent in a red sari. She has ten different weapons of consciousness, and her primary text is the Devi Mahatmyam. Ma Durga is the invincible force of consciousness. She can overcome any forces of regression, negativity, or obstacles that arise, particularly in adult life. Often these are psychological forces, although sometimes they may literally be physical obstacles. It is important during the Durga puja phase to reclaim one's personal energetic magnetic field.

Over the next three nights, a connection is made with Ma Lakshmi, who is the abundant flow of creation in all forms that sustains both our own life and the lives of others—this includes all forms of sustenance: food, money, and vitality. She is often seen seated on a lotus flower, and her primary text is the Sri Lakshmi Sahasranama Sthothra.

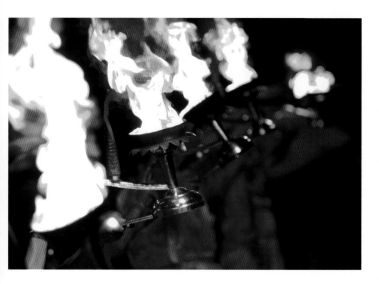

Ya Devi Sarva Bhuteshu Shanthi
Roopaena Samsthitha
Namastasyai Namastasyai
Namastasyai Namo Namah

I bow to the Great Mother who manifests in all beings in the form of peace.

The final three nights are spent worshipping the Mother as Saraswati, the Goddess of wisdom, creation, and intelligence. She is primarily seen with a peacock or swan, and her foremost text is the Saraswati Veda. This final phase of Navaratri is an auspicious time for transformation, manifesting prosperity, creating shifts toward more balance, and feeling supported in academic and literary pursuits.

Honoring Navaratri may include ritual fasting, large or householder-style pujas, daily ritual offering of mantra japa, and deeper study of the different aspects of the Great Mother. Fasts can vary in intensity, from eating just fruit, to fasting with milk, to a kitchari fast. Other ways of fasting include eating vegetarian or vegan foods, or eating just once a day.

FIREKEEPING PRACTICE—AARTI

Aarti is the waving of light at the culmination of one's practice or puja (offering) and derives from the original Vedic-tantric fire ceremonies. You can take a candle or a special aarti lamp with a long handle and wave the flame before your altar while ringing a bell in the left hand, or you can offer with a song. In a temple, aarti is offered in the sandhyas of the sunrise, noon, and sunset, as well as in early morning and late evening. Circulate the light around your altar in a clockwise circle, representing your journey of life illumined by the Source. Aarti during Navaratri often accompanies the following hymn to Devi or the Goddess. You can walk around your whole house to bless your space with the aarti, and offer it to other family members so they may bless themselves with the light.

Ya Devi Sarva Bhuteshu Vishnumaayeti
Shabdita Namastasyei Namastasyei
Namastasyei Namo Namah

Salutations to Divine Mother—Shakti Devi,
 The power of Lord Vishnu, who abides in all beings.
 Who abides as the eternal consciousness in all beings.
 Who manifests as power in all beings.
 Who abides in all beings in the form of forgiveness.
 Who manifests in all beings in the form of peace.
 Who manifests in all beings in the form of faith.
 Who abides in all beings in the form of beauty.
 Who abides in the form of compassion in all beings.
 Who abides in all beings in the form of delusion.
 The ruler of all senses and sensation.
 The ruler of all elements.
 The ruler of all creation and beings.
 To This Divine Mother, My Heartfelt Salutations.
 Shakti Devi pervades this entire universe and abides in
 all beings in the form of consciousness.
 Salutations to Her again and again.

—DEVI MAHATMYAM[2]

vitality rhythm and flow— ayurvedic wisdom for fall season

Ayurveda's emphasis on purification in balance with regeneration, activity and rest, and stimulation and restoration is a perfect complement to the fall season when we begin our journey by being honest with what is happening as we enter the cycle of the new year.

During the fall season, vata dosha is the aspect of nature that is predominant. Made up of the ether and air elements, vata is the generation of movement within the universe, which initiates all motion inside and outside of the body. Thus vata and prana, our vital life-energy, are connected, for life is movement and movement is the sign of life. Vata orchestrates all forms of circulation, from physical movement (actions), to mental activity (perception, thoughts, insights), to communication (words), to respiration, to the pulse and function of our heart and the flow of our nervous system. Vata brings the positive mobile qualities of inspiration, creativity, spontaneity, and initiation, which when disturbed become insecure, anxious, worried, fearful, and overwhelmed—all qualities that can become exacerbated under stress.

This is why the other elements of fire (for warmth), water (for lubrication), and earth (for grounding) are so vital to the fast-moving pace of fall's predominant air and space elements. Fall is the time to balance and nourish ourselves wisely for the coming season of darkness and shadows as the earth regenerates in the northern hemisphere. Staying close to the earth is reflected in completing the harvest of one's creativity from the beginning of the year with the steady, calm, grounded qualities that are so healing to vata.

The gunas, or qualities, of vata that we seek to balance are:

> Dry with lubrication
> Cold with warmth
> Light with guru (heavy, in the positive sense)
> Subtle with presence
> Rough with smooth for the nervous system
> Mobile with steadiness and grounding

When these qualities are in a balanced state, the vata season can be enjoyed with its celebrations, changes, and insights from inner work.

When out of balance, vata qualities build up within the body and mind due to aggravating lifestyle choices. This may be experienced as constipation, bloating, dry skin, insomnia, joint pain, and stress. Harmonizing vata during the cooling, dry fall season is an art that can be cultivated through wisely tending the fire of your life force.

FIVE ANCHORS FOR THE FALL

1. Slow down: try not to eat on the run or multitask, but rather stay present and move mindfully and consciously.

2. Keep grounded: enjoy activities and food that keep you connected to the earthy and heavy qualities. Keep to your routine—to your daily rituals.

3. Protect the body from cold and wind: wear a hat and scarf to protect from excess vata in the head (ears), and keep the lower back covered so that excess vata does not build up in the pelvis nor the colon.

4. Eat moist and warm foods: stay away from cold and raw foods.

5. Make oil your best friend: oil the entire body from head to toe to prevent dry, rough skin.

FOOD RHYTHM

Autumn is an ideal time for using more healthy oils in foods. (Ghee, coconut oil, sesame oil, olive oil, and hempseed oil are all oils I recommend.) Oils create inner lubrication, which keeps us in balance during this time when our bodies and the earth begin to dry up during the dessicating winds of the season.

> Teas: fenugreek, star anise, and cinnamon

> Special "vata" tea: four cups water, one teaspoon fennel seeds, one teaspoon coriander seeds, one teaspoon cardamom. Boil water in a pot. Add slightly crushed fennel seeds, coriander seeds, and cardamom pods. Boil for two more minutes. You can add honey or Sucanat to sweeten. Serve hot. Or you can try another warming digestive tea of fresh-cut ginger (about an inch), cardamom, and cinnamon.

> Sipping warm water and herbal teas throughout the day enhances warmth and hydration.

> As for foods, try to add oily, lubricating foods to your diet.

> Eat foods that are warming, grounding, predominately cooked, sweet, salty, sour, and in season. Soups and stews can be made from carrots, beets, yams, pumpkins, root vegetables, rice, quinoa, and mung beans. Be aware of bitter tastes such as from too much dark, leafy greens or heavy beans or gassy foods, which can aggravate vata. Eat warm and moist oatmeal, rice, or whole grains for breakfast rather than toast or cold cereal. Other good grains for fall include basmati rice, wheat (unless you're gluten intolerant), oats, quinoa, and amaranth.

> Sweet fruits like banana, apricot, apples, pears, peaches, and red grapes are good. Steam or sauté veggies—and prepare them with olive oil, ghee, or almond oil.

> Use mild spices for your food, such as cumin, coriander, ginger, cinnamon, mint, sage, spearmint, or thyme. Better herbs include ajwan, cinnamon salt, ginger, black pepper, hing, rosemary, thyme, oregano, and basil.

> Triphala Guggulu is a very good herb for regularity with elimination, to prevent constipation.

> Chywanprash is a great herbal jam that is healing for all, irrespective of age and gender. It creates a harmonious synergy in the body leading to better metabolism.

> Avoid dry and bloating foods such as popcorn, toast, rice cakes, junk food, and too much alcohol, cold salads, cold water, cold juices, and ice cream.

BODY RHYTHM

One of the most important ways to keep vata in balance is through a regular rhythm of your dinacharya (flow of the day). The primary way to pacify vata is by balancing times for sleep, eating, yoga, love, and work. Look at the rhythm and flow of your daily, weekly, and lunar rhythm for two-week periods. Beginning with the fall equinox or amavasya, maintain a commitment to all of these areas. If your life rhythm is going through a high-intensity phase, try to focus on making one time cycle steady.

> **Waking rhythm:** It's best to wake before 6 a.m. to maintain a good flow. If you need to rest on a weekend or after travel, then make that a loving sadhana for you and your family. The best time to wake up is forty-five minutes to one hour before sunrise.

> **Sleeping rhythm:** Turn your home into a *shantishala*—house of peace.

> **Eating rhythm:** Eat breakfast and dinner, but lunch is the most important meal.

> **Rest rhythm:** Energy-Sabbath days—choose your half-day or full-day retreat times during the ritual times of new and full moon—Navaratri, Rosh Hashanah, or Yom Kippur—for unplugging and tuning in to your and your family's deeper rhythm.

> **Work rhythm:** Place boundaries around working time in the evenings (unless you are in an unusually creative cycle) in order to create sacred bonding time for being with yourself, family, and community.

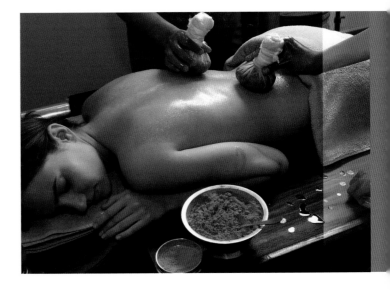

MASSAGE FOR THE FALL SEASON

> *Snehana*—Enjoy a morning full-body massage, done slowly and lovingly, before taking a shower or bath. After dry-brushing, heat sesame oil to use as a warming and deeply nourishing massage oil by placing it in a glass of hot water or a copper pan similarly filled. Essential oils for pacifying vata include jatamamsi, ginger, and lavender. Add geranium, orange, and ylang ylang.

ENERGETIC VINYASA FOR THE FALL SEASON

Kala—The fall season is the time to synch with the setting sun, the season of culmination and letting go; balance stronger practice with the waxing moon and more restorative practice with the waning energy of the moon.

Desa—Begin to move inward, drawing earth colors and the harvest seasons around you; follow the earth's inward pull toward the darkest final six weeks of the year before the winter solstice.

Bhava—Cultivate wisdom in action, fullness with awareness of allowing change, equanimity, ability to stand in your truth.

Dosha—The fall season is the most vulnerable time for those with wavering fire or vishama agni. Vata and pitta dosha can feel imbalanced from the quick changes and stress of the vata season.

Yoga Practice—Cultivate Sringara and Shanti Rasa practices, a balance of solar energy moving toward more lunar energy in your namaskars and practice. Practice softening your lower abdominal cavity, grounding your feet into the earth, building strength and stability, and allowing yourself sufficient rest after your practice. Enjoy standing balance and lower-hip openers to release tension from the lower pelvis and thighs—the main sites of vata dosha.

Remember to move smoothly and slowly and stay grounded and centered in your daily flow, to bring the year to the most auspicious close.

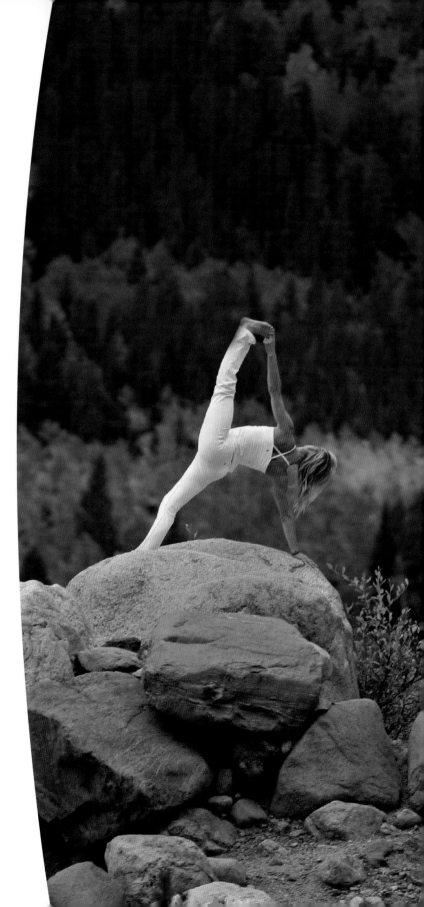

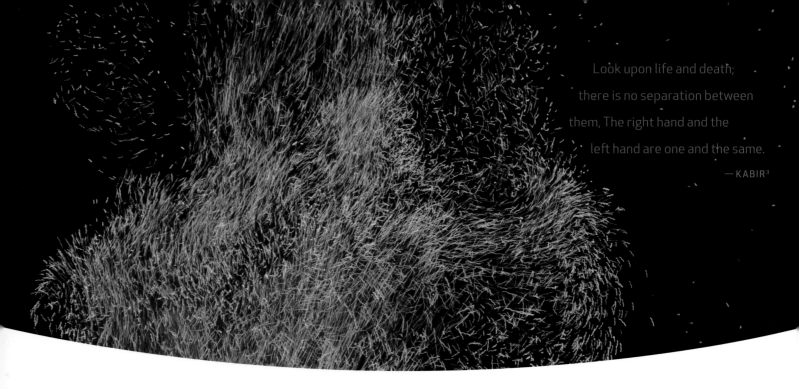

samhain—oct 31, halloween

The great wheel turns, another year

Old, bright gold with death.

Bare branches now,

the Old Lord's limbs,

Chill wind the Old Lord's breath.

Like dancing leaves on sleeping branches

The dark tide of memory is stirred.

The deepest thought-flame now is kindled,

Consuming, the fire in ancient words.

— KENNY KLEIN[4]

Samhain marks the last six-week period of the year, when the veil between the worlds is penetrated and we are able to communicate with the departed. Celtic peoples observed the "Feast of the Dead" by leaving offerings of food for the dead, a practice still alive throughout the United Kingdom and reminiscent of the exchange of candy and the dressing up of Halloween. The Celtic peoples also left any unpicked crops as offerings to nature spirits.

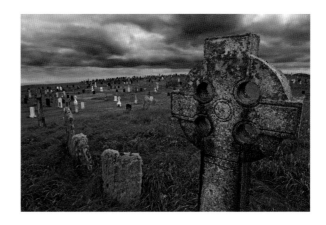

día de los muertos

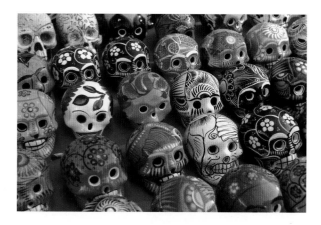

El Día de Los Muertos originated with the Olmecs in Mexico, possibly as long as three thousand years ago, as a way to honor the relationship of the living and the dead reflected in the earth cycle.

A ritual to honor children who have passed on takes place on November 1 and is called Día de los Muertos Chiquitos. The following day is Día de los Muertos, and this marks the return of the spirits of the dead. Observers of the holiday bring food and drink to ancestors' graves, in part for themselves and in part as offerings to their deceased loved ones. It is a festive time for remembering departed family members with love and joy.

> I too have heard the dead singing and they
> tell me that this life is good.
>
> They tell me to live it gently with fire,
> and always with hope.
> There is wonder here and there is surprise—
> in everything the unseen moves.
> —BEN OKRI[5]

FIREKEEPING PRACTICE— TRANSFORMING THE OLD

As we enter into the last six weeks of the year, that which is dying and longing to be released calls for us to let go and allow it to be transformed, like dry stalks into the fire of winter's rebirth. Create a fire in your fireplace, outdoors, or in a "cauldron" or iron pot that can withstand the flames—or even use a candle—to make an offering on Samhain or during the waning nights before the new moon or in the last days of Navaratri. In this way you can experience the liberation that death can bring as the closed fist lets go of what it has been holding on to: an old habit, thought, relationship, or process that is calling to be transformed. Write it down on a piece of paper, or symbolically infuse your offering into herbs from the land, such as sage or dried rosemary. Watch the offering burn all the way to ash.

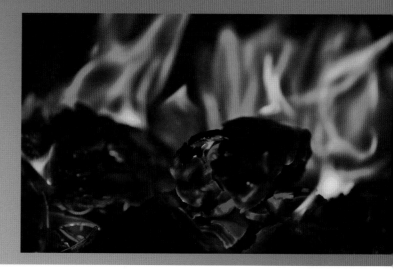

festivals of light

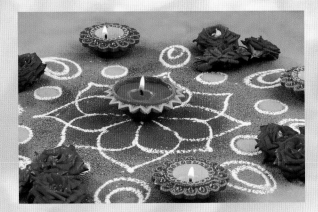

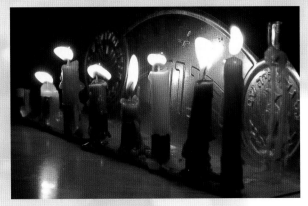

DIWALI

Diwali is a famous Hindu festival of light, and its name is derived from the earthenware oil lamps called *diyas* that are found everywhere at this time.

Lakshmi, the goddess of wealth, is often honored during Diwali, through prayers and lights, for business success and other forms of prosperity.

> Cleaning the home

> Wearing new clothes

> Exchanging gifts (often sweets and dried fruits) and preparing festive meals

> Decorating buildings with fancy lights

> Huge fireworks displays

> Leaving the windows and doors of the house open so that Lakshmi can come in

> Making *rangoli* or yantras by drawing on the floors using rice flour. Rangoli are patterns, and the most popular subject is the lotus flower.

HANUKKAH

The menorah candelabra is a central focus of the celebration of Hanukkah, which celebrates the Israelites' victory over foreign invaders and their restoration of the Temple. It commemorates a miracle: one day's worth of oil burned brightly in the Temple for eight days.

Om Subhajayai Namah
I bow to the Source of Prosperity

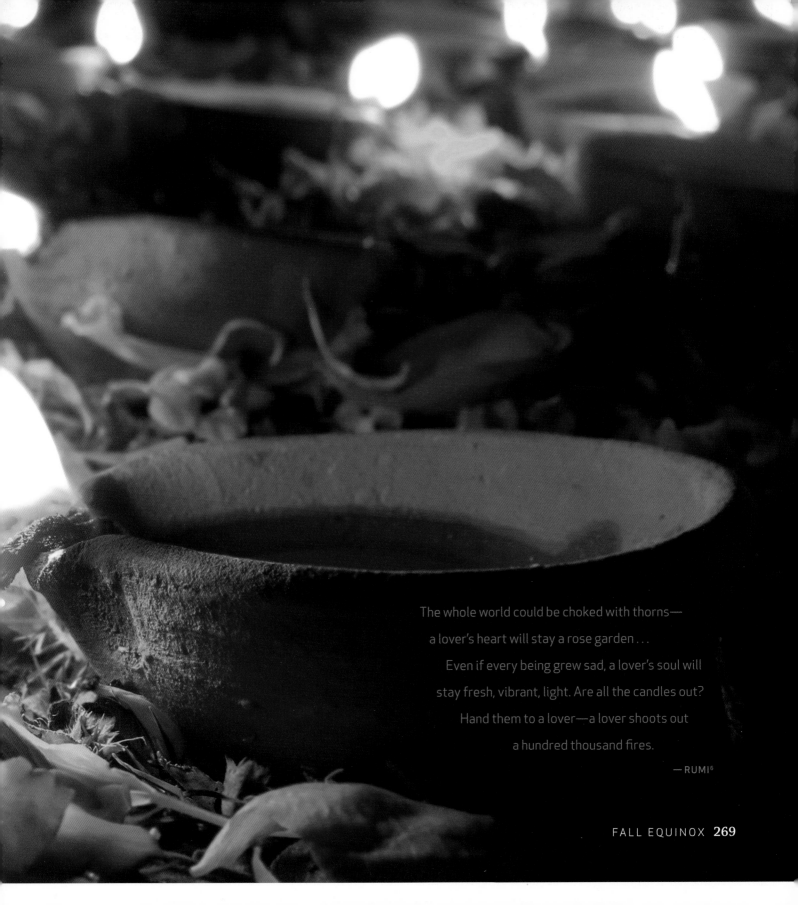

The whole world could be choked with thorns—
a lover's heart will stay a rose garden . . .
Even if every being grew sad, a lover's soul will
stay fresh, vibrant, light. Are all the candles out?
Hand them to a lover—a lover shoots out
a hundred thousand fires.

— RUMI[6]

FIREKEEPING RITUAL—
FILLING YOUR HOUSE WITH LIGHT

It is beautiful to participate in the fall cross-cultural rituals of filling your outer and inner house with light. Our family celebrates this way at every opportunity, beginning with Diwali, Hanukkah, winter solstice, and Christmas. Starting three days before Diwali (usually around the new moon of November), clean your home of any old dust or clutter as a mirror of your own inner process at the close of the year. On the sunrise or sunset of the new moon of Diwali, as well as the other festivals of light, illuminate the doorway of your home and hang lights outside. (We love solar lights.)

The inward and the outward become

as one sky, the Infinite

and the finite are united: I am drunken

with the sight of this All!

This Light of Thine fulfills the universe:

the lamp of love burns on the fuel of knowledge.

— KABIR[7]

Ignite candles in every room of your house, particularly on altars or altarlike spaces, from your central altar to every room of your house. Make sure that these lights are well protected in votive containers, and ignite them with a prayer of goodwill in your heart. The lighting can be accompanied by ringing a bell, burning incense, sprinkling water and rose petals. You can include other family members and make a procession through your house. You may leave the candles lit all night (again, ensuring they are safe and well protected). Or you can extinguish them by waving the flames out with your hand or using a candle dampener a few hours after the sunrise or sunset sandhya has passed. You may enjoy this ritual every new and full moon at any time of the year, but it is incredibly satisfying during the waning light as a triumph of the spirit, goodwill, and sacred space.

mevlana's wedding night

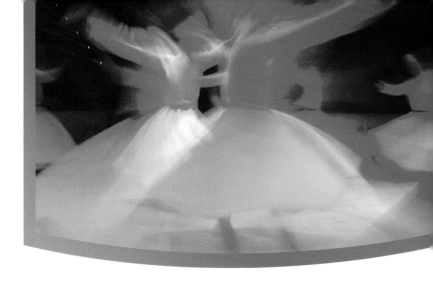

The world celebrates December 13th as the auspicious birthday of Mevlana Jelalluddin Rumi, the great dancing mystic whose passionate poems have been sung, whispered, roared, remembered, revered, and echoed in the hearts of millions. Every being awakened by one of Rumi's poems has experienced his words of tender wisdom and the fire of love in them that blazes across centuries, cultures, and religions. We feel the shaking off of ho-hum living with his call to live life fully.

Perhaps, in an age of contradictions, Rumi reflects a way of being on the spiritual path as a firekeeper that embraces and integrates the full spectrum of the human experience. He expresses devotion with nakedness—exposing his wounds, despair, and longing together with his ecstatic celebration, which is fully alive, passionate, and a practice of Sema, the whirling of the Dervishes in unbroken tradition for the last eight hundred years.

RUMI AND THE HEART FIRE—CLOSING

Rumi's burning, openly ecstatic love songs emerged from the same sparks of life, the same fire that liberates us from detours and frees us to follow our evolutionary path. Do we dare to live our lives with the full passion of the mystic firekeeping Rumi?

What ways of being are covering or dampening our true radiance? How are we holding back from the transforming fire of love? What turns our own sparks into a bonfire of love?

Tending the Heart Fire is not like some fanciful poetry. Like Rumi's passionate songs, it is a real entryway into our truth, deepest love, vision, and wisdom in action. Rumi's poems are the sacred fuel that is kindled in our moment-to-moment living—in the ways we see, touch, taste, hear, feel, and dance with life in its everyday rhythms and its most sublime expressions. Rumi the passionate, Rumi the divine rascal, Rumi the embodiment of blazing, liberating truth, encourages those of us who tend the Heart Fire:

> Your heart is a temple
> Your essence is gold hidden in dust.
> To reveal its splendor you need to
> burn in the fire of love.
>
> — RUMI[8]

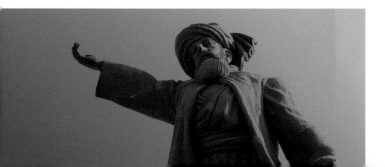

firekeeping call— a parting message

We are the firekeepers, and our heart helps us navigate through all of life's challenges and uncertainties by connecting to the true source of power. Life is change, and our heart is intimately attuned to the modulation, being a continual pulsation of life itself.

Tending our Heart Fire turns everything into sadhana, a process of integral alignment. Like Shakti riding her sacred tiger, our Heart Fire's presence can be fierce and loving simultaneously.

Life in essence is still the savannah where the gazelles must join the herd within an hour of being born.

To be born is to learn to walk in rhythm on your own, to be part of the tribe, to move together, hold your own, and give back.

Firekeeping requires primal power and rhythm in order to be integrated into the fabric of our life. We must kindle our ancestral qualities of humility, stamina, steadiness, and ingenuity.

To tend the Heart Fire is to create a sacred expression of our life.

Our inner fire is connected to all the elements. Earth grounding us. Water nourishing our lives. Our heart transforming ordinary work into a living yoga. Space as a realization of the vast field that holds all of life.

—SHIVA REA

Humankind is being led along an evolving course through this migration of intelligences and though we seem to be sleeping there is an inner wakefulness that guides the dream that will eventually startle us back to the truth of who we are.

— RUMI[9]

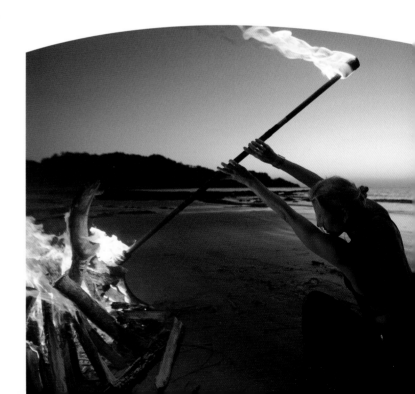

My family and friends—I adore you. Thank you from my heart: Jai, Demetri, Papouzi Kevin Rea, Mama Vicki (in the spirit world), the writers in my family—Grandma & Grandpa Furr, Aunt Ann, Julian, Kiera, Layla, Nikos, Janelle—and all of my dear friends over the past two years who were so patient with me when in the midst of a full life I would dive in the writing cave.

To the teachers who have offered translations, quotes, and inspirations that guided deep reflection on the Heart Fire: Andrew Harvey—mystic mentor and sacred activist—for your initiatory guidance, Daniel Odier—my root teacher of Tandava—for the wisdom of the spandafied translations of the Vijnana Bhairava Tantra, Christopher Tompkins for being there from the beginning with depth translations and teachings of the early Tantras—as well as years of collaboration to bring forth the cosmic vinyasa, Sally Kempton for your revivifying wisdom, teachings, and blessings of the foreword, Coleman Barks for your soulful transmission of Mevlana Jelalluddin Rumi, Dr. Vasant Lad for the inclusion of your ayurvedic wisdom quotes, Sreedevi Bringi for guidance in puja and the ways of the Mother, Paul Muller-Ortega for your inspiration of the Triadic Heart, and the Institute of HeartMath for the science and wisdom of the energetic heart.

To my heroine Tami Simon, for planting the seed invitation of publishing a visual book with Sounds True. To my passionate and patient editor Haven Iverson, for holding the vision with practical enthusiasm. To Sheridan McCarthy, for your timely contributions, and to the Sounds True production team—Karen Polaski, Jennifer Y. Brown, Lisa Kerans, and Jennifer Holder. To the extraordinary design artist Amy Hayes: I am forever grateful for your enlightened creativity. Thank you for trusting and giving me the creative freedom to be involved every step of the way.

To the Samudra Global School of Living Yoga team, and research assistant and Living Yoga Sadhana coordinator Kristen Townsend, who was there from the beginning and dedicated to the end like a pollinating bee. To Maria Garre for your dedicated assistance with the Living Ayurveda, Lisa Firefly for your amazing initial design chart inspirations and collaboration with the Solar-Lunar Calendar of the Year. To Glenisse Pagan, Natalie Sheets, Julian Rea—thank you for your contributions. To all the firekeepers in the Living Yoga Sadhana program, thank you for the openness to apply the teachings of living vinyasa.

To the amazing artists and photographers who made the book come alive (please see art credits): Jenay Martin—darling of the Universe who, along with my beloved Demetri Velisarius, formed most of the images of the book. James Wvinner, Amir Magal, Bill Tipper, Rich Van Every, Mario Covic, Lakshmi Grace, Maria Garre—thank you for your collaboration over the years and for visually

273

imparting the energetic power of nature and the moving body. I am grateful for the permission to include your art: Sarah Tomlinson (sacred yantras), Shakti de Sousa (drawings of namaskar and rasas), Pan Trinity (Firekeeper Montage), Alex Linghorn (Sadhu Tandava), Radisha (108 Saints), Jeff Waters (Burning Man Temple).

For my heart mandala and the teaching lineage that is an ocean, please see the book website, tendingtheheartfire.com. I am eternally grateful for all my teachers and mitras—friends on the path—for you are the fuel, the circle, the sacred exchange that keeps my heart blazing. A bow to you all . . .

EPIGRAPH

1. Translated by Esmeralda Lamas. © Esmeralda Lamas.

INTRODUCTION

1. Jelalluddin Rumi, *The Big Red Book: The Great Masterpiece Celebrating Mystical Love and Friendship,* trans. Coleman Barks (New York: HarperCollins, 2010), 186.
2. Stephen Buhner, *The Secret Teachings of Plants: The Intelligence of the Heart in the Direct Perception of Nature* (Santa Fe: Bear & Co, 2004), 95.
3. Renee Levi, "The Sentient Heart: Messages for Life" (online article) on ResonanceProject.org, April 23, 2001.
4. Statistic from "The Human Heart" on the Franklin Institute website: www.fi.edu. Also cited in: KD Kochanek, JQ Xu, SL Murphy, AM Miniño, HC Kung, "Deaths: final data for 2009," *National vital statistics reports.* 2011; 60(3).
5. Frances Burton, *Fire: The Spark That Ignited Human Evolution* (Albuquerque: University of New Mexico Press, 2009), 15.
6. Paul E. Muller-Ortega, *The Triadic Heart of Śiva: Kaula Tantricism of Abhinavagupta in the Non-dual Shaivism of Kashmir* (Albany: State University of New York Press, 1989), 159.
7. Personal interview with tantric scholar Christopher Tompkins in Santa Monica, CA, on November 12, 2012.
8. Andrew Harvey, *Radical Passion: Sacred Love and Wisdom in Action* (Berkeley, CA: North Atlantic Books, 2012), xv.
9. Daniel Odier, *Yoga Spandakarika: The Sacred Texts at the Origins of Tantra* (Rochester, VT: Inner Traditions, 2005), 103.

CHAPTER ONE

1. Andrew Harvey and Karuna Erickson, *Heart Yoga: The Sacred Marriage of Yoga and Mysticism* (Berkeley, CA: North Atlantic Books, 2010), 71.
2. Mechthild of Magdeburg, *The Flowing Light of the Godhead,* trans. Frank Tobin (Eastford, CT: Martino Fine Books, 2012).
3. Jelalluddin Rumi, *The Book of Love: Poems of Ecstasy and Longing,* trans. Coleman Barks (New York: HarperCollins, 2003), 178.
4. Andrew Harvey and Anne Baring, *The Mystic Vision: Daily Encounters with the Divine* (New York: HarperCollins, 1995).

5. "Bridget Bright," a poem for Imbolc by Hedgewytch, can be found at www.angelfire.com/magic2/imbolc.
6. From a personal interview with shamanic expert Dr. Alberto Villoldo, December 21, 2011.
7. Muller-Ortega, *The Triadic Heart of Śiva,* 65.
8. Translated by Sanskrit scholar Christopher Tompkins. © Christopher Tompkins.
9. Translated by Christopher Tompkins. Sacred texts written by various sages evolved from the Vedas that form the basis of contemporary Vedanta.
10. Translated by Sanskrit scholar Christopher Tompkins. © Christopher Tompkins.
11. The first/source innovative ritual system called "Tantra" is also known as Kashmir Shaivism (from its origins in Kashmir) or *Tantric Shaivism* (Tantra which focuses on the Hindu deity Shiva [male], a.k.a. the personification/symbol omnipresent source Intelligence of the universe, and Shakti [female], the power or energy of Universal Consciousness, or Shiva) as One inseparable from creation. Hence the description of Tantra as a nondual path.
12. Muller-Ortega, *The Triadic Heart of Śiva,* 82.
13. Stephen Amidon and Thomas Amidon, *The Sublime Engine* (Emmaus, PA: Rodale, 2012), 44.
14. St. Augustine of Hippo, *The Confessions.*
15. Amidon and Amidon, 80.
16. Paul Pearsall, *The Heart's Code: Tapping the Wisdom and Power of Our Heart Energy* (New York: Broadway Books, 1999), 68.
17. Renee Levi, "The Sentient Heart: Messages for Life" (online article) on ResonanceProject.org, April 23, 2001.
18. Brian Swimme, *The Universe Is a Green Dragon: A Cosmic Creation Story* (Rochester, VT: Bear & Company, 1984), 169–70.
19. Burton, *Fire,* 15.
20. These statistics are from the U.S. Energy Information Administration in its online article: "Use of Energy in the United States Explained" at www.eia.gov.
21. Statistic from "The Human Heart" on the Franklin Institute website: www.fi.edu.
22. KD Kochanek, JQ Xu, SL Murphy, AM Miniño, HC Kung, "Deaths: final data for 2009," *National vital statistics reports.* 2011; 60(3).
23. The Franklin Institute, www.fi.edu.

24. U.S. Environmental Protection Agency, 1989, Report to Congress on indoor air quality, volume 2.

25. Firekeeping Timeline citations follow:

   a. "Beginning of Time: Connection," *Popular Science,* April 1991, 92.

   b. Ron Cowen, "The Solar System's Big Bang," *Science News,* February 14th, 2009 (vol.175, no. 4), 26.

   c. "Early Pliocene Hominids from Gona, Ethiopia," *Nature* v. 433, no. 7023.

   d. Burton, *Fire,* 171.

   e. Goren-Inbar, et al., "Evidence of Hominid Control of Fire at Gesher Benot Ya`aqov, Israel," *Science,* April 30, 2004, 725–7.

   f. David Price, "Energy and Human Evolution," *Population and Environment: A Journal of Interdisciplinary Studies* 16, no. 4, March 1995: 301–19.

   g. Carey K. Morewedge, Young Eun Huh, and Joachim Vosgerau, "Thought for Food: Imagined Consumption Reduces Actual Consumption," *Science,* 10 December 2010: 1530–1533.

   h. P. Karkanas, et al., "The earliest evidence for clay hearths: Aurignacian features in Klisoura Cave 1, southern Greece," *Antiquity* 78(301):513–525.

   i. "Bulgarian Archaeologist Discovers World's Likely Oldest Sun Temple," *Archaeology,* December 16, 2010.

   j. "Hinduism From Ancient Times," April/May 2007, Himalayan Academy, 2013, www.hinduismtoday.com.

   k. Ian Shaw, ed., *The Oxford History of Ancient Egypt* (Oxford University Press, 2000), 480.

   l. 1200 BCE is cited as the approximate date of the exodus of the Israelites from Egypt (the first Passover) at http://jewishindependent.ca.

   m. "The History of Parsees of India," a paper written by P. P. Balsara.

   n. James Burke, *Connections* (New York: Little, Brown and Co., 1978/1995), 159.

   o. Lewis Mumford, *Technics and Civilization* (New York: Harcourt, Brace & Company, 1934).

   p. François Crouzet, "France" in Mikuláš Teich and Roy Porter, eds., *The Industrial Revolution in National Context: Europe and the USA* (Cambridge: Cambridge University Press, 1996), 45.

   q. John Perlin, *From Space to Earth: The Story of Solar Electricity* (Ann Arbor, MI: Aatec Publications, 1999).

   r. Program description for "Edison's Miracle of Light: The Film & More," www.pbs.org

   s. "The History of Spindletop Texas," Paleontological Research Institution's Museum of the Earth online article: www.museumoftheearth.org.

   t. U.S. Energy Information Administration in its online article: "Use of Energy in the United States Explained" at www.eia.gov.

   u. U.S. Energy Information Administration in its online article: "Petroleum Timeline," www.eia.doe.gov.

   v. From the online article, "Exploration," www.nasa.gov.

   w. "Historic Wind Development in New England: The Age of PURPA Spawns the Wind Farm," www1.eere.energy.gov.

   x. "History of Energy in the United States: 1635–2000," www.eia.doe.gov.

   y. "Small Group of House Republicans Derails ANWR Drilling," November 10, 2005, www.nationalcenter.org

   z. "USDA & DOE Release National Biofuels Action Plan," Oct. 7, 2008, www.energy.gov.

   aa. Sebastian Oberthur and Rene Lefeber, "Holding Countries to Account: The Kyoto Protocol's Compliance System Revisited After Four Years of Experience," *Climate Law* 1 (2010), 133–158.

   bb. "Estimated Energy Use in 2011: 97.3 Quads," Lawrence Livermore National Laboratory and the Department of Energy, Oct 2012, https://flowcharts.llnl.gov.

   cc. "Renewables 2011: Global Status Report," 17–18, www.map.ren21.net.

   dd. Ben Sills, "Solar May Produce Most of World's Power by 2060, IEA Says," *Bloomberg* online (Aug 29, 2011).

26. Brian Swimme interview: "Episode 40: Brian Swimme—Love in the Cosmos" of Personal Life Media's Sex, Love, and Intimacy Series, http://podcasts.personallifemedia.com.

CHAPTER TWO

1. This excerpt from the Bhagavad Gita is translated by Christopher Tompkins. © Christopher Tompkins. My understanding of this excerpt from the Bhagavad Gita is supported by Paul Muller-Ortega's work on the Tantric heart and by translator Christopher Tompkins's in-depth research on the cosmic breath cycles within Tantra.

2. This excerpt from the Shiva Samhita is translated by Christopher Tompkins. © Christopher Tompkins.

3. This excerpt of the Tirumanitram is translated by Christopher Tompkins. © Christopher Tompkins.

4. Sambhu Natanam by Patanjali, translation and commentary by H. H. Swamini Sarada Priyananda, in Lakshmi Bandlamudi, *Movements with the Cosmic Dancer: On Pilgrimage to Kailash Manasarovar* (New Delhi: New Age Books, 2006), 21.

5. Ibid.

6. This excerpt of the Purusha Sukta is translated by Christopher Tompkins. © Christopher Tompkins.

7. Vasant Lad, *Textbook of Ayurveda: Fundamental Principles* (Albuquerque, NM: The Ayurvedic Press, 2002), 26.

8. Patanjali in Bandlamudi, *Movements with the Cosmic Dancer,* 21.

9. Ibid.

10. Translated by Christopher Tompkins. © Christopher Tompkins.

11. Translated by Christopher Tompkins. © Christopher Tompkins.

12. Translated by Christopher Tompkins. © Christopher Tompkins.

13. Translated by Christopher Tompkins. © Christopher Tompkins.

14. Swami Tapasyananda, trans., *Saundarya-Lahari of Sri Sankaracarya* (Madras, India: Sri Ramakrishna Math Press, 1987).

15. Madhu Khanna, *Yantra: The Tantric Symbol of Cosmic Unity* (New York: Thames and Hudson, 1979), 77.

16. This revelation about kundalini shakti being located in the heart is made known to us today through a translation by Christopher Tompkins. © Christopher Tompkins.

17. Translation by Sanskrit scholar Christopher Tompkins. © Christopher Tompkins.

18. Ibid.

19. *The Bhagavad Gita* (second edition), trans. Eknath Easwaran (Berkeley, CA: Nilgiri Press, 2007).

20. Translation by Christopher Tompkins. © Christopher Tompkins.

21. Sri Abhinavagupta's "Hymn to Bhairava" (Bhairava Stotra) from Lorin Roche, *Radiance Sutras.*

22. Translation of Baul Song by Christopher Tompkins. © Christopher Tompkins.

23. Translation by Christopher Tompkins. © Christopher Tompkins.

CHAPTER THREE

1. Patricia Daniels, et al., *Body: The Complete Human* (Washington, D.C.: National Geographic Society, 2007).

2. Doc Childre and Howard Martin, *The HeartMath Solution* (New York: HarperCollins, 1999), 30.

3. Rollin McCraty, *The Energetic Heart: Bioelectromagnetic Interactions Within and Between People* (Boulder Creek, CA: Institute of Heart Math, 2003).

4. Renee Levi, "The Sentient Heart: Messages for Life" (online article) on ResonanceProject.org, April 23, 2001).

5. Stephen Buhner, *The Secret Teachings of Plants: The Intelligence of the Heart in the Direct Perception of Nature* (Santa Fe: Bear & Co, 2004), 85.

6. Ibid.

7. The Hafiz poem is from *I Heard God Laughing: Renderings of Hafiz,* trans. Daniel Ladinsky (Walnut Creek, CA: Sufism Reoriented, 1996), 73.

8. Lawrence Chilnick, *Heart Disease: An Essential Guide for the Newly Diagnosed* (Philadelphia: Perseus Books Group, 2008).

9. Childre and Martin, 35.

10. Buhner, 84.

11. Buhner, 85.

12. Childre and Martin, 58.

13. Childre and Martin, 55.

14. Childre and Martin, 15.

15. Childre and Martin, 54.

16. Childre and Martin, 61.

17. Childre and Martin, 90–91.

18. Childre and Martin, 139.

19. Childre and Martin, 161.

20. Conrad Pritscher, *Einstein and Zen: Learning to Learn* (New York: Peter Lang Publishing, 2009), 36.

21. Marcel Zentner and Tuomas Eerola, "Rhythmic engagement with music in infancy" in *Proceedings of the National Academy of Sciences* (early online edition), March 19, 2010.

22. Rumi, *The Big Red Book,* 186.

23. The power of our hand upon our bodies (*mudra*); the resting of our gaze (*dristi*); the listening to our pulse (*mantra*); and the transmutation of dissonant, stuck emotions or thought patterns into a more unified state of meditation is the essence of a universal yoga process mirrored in many of the world's meditative traditions— including the Institute of HeartMath's "heart lock-in" technique. This technique teaches people to keep their focus in their heart region and transform stress and negative emotions into the highly coherent states of gratitude and love that can encompass anything that arises. Childre and Martin, *The HeartMath Solution,* 211.

CHAPTER FOUR

1. This poem is inspired by a south Indian artist song published in: Madhu Khanna, *Yantra: The Tantric Symbol of Cosmic Unity* (New York: Thames and Hudson, 1979), 129–131.

2. Rumi, from "Birdsong from Inside the Egg" in *The Book of Love,* 162.

3. References to the connection of Shiva with the rise of dance and music is found within Natya Shastra and the oral traditions connected to the Chidambaram temple, which shows the 108 karanas of Shiva. The Gheranda Samhita attributes 8.4 million asanas to Shiva.

4. Nitin Kumar, "The Rhythm of Music: A Magical and Mystical Harmony," in *Exotic India,* September 2003, exoticindia.com.

5. For example, the Pashupata Sutra, a work of the Atimarga ("Direct Path"), a Shaiva school of early Tantric Shaivism that dates to around the fourth century CE, instructs its *sadhakas* (initiated yogis) to perform a dance to a specific tempo known as Rangava in order to magically ward off the impending death of others: "For those in sudden danger of death and so on, the sādhaka (yogī) enacts a dance that follows the common 'Rangava' tempo for the continuation of life. Hence, in this case the appropriate way for the sadhaka to conduct himself is to physically enact the gestures of a dancer." —*Pashupata Sutra III.2* (trans. Christopher Tompkins)

6. This early understanding of vinyasa is based on a translation by Christopher Tompkins of the Nishvasa Tantra (chapter 1 of the Naya Sutra section). The Jayadrathayamala Tantra is based on the translation of Alexis Sanderson, from his "The Shaiva Exegesis of Kashmir," in *Tantric Studies in Memory of Hélène Brunner,* eds. Dominic Goodall and André Padoux (Pondicherry, India: Institut français d'Indologie/École française d'Extrême-Orient, 2007), 285–291.

7. From a translation by Christopher Tompkins of the Jayadrathayamala Tantra, (as referenced in note 6 above), which describes the poses performed by Kaula (Tantric) practitioners as *karanas*.

8. Anandamayi Ma and Joseph Fitzgerald, *The Essential Sri Anandamayi Ma: Life and Teaching of a 20th-Century Indian Saint* (Delhi: Motilal Banarsidass Publishers, 2007), 96.

9. Miranda Shaw, *Passionate Enlightenment* (Princeton, NJ: Princeton University Press, 1995), 189.

10. Bhumi Pranam prayer translated by Kristen Vrinda Seth.

11. Translated by Christopher Tompkins.

12. Transliteration by Christopher Tompkins. © Christopher Tompkins.

13. Kabir poem translated by Christopher Tompkins. © Christopher Tompkins.

14. Daniel Odier, *Vijnana Bhairava Tantra* (in French) (Paris: Albin Michel, 1998).

15. Richard Lannoy, *Anandamayi: Her Life and Wisdom* (Rockport, ME: Element Books Ltd, 1996), 26.

16. Shaw, 189.

17. Translated by Christopher Tompkins. © Christopher Tompkins.

18. Translated by Christopher Tompkins. © Christopher Tompkins.

19. Translated by Christopher Tompkins. © Christopher Tompkins.

20. Harvey and Erickson, *Heart Yoga,* 67.

21. Rumi, from "Burnt Kabob" in *A Year With Rumi,* 122.

CHAPTER FIVE

1. Jelalluddin Rumi, *The Love Poems of Rumi,* ed. Deepak Chopra, trans. Fereydoun Kia (New York: Harmony, 1998), 28.

2. Swami Sivananda, *Bhakti Yoga* (Fremantle, Australia: Divine Life Society, 1987).

3. Translation of Shri Abhinavagupta's "Light on Tantra" by Christopher Tompkins. © Christopher Tompkins.

4. Bhaskar Bhattacharyya, *The Path of the Mystic Lover: Baul Songs of Passion and Ecstasy,* ed. Nik Douglas (Rochester, VT: Destiny Books, 1993), 184.

5. Rumi, *A Year With Rumi,* 122.

6. Kabir poem translated by Christopher Tompkins. © Christopher Tompkins.

CHAPTER SIX

1. Swami Sivananda, *Bhakti Yoga* (Fremantle, Australia: Divine Life Society, 1987).

2. Mata Amritanandamayi Math, *Amritapuri Archana Book with English Translations* (Kerala India: Mata Amritanandamayi Trust, 2008), line 596, p. 110.

3. Bhattacharyya, *The Path of the Mystic Lover,* 8.

4. Lines from a Kabir poem translated by Christopher Tompkins. © Christopher Tompkins.

5. Math, line 204, p. 60.

6. Lannoy, *Anandamayi,* 138.

7. Lines from a Kabir poem translated by Christopher Tompkins. © Christopher Tompkins.

8. Odier, *Vijnana Bhairava Tantra.*

9. Ibid.

10. Ibid.

11. Excerpt from the Upanishads translated by Christopher Tompkins. © Christopher Tompkins.

12. Odier, *Vijnana Bhairava Tantra.*

13. Ibid.

CHAPTER SEVEN

1. Translated by Christopher Tompkins. © Christopher Tompkins.
2. Translated by Christopher Tompkins. © Christopher Tompkins.
3. Translated by Christopher Tompkins. © Christopher Tompkins.
4. Lad, 28.
5. Translated by Christopher Tompkins. © Christopher Tompkins.
6. Translated by Christopher Tompkins. © Christopher Tompkins.
7. Lad, 216.
8. Ibid.
9. Translated by Christopher Tompkins. © Christopher Tompkins.
10. Lad, 220.
11. Lad, 224.
12. Lad, 225.
13. T.K.V. Desikachar, oral tradition.

CHAPTER EIGHT

1. Deepak Chopra, *The Essential Spontaneous Fulfillment of Desire* (New York: Harmony, 2007), 40.
2. Bhattacharyya, 44.
3. Hafiz, "Cast All Your Votes for Dancing" in *I Heard God Laughing: Renderings of Hafiz,* trans. Daniel Ladinsky (Walnut Creek, CA: Sufism Reoriented, 1996), 17.
4. Kabir poem translated by Christopher Tompkins. © Christopher Tompkins.
5. Shiva Kumar, oral tradition.
6. Odier, *Yoga Spandakarika.*
7. Harvey and Erickson, 57.
8. "The Male Reproductive Cycle," online article by the Palo Alto Medical Foundation, 2013. www.pamf.org.
9. Bhattacharyya, 65.
10. Odier, *Vijnana Bhairava Tantra.*
11. Bhattacharyya, 50.
12. Odier, *Vijnana Bhairava Tantra.*
13. Lad, 32.
14. Roger P. Briggs, Robert J. Carlisle, and Barbara B. Poppe, *Solar Physics and Terrestrial Effects* (Boulder, CO: Space Environment Laboratory, National Oceanic and Atmospheric Administration, 1993), 8, 11.
15. "Solar System Exploration: Sun," an online data sheet: National Aeronautics and Space Administration (NASA), June 11, 2008. solarsystem.nasa.gov.
16. Hafiz, "The Sun Never Says," in *The Gift: Poems by Hafiz, the Great Sufi Master,* trans. Daniel Ladinsky, (New York: Penguin, 1999), 34.

CHAPTER NINE

1. Ecclesiastes 3:2
2. Harvey and Baring, *The Mystic Vision.*
3. These basic puja steps are offered from the guidance of Sreedevi Bringi, a teacher and my dear mentor in Tantric bhakti teachings for householders. Her website is shaktiinstitute.com.
4. Roger Boese, "What's Up with 108?" in *The Empty Step,* Issue 2, September 1, 2009.
5. Excerpt from the Mundaka Upanishads translated by Christopher Tompkins. © Christopher Tompkins.
6. Lawrence Livermore National Laboratory: U.S. Energy Flowchart, 2009.

PART FOUR

1. Bhattacharyya, 163.
2. Hafiz, *The Subject Tonight Is Love: 60 Wild and Sweet Poems of Hafiz,* trans. Daniel Ladinsky (New York: Penguin, 2003), 4.

CHAPTER TEN

1. Sydney Bertram Carter, songwriter, wrote the lyrics for "Lord of the Dance" during the 1960s to accompany a Shaker folk tune. Elektra EPK 801, 1965.
2. John Matthews, *The Winter Solstice: The Sacred Traditions of Christmas* (London: Godsfield Press, 1998), 52.
3. Susan Cooper, *The Dark Is Rising* (New York: Margaret K. McElderry Books, 1999).
4. Pauline Campanelli and Dan Campanelli, *Wheel of the Year: Living the Magical Life* (St. Paul, MN: Llewellyn Publications, 1989), 1–16.
5. Ibid.
6. Translated by Christopher Tompkins and Shiva Rea. © Christopher Tompkins and Shiva Rea.
7. Aleaf Bacharous, "Oimelc," a poem published online: www.angelfire.com/magic2/imbolc.

CHAPTER ELEVEN

1. Lad, 215.
2. Rumi, "On the Turn," in *The Essential Rumi: New Expanded Edition,* trans. Coleman Barks (New York: HarperCollins, 2004), 280.

3. Kaaren Whitney, "Beltane Fires," published online at White Trinity Witch website: whitetrinitywitch.co.uk.

4. Larry Chang, ed., *Wisdom for the Soul: Five Millennia of Prescriptions for Spiritual Healing* (Washington, D.C.: Gnosophia Publishers, 2006), 400.

CHAPTER TWELVE

1. Odier, *Vijnana Bhairava Tantra*.

2. "Sun and the Summer Solstice," published online at http://mikonmark.wordpress.com/category/symbolic-meaning/

CHAPTER THIRTEEN

1. John de Kadt, poet and musician

2. Devi Mahatmyam translated by Christopher Tompkins. © Christopher Tompkins.

3. Kabir poem translated by Christopher Tompkins. © Christopher Tompkins.

4. Kenny Klein, "Samhain," The Pagan Library (online), paganlibrary.com/music_poetry/samhain.php.

5. Ben Okri, "An African Elegy" in *An African Elegy* (London: Jonathan Cape Ltd, 1992).

6. Jelalluddin Rumi, "Love's Horse Will Carry You Home" in *Light Upon Light: Inspirations from Rumi,* trans. Andrew Harvey. (Berkeley, CA: North Atlantic, 1996), 178.

7. Kabir poem translated by Christopher Tompkins. © Christopher Tompkins.

8. Rumi, *The Love Poems of Rumi,* 28.

9. Rumi, "The Dream That Must Be Interpreted" in *The Essential Rumi,* 113.

Amidon, Stephen and Thomas Amidon. *The Sublime Engine: A Biography of the Human Heart.* Emmaus, PA: Rodale, 2012.

Anandamayi Ma and Joseph Fitzgerald. *The Essential Sri Anandamayi Ma: Life and Teaching of a 20th-Century Indian Saint.* Delhi: Motilal Banarsidass Publishers, 2007.

Avraham, Regina. *The Circulatory System.* Philadelphia, PA: Chelsea House Publishers, 2000.

Bandlamudi, Lakshmi. *Movements with the Cosmic Dancer: On Pilgrimage to Kailash Manasarovar.* New Delhi: New Age Books, 2006.

Barron's Essential Atlas of Physiology. Hauppauge, NY: Barron's Educational Series, Inc., 2005.

Berendt, Joachim-Ernst. *The World Is Sound: Nada Brahma: Music and the Landscape of Consciousness.* Rochester, VT: Destiny Books, 1991.

The Bhagavad Gita (second edition). Translated by Eknath Easwaran. Berkeley, CA: Nilgiri Press, 2007.

Bhattacharyya, Bhaskar. *The Path of the Mystic Lover: Baul Songs of Passion and Ecstasy.* Edited by Nik Douglas. Rochester, VT: Destiny Books, 1993.

Buhner, Stephen Harrod. *The Secret Teachings of Plants: The Intelligence of the Heart in the Direct Perception of Nature.* Santa Fe: Bear & Co, 2004.

Burton, Frances. *Fire: The Spark That Ignited Human Evolution.* Albuquerque: University of New Mexico Press, 2009.

Busia, Kofi, ed. *Iyengar: The Yoga Master.* Boston: Shambhala Publications, 2007.

Campanelli, Pauline and Dan Campanelli. *Wheel of the Year: Living the Magical Life.* St. Paul, MN: Llewellyn Publications, 1989.

Carr-Grom, Phillip. *Druid Mysteries: Ancient Wisdom for the 21st Century.* London: Random House UK, 2003.

Chang, Larry, ed. *Wisdom for the Soul: Five Millennia of Prescriptions for Spiritual Healing.* Washington, D.C.: Gnosophia Publishers, 2006.

Childre, Doc and Howard Martin. *The HeartMath Solution.* New York: HarperCollins, 1999.

Chilnick, Lawrence. *Heart Disease: An Essential Guide for the Newly Diagnosed.* Philadelphia: Perseus Books Group, 2008.

Chopra, Deepak. *The Essential Spontaneous Fulfillment of Desire.* New York: Harmony, 2007.

Csikszentmihalyi, Mihaly. *Creativity: Flow and the Psychology of Discovery and Invention.* New York: Harper Perennial, 1996.

Dale, Cyndi. *The Subtle Body: An Encyclopedia of Your Energetic Anatomy.* Boulder, CO: Sounds True, 2009.

Daniels, Patricia, et. al. *Body: The Complete Human.* Washington, D.C.: National Geographic Society, 2007.

Davis, Goode P., and Edwards Park. *The Heart: The Living Pump.* Washington D.C.: U.S. News Books, 1981.

Dyczkowski, Mark S.G. *The Doctrine of Vibration: An Analysis of the Doctrines and Practices of Kashmir Shaivism.* Albany: State University of New York Press, 1987.

Hafiz. *The Gift: Poems by Hafiz, the Great Sufi Master.* Translated by Daniel Ladinsky. New York: Penguin, 1999.

_____. *I Heard God Laughing: Renderings of Hafiz.* Translated by Daniel Ladinsky. Walnut Creek, CA: Sufism Reoriented, 1996.

_____. *The Subject Tonight Is Love: 60 Wild and Sweet Poems of Hafiz.* Translated by Daniel Ladinsky. New York: Penguin, 2003.

Harvey, Andrew. *The Essential Mystics: Selections from the World's Great Wisdom.* New York: HarperOne, 1997.

_____. *The Hope: A Guide to Sacred Activism.* Hay House, 2009.

_____. *Radical Passion: Sacred Love and Wisdom in Action.* Berkeley, CA: North Atlantic Books, 2012.

Harvey, Andrew and Karuna Erickson. *Heart Yoga: The Sacred Marriage of Yoga and Mysticism.* Berkeley, CA: North Atlantic Books, 2010.

Harvey, Andrew and Anne Baring. *The Mystic Vision: Daily Encounters with the Divine.* New York: HarperCollins, 1995.

Heinberg, Richard. *Celebrate the Solstice: Honoring the Earth's Seasonal Rhythms through Festival and Ceremony.* Wheaton, IL: Quest Books, 1993.

Hobday, Richard. *The Healing Sun: Sunlight and Health in the 21st Century.* Forres, Scotland: Findhorn Press, 1999.

Khanna, Madhu. *Yantra: The Tantric Symbol of Cosmic Unity.* New York: Thames and Hudson, 1979.

Kumar, Nitin. "The Rhythm of Music: A Magical and Mystical Harmony." In Exotic India, September 2003. (exoticindia.com)

Lad, Vasant. *Textbook of Ayurveda: A Complete Guide to Clinical Assessment.* Albuquerque, NM: The Ayurvedic Press, 2007.

_____. *Textbook of Ayurveda: Fundamental Principles.* Albuquerque, NM: The Ayurvedic Press, 2002.

_____. *Textbook of Ayurveda: General Principles of Management and Treatment.* Albuquerque, NM: The Ayurvedic Press, 2012.

Liberman, John. *Light: Medicine of the Future.* Santa Fe, NM: Bear & Company, 1991.

Math, Mata Amritanandamayi. *Amritapuri Archana Book with English Translations.* Kerala, India: Mata Amritanandamayi Trust, 2008.

Matthews, John. *The Winter Solstice: The Sacred Traditions of Christmas.* London: Godsfield Press, 1998.

McCraty, Rollin. *The Energetic Heart: Bioelectromagnetic Interactions Within and Between People.* Boulder Creek, CA: Institute of Heart Math, 2003.

Mechthild of Magdeburg. *The Flowing Light of the Godhead.* Translated by Frank Tobin. Eastford, CT: Martino Fine Books, 2012).

Menon, T. V. Narayana. *The Thousand Names of the Divine Mother: Sri Lalita Sahasranama with Commentary.* Translated by M. N. Namboodiri. Kerala, India: Mata Amritanandamayi Center, 1996.

Muller-Ortega, Paul E. *The Triadic Heart of Śiva: Kaula Tantricism of Abhinavagupta in the Non-dual Shaivism of Kashmir.* Albany: State University of New York Press, 1989.

Nanda, Vivek with George Mitchell. *Chidambaram: Home of Nataraja.* Gaithersburg, MD: Marg Publications, 2004.

Odier, Daniel. *Desire: The Tantric Path to Awakening.* Rochester, VT: Inner Traditions, 2001.

_____. *Vijnana Bhairava Tantra (in French).* Paris: Albin Michel, 1998.

_____. *Yoga Spandakarika: The Sacred Texts at the Origins of Tantra.* Rochester, VT: Inner Traditions, 2005.

Oschman, James. *Energy Medicine: The Scientific Basis.* Philadelphia: Churchill Livingstone, 2000.

Panikkar, Raimundo. *The Vedic Experience: Mantramanjari.* New Delhi, India: Motilal Banarsidass, 2001.

Pearsall, Paul. *The Heart's Code: Tapping the Wisdom and Power of Our Heart Energy.* New York: Broadway Books, 1999.

Pennick, Nigel. The Pagan Book of Days: A Guide to the Festivals, Traditions, and Sacred Days of the Year. Rochester, VT: Destiny Books, 2001.

Poonjaji, H. W. L. *Wake Up and Roar.* Ashland, OR: Gangaji Foundation, 1993.

Pritscher, Conrad. *Einstein and Zen: Learning to Learn.* New York: Peter Lang Publishing, 2009.

Reader's Digest: The Heart and Circulatory System. Pleasantville, NY: The Reader's Digest Association, Inc., 2000.

Rumi, Jelalluddin. *The Big Red Book.* Translated by Coleman Barks. New York: HarperCollins, 2010.

_____. *The Book of Love: Poems of Ecstasy and Longing.* Translated by Coleman Barks. New York: HarperCollins, 2003.

_____. *The Essential Rumi: New Expanded Edition.* Translated by Coleman Barks. New York: HarperCollins, 2004.

_____. *Light Upon Light: Inspirations from Rumi,* Translated by Andrew Harvey. Berkeley, CA: North Atlantic, 1996.

_____. *The Love Poems of Rumi.* Edited by Deepak Chopra. Translated by Fereydoun Kia. New York: Harmony, 1998.

_____. *A Year With Rumi: Daily Readings.* Translated by Coleman Barks. New York: HarperCollins, 2006.

Satyananda Saraswati. *Asana Pranayama Mudra Bandha.* Munger, India: Bihar School of Yoga, 2008.

Saundarya-Lahari of Sri Sankaracarya. Translated by Swami Tapasyananda. Madras, India: Sri Ramakrishna Math Press, 1987.

Schwartz, Gary E. *The Sacred Promise: How Science Is Discovering Spirit's Collaboration with Us in Our Daily Lives.* New York: Atria Books/Beyond Words, 2011.

Shaw, Miranda. *Passionate Enlightenment.* Princeton, NJ: Princeton University Press, 1995.

Stein, Diane. *Casting the Circle: A Women's Book of Ritual.* Berkeley, CA: Crossing Press, 1990.

Swimme, Brian. *The Universe Is a Green Dragon: A Cosmic Creation Story.* Rochester, VT: Bear & Company, 1984.

Teilhard de Chardin, Pierre. *Toward the Future.* Translated by René Hague. New York: Mariner Books, 2002.

Tsiaras, Alexander. *The InVision Guide to a Healthy Heart.* New York: HarperCollins, 2005.

The Upanishads, second edition. Translated by Eknath Easwaran. Berkeley, CA: Nilgiri Press, 2007.

Vanamali. *Shakti: Realm of the Divine Mother.* Rochester, VT: Inner Traditions, 2006.

Wallis, Christopher. *Tantra Illuminated: The Philosophy, History, and Practice of a Timeless Tradition.* The Woodlands, TX: Anusara Press, 2012.

Listed by page number

DEDICATION

v. Ganga offering, © Jenay Martin, Anjenaya Imagery, anjenayaimagery.com.

EPIGRAPH

vii. Crescent Heart Fire, © Jenay Martin, Anjenaya Imagery, anjenayaimagery.com.

INTRODUCTION

2. Shiva and Mother, © Shiva Rea.

CHAPTER ONE

11. Fire offering, Collage by Amy Hayes | Origin. Photo of Shiva Rea © Demetri Velisarius. Abstract light photo from Shutterstock, by CS Stock.

13. Heartfire, Collage by Amy Hayes | Origin. Fire image from Shutterstock, by Ozerina Anna and Sacred Heart photo by Lucien Renjilian-Burgy.

14–15. Crescent Heart Fire, © Jenay Martin, Anjenaya Imagery, anjenayaimagery.com. Brush circle, Shutterstock, by Alena P.

16. Sacred Heart of Jesus, Shutterstock, Andrew F. Kazmierski.

16. Sacred Heart of Jesus, Shutterstock, by Zvonimir Atletic.

17. Flaming Sufi Heart, binashah.blogspot.com/2012/07/the-religion-of-heart.html.

17. Winged-Heart Calligraphy, © Hafizullah Chishti, illuminedliving.com.

17. Kabbalah Heart Fire, sacred-texts.com/eso/sta/sta17.htm.

18. Neijingtu Diagram, djwx.com.

18. Celtic Spirals, Shutterstock, by art_of_sun.

19. Beach fire, Shutterstock, by Shironina.

19. Tantric Buddhism, Shutterstock, by Pawel Kowalczyk.

20. Shiva meditating illustration, © Shakti de Souza, shakticards.com.

21. Tantric Shaivism, Collage by Amy Hayes | Origin. Shiva/Shakti photo, Shutterstock, by Boris Stroujko. Sunset photo, Shutterstock, by Djgis.

21. Diwali Lamps, Shutterstock, by anshu18.

22. Heart in the Cross, Lucien Renjilian-Burgy. Taken on Pilgrimage to the Kilree High Cross, Co. Kilkenny, Ireland. Collage by Amy Hayes | Origin.

23. Funerary papyrus of Djedkhonsouefankh depicting the judgement of the deceased, Third Intermediate Period (papyrus), Egyptian 21st Dynasty (c.1069-945 BC) / Egyptian National Museum, Cairo, Egypt / Giraudon / The Bridgeman Art Library

23. Statue of Plato, Shutterstock, by Anastasios71.

24. Vitruvian Man by Leonardo da Vinci, Shutterstock, by Janaka Dharmasena.

24. Mechanical Chrome Heart, Shutterstock, by GrandeDuc.

25. Energetic Heart, Collage by Amy Hayes | Origin. X-ray Heart Anatomy, Shutterstock, by CLIPAREA | Custom Media. Abstract Mandala Background, Shutterstock, by Mahesh Patil.

26. Fire wilderness, © LakshmiGrace, lakshmigracedesigns.com.

27. Ancestral Flame, Shutterstock, by Mona Makela.

28. Modern Office, Shutterstock, by Terekhov Igor.

29. Ancient Symbols, Shutterstock, by MBPROJEKT MaciejBledowski.

30. Cosmic fireball, Shutterstock, by Alin Brotea.

31. Firekeepers: Neem Karoli Baba, Dalai Lama, Gandhi, Anandamayi Ma, Martin Luther King Jr., Amma; illustration, © Pan Trinity Das, pantrinitydas.net.

CHAPTER TWO

33. Shiva Rea in Nataraja; © Jenay Martin, Anjenaya Imagery, anjenayaimagery.com.

34–35. Cosmic Dance, Collage by Amy Hayes | Origin. Gnawai Sunset Lila, Morocco; © Amir Magal, Amirimage, amirimage.com. Stars of a planet and galaxy in a free space, Shutterstock, by Maria Starovoytova.

35. Meenakshi Temple, Madurai; Shutterstock, by VLADJ55.

36. Chidambaram Temple, Shutterstock, by Msankar4.

37. Temple image, © Maria Garre.

37. Temple image, © Maria Garre.

37. Shiva Rea in Nataraja at Chidambaram, © Maria Garre.
38. Vastu Purusha grid, © Amy Hayes | Origin.
39. Fire altar, Shutterstock, by Andrey Armyagov.
39. Agni Hotra Offering, Collage by Amy Hayes | Origin. Altar Photo, Shutterstock, by Nadina.
40–41. Sun-Moon Breath, © Jenay Martin, Anjenaya Imagery, anjenayaimagery.com. Design by Lisa Johnston, Firefly Artists.
42. Sri Yantra, Collage by Amy Hayes | Origin.
42. Small image and yantra, © James Wvinner. Design by Lynda Carre.
43. Shiva-Shakti Khajuraho, iStock, by Jpll2002.
43. Double Spiral, Shutterstock, by Diego Barucco.
43. Yantra Illustration, © Amy Hayes | Origin.
44. Kundalini Shakti Tantric painting, © Christopher Tompkins.
45. Shiva-Shakti in Union, Shutterstock, by Txanbelin.
46. Sri Radha-Krishna, © B. G. Sharma, Mandala Publishing.
47. Sri Chaitanya in Kirtan dance, © Mandala Publishing.
48. Guru Mandala, © Radisha, radisha.com.
49. Shiva Rea and Rishikesh Moon, © Jenay Martin, Anjenaya Imagery, anjenayaimagery.com.

CHAPTER THREE

51. Embodied Heart, Collage by Amy Hayes | Origin. X-ray Heart Anatomy, Shutterstock, by CLIPAREA | Custom Media.
52. Sunset Backbend, Collage by Amy Hayes | Origin. Shiva Rea photo, © Demetri Velisarius. Sunburst, Shutterstock, by S. Ragets. Blazing heart, Shutterstock, by Ozerina Anna.
53. Fetus Heart Pulse, Collage by Amy Hayes | Origin. Fetus, Shutterstock, by Mopic. Abstract Background, Shutterstock, by balounm.
54. Embodied Heart, Collage by Amy Hayes | Origin. X-ray Heart Anatomy, Shutterstock, by CLIPAREA | Custom Media.
55. Malasana, India; © Jenay Martin, Anjenaya Imagery, anjenayaimagery.com.
56. Energetic Heart, Collage by Amy Hayes | Origin. Human Heart, Shutterstock, by Sebastian Kailitzki. Bright Fractal Sun Flower, Shutterstock, by cycreation.
56. Coherent Heart Rhythm graph, Based on charts © Institute of HeartMath Research Center.
57. Dissonant Heart Rhythm graph, Based on charts by Institute of HeartMath Research Center, © 1998.

57. Cell mitosis, Shutterstock, by fusebulb.
57. Cardiac muscle cells, iStock, by BeholdingEye.
58. Heart and Brain Coherence, Collage by Amy Hayes | Origin. Heart & brain illustrations, Shutterstock, by Sebastian Kaulitzki.
58. Heart Rhythm and Brainwaves in Synch, Based on charts © Institute of HeartMath Research Center.
59. Energy Mandala, Shutterstock, by balounm.
60. Busy City Business People, Shutterstock, by Pan Xunbin.
61. Dissonant Heart and Brainwave Rhythm, Based on charts © Institute of HeartMath Research Center.
62. Lovers Sunset, Collage by Amy Hayes | Origin. Young Lovers, Shutterstock, by Dudarev Mikhail. Geometric mandala, Shutterstock, by Lucy Ya.
63. Father and baby, Shutterstock, by itsmejust.
64. Collective Dance at Wanderlust, © Rich Van Every.
64. Bob Wisdom drumming, © Jenay Martin, Anjenaya Imagery, anjenayaimagery.com.
64. Chant4Change, © Gaura Vani.
65. Children dancing, © Jenay Martin, Anjenaya Imagery, anjenayaimagery.com.
65. Collective Heart Mandala, © James Winner.
66. Hands flame, Shutterstock, by Elena Ray.
68. Shiva Rea and Demetri Velisarius with Staff, © Jenay Martin, Anjenaya Imagery, anjenayaimagery.com.

CHAPTER FOUR

69. Costa Rica bonfire, © Demetri Velisarius.
71. Nataraja, Collage by Amy Hayes | Origin. Shiva Statue, Shutterstock, by Dudarev Mikhail.
72–73. Kalari Ocean, © Jenay Martin, Anjenaya Imagery, anjenayaimagery.com.
73. Temple Sahaja, © Erik Paulsrud.
74. Prostrations, Shutterstock, by Pius Lee.
74. Kodo drummers, Shutterstock, by Alan49.
75. Davening, Shutterstock, by Kobby Dagan.
75. Qigong, Shutterstock, by Mojca Odar.
75. Kecak, Shutterstock, by deamles.
75. Sema, Shutterstock, by mehmetcan.
76. Shiva-Shakti dancing, © Exotic India, by Kailash Raj.
77. Shiva-Shakti music, © Exotic India, by Kailash Raj.
78. Harappan Seal of Siva, en.wikipedia.org/wiki/File:Shiva_Pashupati.jpg, columbia.edu/itc/mealac/pritchett/00routesdata/bce_500back/indusvalley/protoshiva/protoshiva.jpg.
78. Vedic surya namaskar, © Exotic India.
78. Nath Sadhu, © Lex Linghorn MMX, lexphoto.co.uk.

216. Earth turning, Shutterstock, by Molodec.
217. Newgrange spirals, Shutterstock, by S. Hanusch.
217. Stonehenge, Shutterstock, by gary718.
218. Thailand fire lanterns, Shutterstock, by Neung Stocker.
219. Yule fire, Shutterstock, by Andris Tkacenko.
220. Flowers and candles, Shutterstock, by indianstockimages.
220. Festival in India, Shutterstock, by AJP.
221. Beach labyrinth, © Shiva Rea.
222. Candle, Shutterstock, by Bank2Cool.
222. Candle between hands, Shutterstock, by Pincasso.
223–224. Chakra illustrations, Shutterstock, by Mauritania.
224. Flower Mandala, Shutterstock, by Migelito.
225. Winter Sunrise, Shutterstock, by Sandy MacKenzie.
226. Ayurvedic herbs, Shutterstock, by p.studio66.
227. Ayurveda, Shutterstock, by Quintanilla.
228. Fire, Shutterstock, by yuriy kulik.
228. Candles and rose petals, Shutterstock, by Africa Candles.
229. Saraswati, Shutterstock, by Desiree Walstra.
230. Shiva lingam, Shutterstock, by Amith Nag.
231. Shiva Nataraja statue, © Jenay Martin, Anjenaya Imagery, anjenayaimagery.com.

CHAPTER ELEVEN

233. Buddha at sunrise, Shutterstock, by somchaij.
234. Pink flower background, Shutterstock, by mythja.
235. Pink flowers, Shutterstock, by Maria Timofeeva.
235. Blowing the shofar at Western Wall, Shutterstock, by Mikhail.
236. Easter at Church of the Holy Sepulchre, Jerusalem; Shutterstock, by Mikhail.
236. Chichén Itzá, Shutterstock, by Vaclav Volrab.
237. Hanuman, Shutterstock, by f9photos.
237. Candles, Shutterstock, by Ilya Andriyanov.
238. Abstract Summer Background, Shutterstock, by Mythja.
240. Shiva Rea in handstand, © Jenay Martin, Anjenaya Imagery, anjenayaimagery.com.
241. Beltane May pole, Shutterstock, by Ralf Gosch.
241. Bonfire, Shutterstock, by Lijuan Guo.
242. Monks meditating, Shutterstock, by naihei.
242. Golden Buddha, Shutterstock, by Luciano Mortula.

CHAPTER TWELVE

243. Shiva Poi, © Demetri Velisarius.
244. Stonehenge sunrise, Shutterstock, by Filip Fuxa.
245. Wedding Hands in India, Shutterstock, by Jayakumar.

246–247. Dancers at Burning Man, © Mario Covic.
248. Full moon reflected in water, Shutterstock, by Jens Beste.
249. Mint tea, Shutterstock, by mythja.
250. Fresh Arugula Salad, Shutterstock, by Shebeko.
250. Lavender and jasmine, Shutterstock, by Snowbelle.
251. Montpelier waterfall, © Demetri Velisarius.
252–253. Burning Man temple, © Jeff Walters.
253. Demetri Poi, © Shiva Rea.
254. Raksha Ti, Shutterstock, by intellistudies.
254. Krishna Festival, Shutterstock, by reddees.
254. Rishikesh Ganesh, © Jenay Martin, Anjenaya Imagery, anjenayaimagery.com.

CHAPTER THIRTEEN

255. Fall leaves, Shutterstock, by Tatiana Grozetskaya.
256. Fall forest, Shutterstock, by Hofhauser.
256. Foggy Meadow Morning, Shutterstock, by Milosz_G.
257. Global Mala Project, © Amir Magal, Amirimage, amirimage.com.
257. Japa Mala, Shutterstock, by f9photos.
258. Yom Kippur, Shutterstock, by David Orcea.
258. Shofar, Shutterstock, by blueeyes.
258. Star of David, Shutterstock, by LadyLyonnesse.
258. Shabbat candles with Star of David, Shutterstock, by blueeyes.
259. Ancestor image, Shutterstock, by LiliGraphie.
259. Shabbat candles, Shutterstock, by Anneka.
260. Triple Goddess, courtesy Christopher Tompkins.
261. Aarti, Shutterstock, by Viktor Borovskikh.
262. Autumn background, Shutterstock, by mythja.
264. Ayurvedic massage, Shutterstock, by Valery Kraynov.
265. Fall Vasisthasana, © Bill Tipper.
266. Sparks of Bonfire Night, Shutterstock, by Artur Marfin.
266. Graveyard with Celtic Cross, Shutterstock, by Ronald Sumners.
267. Día de los Muertos skulls, Shutterstock, by Jose Gil.
267. Decaying Coals, Shutterstock, by Anrey.
268–269. Diwali candles, Shutterstock, by TheFinalMiracle.
268. Diwali Rangoli, Shutterstock, by D.Shashikant.
268. Menorah, Shutterstock, by diligent.
270. Votive candles. Shutterstock, by Roman Sinichkin.
271. Rumi statue, Shutterstock, by muratcankaragoz.
271. Whirling Dervishes, Shutterstock, by mehmetcan.
272. Costa Rica bonfire, © Demetri Velisarius.

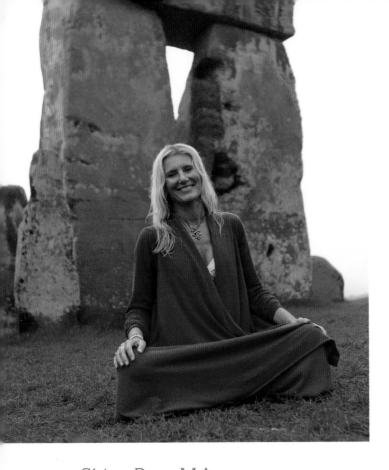

As a pioneering teacher in the evolution of vinyasa and the power of free-form (sahaja) movement for more than twenty years, her home practice DVD and CD workshops, teacher trainings, pilgrimage retreats, and online programs have fertilized the lives of many—from yoga teachers and students to high-level athletes to leaders and artists living around the world. From large-scale festivals to transformative local classes, her energetic "pathways of flow" offer ways to kindle life-force from the heart outward into the world.

Shiva's life bridges healing arts and the science of flow, individual empowerment and collective shifts of consciousness, embodied liberation and sacred activism. Her mission is to awaken and serve our innate intelligence within our bodies and within our lives to achieve a sustainable future for all.

For inspiration, resources, and more information about Shiva's teaching and service activities, please visit tendingtheheartfire.com.

Shiva Rea, MA, has founded the Global Mala Project, Prana Flow-Energetic Vinyasa, and the Samudra Global School for Living Yoga. She bases her work upon her worldwide travels, studies in UCLA's World Arts and Cultures program, and the roots of yoga found in tantra, ayurveda and bhakti. She has learned from: elders in places like Ghana and Kerala; masters of the arts of yoga, kalarippayatu (martial arts), odissi (classical dance), world dance; and from collaborations with DJs and kirtan musicians.

Sounds True is a multimedia publisher whose mission is to inspire and support personal transformation and spiritual awakening. Founded in 1985 and located in Boulder, Colorado, we work with many of the leading spiritual teachers, thinkers, healers, and visionary artists of our time. We strive with every title to preserve the essential "living wisdom" of the author or artist. It is our goal to create products that not only provide information to a reader or listener, but that also embody the quality of a wisdom transmission.

For those seeking genuine transformation, Sounds True is your trusted partner. At SoundsTrue.com you will find a wealth of free resources to support your journey, including exclusive weekly audio interviews, free downloads, interactive learning tools, and other special savings on all our titles.

To learn more, please visit SoundsTrue.com/bonus/free_gifts or call us toll free at 800-333-9185.

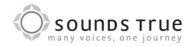

SOUNDS TRUE
many voices, one journey